Nursing in Today's World

CHALLENGES, ISSUES, AND TRENDS

Nursing in Today's World

CHALLENGES, ISSUES, AND TRENDS

FIFTH EDITION

Janice Rider Ellis, RN, PhD
Professor of Nursing
Director of Nursing Education
Shoreline Community College
Seattle, Washington

Celia Love Hartley, RN, MN
Professor of Nursing
Chair, Allied Health and
Director, Nursing Programs
College of the Desert
Palm Desert, California

BISHOP MUELLER LIBRARY
Briar Cliff College
SIOUX CITY, IA 51104

J.B. Lippincott Company
Philadelphia

Sponsoring Editor: Margaret Belcher
Coordinating Editorial Assistant: Emily Cotlier
Project Editor: Amy P. Jirsa
Indexer: Patricia Perrier
Design Coordinator: Melissa G. Olson
Interior Designer: William T. Donnelly
Cover Designer: Ilene Griff
Production Manager: Helen Ewan
Production Coordinator: Kathryn Rule
Compositor: Circle Graphics
Printer/Binder: R.R. Donnelley & Sons Co.
Cover Printer: Lehigh Press Lithographers

5th Edition

6   5   4   3   2   1

Library of Congress Cataloging-in-Publications Data

Ellis, Janice Rider.
      Nursing in today's world : challenges, issues, and trends / Janice Rider Ellis,
   Celia Love Hartley.—5th ed.
         p.   cm.
      Includes bibliographical references and index.
      ISBN 0-397-55177-0
      1. Nursing.   2. Nursing—Practice.   3. Nursing—United States.
   I. Hartley, Celia Love.   II. Title
      [DLNM: 1. Nursing—United States.   WY 16 E47n 1995]
   RT82.E45   1995
   610.73—dc20
   DNLM/DLC
   for Library of Congress   94-32255
                                                                                    CIP

Any procedure or practice described in this book should be applied by the healthcare practitioner
under appropriate supervision in accordance with professional standards of care used with regard
to the unique circumstances that apply in each practice situation. Care has been taken to confirm
the accuracy of information presented and to describe generally accepted practices. However, the
authors, editors, and publisher cannot accept any responsibility for errors or omissions or for any
consequences from application of the information in this book and make no warranty express or
implied, with respect to the contents of the book.

Every effort has been made to ensure drug selections and dosages are in accordance with current
recommendations and practice. Because of ongoing research, changes in government regulations
and the constant flow of information on drug therapy, reactions and interactions, the reader is
cautioned to check the package insert for each drug for indications, dosages, warnings and precautions, particularly if the drug is new or infrequently used.

Preface

The fifth edition of *Nursing in Today's World: Challenges, Issues, and Trends*, like the previous edition, represents an effort on our part to present in an interesting and stimulating format, content essential to nursing practice that is often viewed by students as secondary or less important than the courses with a clinical component. Certainly, the largest segment of the educational preparation of any student pursuing a nursing career is spent developing a theoretical foundation for and applying the clinical aspects of care. The rapidly increasing body of nursing knowledge and the technological advances that have reshaped nursing practice demand that the new graduate have a sound understanding of nursing theory that will guide the critical thinking and related performance of the many psychomotor skills that comprise the art and science of nursing.

It is just as important that individuals who accept the role demanded of today's professional nurse possess an understanding of the development, heritage, and history of nursing as a profession; and the many studies that have been instrumental in shaping our profession. It is also important for the student to be aware of the many struggles and controversies waged with regard to nursing and to be able to recognize the issues to which there are no ready solutions. Many questions are likely to remain unanswered, or can be answered only on an individual basis. It is in consideration for this aspect of nursing that *Nursing in Today's World* is written. Our challenge has been to present this content in a format that will provoke the students' curiosity and provide incentive to explore these issues in greater depth.

Students need to know how nursing relates to society as a whole. What impact does nursing have on society and, conversely, what impact does society have on the practice of nursing? What are the effects of legal, ethical, bioethical, legislative, and political concerns? What type of image does the public hold of nurses and nursing? How should this image be changed? What will be the role of the nurse in a health care delivery system reshaped by health care reform? What education best prepares for those roles? What avenues of education are available to today's student?

Students can benefit additionally from information that will help them into the nursing profession. This includes knowledge of opportunities in nursing as well as the specifics of applying and interviewing for positions, understanding the hospital environment and how it is structured, anticipating conflicts that may occur in their professional roles, and understanding the organizations that represent nursing. Students with this preparation will be in a better position to practice nursing as it exists today and to influence the development of future nursing practice.

We have written this book as an introduction to those responsibilities. It is our hope that it will assist you with your course in "Issues," "Trends," or "Professional Adjustments," or with such material integrated into other courses. Each chapter is preceded by a list of general objectives designed to guide you to an understanding of the information that follows. A summary of key concepts concludes each chapter. Exercises that will permit you to apply critical thinking to topics covered in the chapter follow. Additional bibliographical references at the end of each chapter lend direction to those seeking a more in-depth exploration of a given topic.

We recognize that many of the topics presented in the context of this book have enough subject matter to fill an entire textbook or, in cases such as bioethical issues, an entire encyclopedia. Our purpose is to provide you with an overview of basic information necessary to move into the nursing role, while at the same time stimulating a desire for further reading. Changes in our society occur so rapidly that many of our most heavily and heatedly debated issues are history by the time they can be placed in a textbook. While time adds perspective, day-to-day reading of newspapers and periodicals is vital to remain informed; thus, we encourage students using this book to read additional materials to be completely up to date.

With each edition we have tried to make this book more responsive to your needs. Nursing education, as it responds to the changing world of work, is a dynamic process. Today some leaders in nursing curriculum development and teaching are encouraging the art of story-telling as a valuable teaching technique. As you examine *Nursing in Today's World*, we hope you will value the stories used to illustrate our points of emphasis–stories of real people and their problems, stories of legal challenges, and stories of some of the individuals who have helped to paint the kaleidoscope of nursing history. Through the cartoon-like illustrations, we hope you will gain a varied visual introduction to nursing issues that will provide some humor, as well as gratification, to your commitment of nursing.

In accomplishing our task, many thanks are in order, and we hesitate for fear of omitting anyone. Certainly we need to acknowledge the support of our colleagues who continue to bring new issues to our attention. As we worked at perfecting the content of the fifth edition, we have appreciated the comments of fellow educators throughout the United States who have used our text and offered enthusiastic support and constructive criticism of the content. Likewise, your suggestions and recommendations regarding this edition will be valued. We also thank these individuals for their continued selection of this text for their classes. We are well aware of the number of books published since the first edition of *Nursing in Today's World* from which you can choose. Many address issues and trends with a similar design and approach. In this very competitive market we are appreciative of your support. We also need to thank our students, who provide one of the best audits of our ability to set forth this content clearly and interestingly.

Certainly our list of acknowledgments would be incomplete if we did not express our heart-felt thanks for the emotional support provided by our respective husbands, Ivan and Gordon, both of whom have moved into semi-retirement since the fourth edition was published, putting them in a very special position to receive and post express mail, attend to extra housekeeping, shopping, and a myriad of other duties that have allowed us to put the book first when necessary. And last, but not least, we thank the editors of J.B. Lippincott Company for their help with this text.

Janice Rider Ellis, PhD, RN

Celia Love Hartley, MN, RN

Contents

Nursing in Today's World

CHALLENGES, ISSUES, AND TRENDS

I Understanding the Development of Nursing as a Profession

As you embark on a career in nursing you can best appreciate the role and responsibilities you are learning to assume if you have an understanding of the history and development of the profession. Nursing is considered a relatively young profession by many people. Others challenge that it has yet to achieve professional status. The educational processes by which we prepare nurses continue to experience change and modification. Are you interested in how this might affect you and your career in nursing? In this unit we present a history of nursing that describes its growth from an apprentice-type training to a profession that encompasses doctoral degrees. We also discuss the various educational routes by which you can prepare for a role as a nurse and conclude with a discussion of the future of nursing education.

1 | Nursing as a Developing Profession

Objectives

After completing this chapter, you should be able to

1. Discuss the reasons the profession has had difficulty defining nursing.

2. Give a definition of nursing and identify a theorist who defines nursing similarly.

3. Using the formal characteristics provided, determine whether you believe nursing is a profession.

4. Describe the health care practices of early civilizations.

5. Discuss the three major historical images of the nurse.

6. Describe how each of these historical images has influenced the development of nursing as a profession.

7. Explain the significance of the "Dark Ages of Nursing" to the development of the nursing profession.

8. Discuss the contribution of Florence Nightingale to the development of nursing as a profession.

9. List some early hospitals established in the Americas.

10. Describe the early development of nursing schools in the United States.

11. Discuss factors that have affected the image of nursing today.

12. Identify at least three studies about nursing and explain why each is important.

What is nursing? Is nursing an art or a science? If both, which should receive the primary emphasis? How should or can "hunches," "gut feelings," and "intuition" exist in a world surrounded by scientific rationale and steeped in protocol? Should nursing be considered a profession or an occupation? What factors are affecting the emergence of nursing as a profession? Does nursing possess a unique body of knowledge? Is the nurse a professional? If so, what educational background qualifies the nurse for professional standing? Should the educational preparation for nursing occur in a variety of settings that award differing degrees? How will the skills of graduates from various programs be differentiated in practice? Do differing levels of competence exist in the practice of clinical nursing? What is the position of the nurse in relation to other members of the health care team? What is the exclusive role of the nurse? What forces have had a hand in the development of that role? What is the future of that role? What should we remember from our past that will assist with the development of nursing for the future? These are only some of the questions being asked by nurses about nurses and nursing today. Not all the questions have clear answers. Some of the answers given provide the basis for debate and dialogue among nurses, health care providers, and the public as health care consumers. As a novice, joining the ranks of those who have preceded you, you will need a grasp of the issues that have challenged, and in some instances plagued, nursing over the years to participate effectively in the debate. As the nurse of the 21st century, you may have a direct impact on some of the answers to these questions.

Nursing Defined

Defining nursing is difficult. Nurses themselves cannot agree on a single definition, partly because of nursing's historical background. Little is known other than by inference about the work of the nurse in prehistory. Yet Donahue (1985, p 2) writes, "From the dawn of civilization, evidence prevails to support the premise that *nurturing* has been essential to the preservation of life. Survival of the human race, therefore, is inextricably intertwined with the development of nursing."

DISTINGUISHING NURSING FROM MEDICINE

Clear and concise definitions of nursing are also impeded by the lack of separation or an obvious distinction from medicine. For example, it is not unusual to hear a prospective nursing student say, "I've always been interested in the medical field, so I decided to go into nursing." Something of an interdependence exists between the two professions, medicine and nursing, and they have somewhat paralleled one another in historical development. However, anyone who has been involved in the profession of nursing for any period of time will be quick to assure you that distinct differences exist. Primarily these are focused on the major goal of each profession and the educational preparation needed to fulfill the role. In general, medicine is concerned with the diagnosis and treatment (cure when possible) of disease. Nursing is concerned with caring for the person in a variety of health-related situations. Thus, we think of medicine being involved in the cure of the patient and nursing with the care of that patient. This care involves significant roles in health teaching and the prevention of illness as well as the care of the ill individual.

With the advancing technology in the health care fields, the varying areas of specialization, the different routes to educational preparation, and the variety of practice settings and roles occupied by the nurse, it is critical that nurses provide clear information for themselves as well as for the public. To state that you are a registered nurse says little about what you do. It conveys nothing about where you are employed or about your educational background. For example, you could be employed in a community hospital, you might be working in a long-term care facility, you might have earned additional credentials and be working in advanced practice, or you might be a nurse educator.

Thus, you can see that the words "nurse" and "nursing" have been applied to a wide variety of health care activities in many different settings performed by many variously educated people. The old adage "A nurse, is a nurse, is a nurse" is out of place in our highly technical health care delivery system that struggles to keep "high touch" and "high tech" compatible.

THE EFFECT OF TECHNOLOGY
ON THE DEFINITION OF NURSING

Technological advances have significantly affected the definition of nursing and the role of the nurse. This is reflected in the comments made by a colleague after looking in a late-1950s medical-surgical nursing textbook to review the nursing care of a patient diagnosed as having an aortic aneurysm in 1960. She found that nurses did not usually manage such patients because these patients seldom lived long enough to require any nursing care. Today such patients are in intensive care units making a good, although cautious, recovery after careful diagnosis that perhaps requires angiography, sonography, or tomography; delicate surgery to excise and repair the distention of the artery; and specialized critical care nursing. "A nurse is a nurse is a nurse" would certainly not reflect with any specificity the role of the person who would provide care to this patient, the critical thinking skills needed to fulfill the expected behaviors, or the diversity that exists within the profession. Nurses in many positions have been required to assume ever greater levels of responsibility. Paradoxically, they have not always been given the official authority, autonomy, or recognition that would be expected to accompany those responsibilities. Fortunately, in recent years there has been more appreciation of the role nurses are filling in the health care delivery

EARLY DEFINITIONS OF NURSING

Beginning with the simplest definition, a nurse is a person who nourishes, fosters, and protects—a person who is prepared to care for the sick, injured, and aged. In this sense "nurse" is used as a noun and is derived from the Latin *nutrix*, which means "nursing mother." Another early use of the word "nurse" was associated with the meaning of a woman who suckled a child, usually not her own—a wet nurse. Dictionary definitions of nurse also include such words as "suckles or nourishes," "to take care of a child or children," "to bring up; rear." In this way "nurse" is used as a verb, deriving from the Latin *nutrire*, which means "to suckle and nourish." With such an origin it is understandable that people generally have associated nursing with women.

References to "the nurse" can be found in the Talmud and in the Old Testament, although the role of this person is not clearly identified. It was probably more similar to that of the wet nurse than to that of someone who cared for the sick. Slowly, over the centuries, the word "nurse" has evolved to refer to a person who cares for or tends to the needs of the sick. Florence Nightingale, in her *Notes on Nursing: What It Is, and What It Is Not*, described

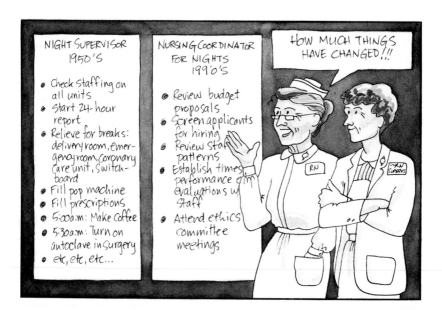

FIGURE 1–1 In recent years there has been more appreciation of the role nurses are filling.

the nurse's role as one that would "put the patient in the best condition for nature to act upon him" (Nightingale, 1860, p 133).

It is more than just a coincidence that the development of nursing as a profession has been inextricably tied to the role that women occupied in a society at that given time and to the forces that were having an impact on that society. People who functioned in the capacity of nurses were undoubtedly more concerned about carrying out the responsibilities of the role than about defining the role. Throughout the years we have seen the concepts of nurse and nursing grow and evolve from one of the nurse as mother, nourishing and nurturing children, to one of the nurse without specific reference to gender and with responsibilities encompassing ever-expanding and challenging services to people needing health care.

DEFINITIONS OF NURSE THEORISTS

As nursing has grown as a profession, various nursing theorists have developed definitions of nursing consistent with their conceptual frameworks.
presents the definitions of some of the theorists.

In 1958, Virginia Henderson was asked by the nursing service committee of the International Council of Nurses to describe her concept of basic nursing. Hers is one of the most widely accepted definitions of nursing:

> The unique function of the nurse is to assist the individual, sick or well, in the performance of those activities contributing to health or its recovery (or to peaceful death) that he would perform unaided if he had the necessary strength, will or knowledge. And to do this in such a way as to help him gain independence as rapidly as possible (Henderson, 1966, p 15).

NURSING AS DEFINED BY ORGANIZATIONS

In 1965, the American Nurses Association (ANA) published the "First Paper on Education for Nursing." Within that paper were identified significant aspects of nursing. It stated "essential components of professional nursing practice include care, cure, and coordination" (American Nurses Association, 1965, p 107).

Others would stress that it is important that any definition of nursing must indicate that it is both an art and a science. It is an art in the sense that it is composed of skills that require expertness and proficiency for their execution. It is a science in the sense that it requires systematized knowledge derived from observation, study, and research.

Again in 1980, the ANA, through its Social Policy Statement, provided yet another definition of nursing: "Nursing is the diagnosis and treatment of human responses to actual or potential health problems" (American Nurses

TABLE 1–1 Definitions of Nursing Developed by Major Theorists

Florence Nightingale (1859)	The goal of nursing is to put the patient in the best condition for nature to act upon him, primarily by altering the environment.
Hildegard Peplau (1952)	Nursing is viewed as an interpersonal process involving interaction between two or more individuals that has as its common goal assisting the individual who is sick or in need of health care.
Virginia Henderson (1966)	Nursing's role is to assist the individual (sick or well) to carry out those activities . . . he would perform unaided if he had the necessary strength, will, or knowledge.
Faye Abdellah (1960)	Nursing is a service to individuals, families, and society based on an art and science that molds the attitudes, intellectual competencies, and technical skills of the individual nurse into the desire and ability to help people cope with their health care needs, and is focused around twenty-one nursing problems.
Ernestine Wiedenbach (1964)	Nursing is a helping, nurturing, and caring service rendered with compassion, skill, and understanding in which sensitivity is key to assisting the nurse to identify the problem.
Ida Jean Orlando (1972)	Nursing's unique and independent role concerns itself with an individual's need for help in an immediate situation for the purpose of avoiding, relieving, diminishing, or curing that individual's sense of helplessness.
Dorothea Orem (1980)	Nursing is concerned with the individual's need for self-care action, which is the practice of activities that individuals initiate and perform on their own behalf in maintaining life, health, and well-being.
Dorothy E. Johnson (1980)	Nursing is an external regulatory force that acts to preserve the organization and integration of the patient's behavior at an optimal level under those conditions in which the behavior constitutes a threat to physical or social health, or in which illness is found.
Imogene M. King (1981)	The focus of nursing is the care of human beings resulting in the health of individuals and health care for groups who are viewed as open systems in constant interaction with their environment.
Betty Neuman (1982)	Nursing responds to individuals, groups, and communities who are in constant interaction with environmental stressors that create disequilibrium. A critical element is the client's ability to react to stress and factors that assist with reconstitution or adaptation.

(continued)

TABLE 1–1 Definitions of Nursing Developed by Major Theorists
(Continued)

Sister Callista Roy (1984)	The goal of nursing is the promotion of adaptive responses (those things that positively influence health) that are affected by the person's ability to respond to stimuli. Nursing involves manipulating stimuli to promote adaptive responses.
Martha E. Rogers (1984)	Nursing is an art and science that is humanistic and humanitarian and directed toward the unitary human and is concerned with the nature and direction of human development.

Association, 1980, p 9). That definition had widespread effect and was realized in the language used in some of the nursing diagnoses we use today.

In 1982, the National Council of State Boards of Nursing (NCSBN) developed a Model Nurse Practice Act. (This document was updated in 1988.) The single most important part of any nurse practice act is the legal definition of nursing practice. This is critical because it provides the foundation and guidelines for education, licensure, scope of practice of the profession, and when necessary, the basis for corrective actions against the person who violates the practice act. The committee that developed the act had difficulty arriving at a precise and succinct definition. It found a lack of consensus within the literature and the profession. The committee was looking for a definition that would clearly differentiate nursing from the practice of any other health care discipline. It was looking for terms that would describe the essential elements unique to nursing but that would be broad enough to include all levels of nurses who should be licensed to practice. In reaching for these goals the committee found that the term *nursing* was not differentiating or limiting and therefore did not use it in the definition. As a working alternative the National Council incorporated currently accepted concepts of the nursing process and proposed that the practice of nursing be defined around these concepts (Pavelka, 1982).

Another factor that has made it difficult to define nursing is that it is taught as encompassing both theoretical and practical aspects, but it is pursued (and continues to be defined) primarily through practice, an area little studied. Benner (1984) states, "Nurses have not been careful record keepers of their own clinical learning. . . . This failure to chart our practices and clinical observations has deprived nursing theory of the uniqueness and richness of the knowledge embedded in expert clinical practice." She further discusses the differences between "knowing that" and "knowing how." When attempting to define nursing we often stumble over these two concepts and how to combine the distinct and unique aspects of both.

As the profession grows and responsibilities change, undoubtedly we will continue to redefine and refine our definition of nursing. In being responsive to changes, nursing becomes even more closely aligned with professions such as law, theology, and education in which changing practices have required greater precision and refinement of definitions of the profession.

Characteristics of a Profession

Since the 1950s, some nursing leaders have been primarily concerned about providing an explicit definition of nursing, whereas others have examined, challenged, and defended nursing's standing as a profession. Certainly at the time nursing and nursing education were evolving in the United States no one asked if nursing qualified as a profession. As a matter of fact, evidence suggests that from an early date the word "profession" was associated with nursing. Strauss (1966) gives as an example a magazine article entitled "A New Profession for Women" that appeared in 1882. The article described nursing reform and carried with it a picture of Isabel Hampton. Strauss (1966) also refers to writings of Lizabeth Price, published in 1892, in which nursing was discussed as a profession.

From a period of time lasting approximately from the 1950s through the 1970s or mid-1980s nursing periodically was reviewed against the characteristics of a profession that had been established in the sociological literature. The activities for which nurses were responsible, the legal ramifications of practice, and particularly the education of future nurses were subjected to the scrutiny of sociologists and nursing leaders who found it challenging to examine nursing against established standards. The characteristics of a profession have been discussed by many (Flexner, 1915; Bixler and Bixler, 1945; Pavalko, 1971). Generally a profession will:

- Possess a well defined and well organized body of knowledge that is on an intellectual level and can be applied to the activities of the group.
- Enlarge a systematic body of knowledge and improve education and service through use of the scientific method.
- Educate its practitioners in institutions of higher education.
- Function autonomously in the formulation of professional policy and in the control of professional activity.
- Develop within the group a code of ethics.
- Attract to the profession individuals who recognize this occupation as their life work and who desire to contribute to the good of society through service to others.
- Strive to compensate its practitioners by providing autonomy, continuous professional development, and economic security.

Some critics challenge that nursing falls short of meeting these criteria. Some of nursing's leaders would also claim that nursing falls short of fulfilling a professional role (Schlotfeldt, 1987; Newman, 1990). In light of that challenge it might be helpful to explore each of the above criteria as it might be applied to

A BODY OF SPECIALIZED KNOWLEDGE

A major criticism often levied at nursing is that nursing has no "body of specialized knowledge" that belongs uniquely to nursing. Critics state that nursing borrows from biologic sciences, social sciences, and medical science, and then combines the various skills and concepts to call it "nursing." Nursing leaders and theorists disagree as to whether nursing is a unique profession

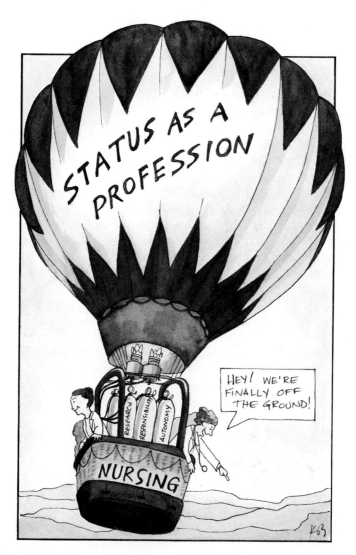

FIGURE 1–2 Some continue to question whether nursing truly can support the title of "profession."

or one borrowed from other disciplines. In fact, this amalgamation and synthesis of some areas with application to another may be one of the unique qualities of nursing. Nursing researchers are also working to develop an organized body of knowledge that is unique to nursing. Even simple tasks, such as the length of time required to get an accurate reading on a rectal thermometer, are being researched and recorded. Other nurses are working to advance the standing of nursing through the development of a code of ethics, standards of practice, and peer review. Nursing theorists are challenging the work of one another in efforts to identify and describe the general principles that govern nursing practice. (See Chapter 3 for more information on nursing theories.) As the results of these efforts become realized, nursing should emerge as a profession with an established body of knowledge.

USE OF THE SCIENTIFIC METHOD TO ENLARGE THE BODY OF KNOWLEDGE

Critical to any profession is its ability to grow and change as the world changes. Equally important is the method by which those changes occur. They cannot take place in a haphazard, random, or hit-or-miss fashion. In other words, they must be well thought out. Data must be systematically gathered and carefully analyzed, the problem(s) must be correctly identified, alternative solutions must be sought, the best approach selected and implemented, and the results thoroughly evaluated. As a student of nursing you already recognize that this has been applied to nursing practice through the nursing process. It is also being applied to nursing research. Through research and practice we add to the established body of nursing knowledge. Tangible proof of this growth can be monitored in the quick turnover in nursing textbooks. One seldom finds a clinical text in use in a quality program that has not been published within the last 4 years. Accreditation criteria set down for nursing programs by the national accrediting agencies require that libraries be stocked with up-to-date texts and periodicals. All of this reflects the continued growth of the body of knowledge in nursing.

EDUCATION WITHIN INSTITUTIONS OF HIGHER EDUCATION

Perhaps no issue in nursing has been any more controversial than the education of its practitioners. Nursing's heritage, like that of medicine, was founded in an apprenticeship beginning. Students were assigned to experienced practitioners who taught the skills with which they were familiar. Once those skills were acquired the student moved into the world of employment. Our earliest programs of education were located in hospitals rather than universities. (See

Chapter 2 for more information on the history of nursing education.) Over time the setting in which nurses are educated has changed. Today by far the majority of nursing programs preparing registered nurses are located in collegiate settings, either the community college or the senior college or university. However, some controversy still exists with regard to 2-year versus 4-year nursing education and to the "technical" aspects of patient care. All these issues will be discussed at length later in this book as we continue to study the profession of nursing.

CONTROL OF PROFESSIONAL POLICY AND PROFESSIONAL ACTIVITY

Most critics reviewing professions against standards for professions place emphasis on the ability of any group to develop its own policy and to function fairly autonomously. To some extent, this has always been a problem for nursing although the current health care reform may assist the profession to achieve the full autonomy it has been seeking. Traditionally the nurse works under the direction of the patient's physician, often in a hospital setting. The physician writes the orders for medical care that are to be implemented by the nurse, and the agency or hospital sets the policies under which that care is delivered. Only in the last 50 years has nursing made significant inroads in defining the unique role of the nurse in "care" as opposed to "cure" of the patient. Today nurses are responsible for planning and implementing the nursing care patients are to receive and are also accountable for the care provided. The practice acts in many states may even provide for an expanded role of the nurse that gives prescriptive authority to nurses who have completed the necessary educational preparation to be so licensed. Nursing diagnosis, once challenged as an inappropriate responsibility for nurses, has become a standard of good nursing care. In some practice settings, nurses are eligible for third-party payment; that is, they can be reimbursed by insurance companies for the care they have provided, a situation that will increase with health care reform. Although nurses continue to carry out the medical regimen outlined by physicians, a more collaborative relationship is beginning to occur and the contribution of the nurse is receiving more recognition.

A CODE OF ETHICS

The general standard for professional behavior of nurses in the United States is the ANA Code for Nurses. This document was developed by the ANA and is periodically revised to address current issues in practice. The International Council of Nurses, housed in Geneva, Switzerland, has also developed a code for nurses that reiterates many of the behaviors outlined in the ANA code.

The international code sets the standards for ethical practice by nurses throughout the world. Copies of both of these codes and more discussion of the ethical conduct of nurses are found in Chapter 6.

NURSING AS A LIFETIME COMMITMENT

Bixler and Bixler (1945) emphasized in their listing of criteria for professions that a profession should attract people of intellectual and personal qualities who exalt service above personal gain and who recognize their chosen occupation as a lifework. Pavalko (1971) also identified as a significant criterion the sense of commitment the members have toward work as a lifetime or at least a long-term pursuit rather than as a stepping stone to another profession. Studies of nursing indicate that most individuals gaining educational preparation for nursing remain within the profession although concern has been voiced regarding the "burnout" that occurs from stress (see Chapter 11). Most individuals who have been nurses continue to identify themselves as such long after they have retired. Of even greater emphasis today is the tendency of individuals to enter the profession of nursing at one educational level and to continue to advance in practice and education by pursuing additional degrees and experience. The concept of "articulation" between variously positioned degree-granting institutions is in the forefront of nursing today. More discussion of articulation in nursing education is found in Chapter 2.

SERVICE TO THE PUBLIC

Various theorists list criteria for professions that discuss concepts of altruism, service to the public, and dedication. Some suggest that altruism, or the desire to provide for the good of society, must be the worker's motivating force. Nurses have long struggled with the ambiguity that can result from this concept. Possessing a history with a strong religious heritage, the giving of oneself at all costs helped frame the image of nursing and nurses. As nursing has come of age as a profession, some of our thinking is changing to recognize that "giving away" one's services should not be considered professional. Because nurses expect appropriate remuneration for services rendered does not suggest that they are less than dedicated to the patients for whom they are caring and the care that is being given. Providing service to the public should not be thought of as requiring the sacrifice of one's financial security. One can list medicine, law, dentistry, and engineering as some examples of other professions in which the practitioners are amply rewarded financially for the services provided. Greater discussion of nurses and collective bargaining is included in Chapter 9.

Differentiating Between the Terms *Profession* and *Professional*

The practice of nursing involves many activities that may be performed by many caregivers. These people include nurse aides or assistants, orderlies, practical nurses, and registered nurses prepared for entry into nursing through any of several educational avenues (see Chapter 2). Each of these caregivers is contributing to nursing as a profession. To meet the nursing needs of the public, it is essential that caregivers function at various levels of practice. This has led to confusion about the use of the terms *profession* and *professional*. Is there a difference in looking at the practice of nursing in its totality and at the practice of professional nursing?

A popular view of a profession involves the approach a person has to an occupation. Most professionals are seriously concerned about their occupation, strive for excellence in performance, and demonstrate a sense of ethics and responsibility in relationship to their career. Such people consider their work a lifelong endeavor rather than a stepping stone to another field of employment. They place a positive value on being termed professional and perceive being termed nonprofessional or technical as an adverse reflection on their status, position, and motivation.

Others consider the attributes of professionalism to have a great deal to do with attitude, dress, conduct, and deportment. Often built into this concept of the professional are the personal values and stereotypes held by the person doing the evaluating. For example, an early perception of the "truly professional" nurse described a person dressed in a starched white uniform and cap, whose hair is off her collar, and whose shoes are freshly polished. Some individuals would continue to support this concept of the "professional nurse." Others may perceive the "professional nurse" as the one who is open and kind in interpersonal relationships, who focuses on the needs of others, and who is tactful and skillful in interview techniques.

In at least one instance, federal legislation has helped to establish a list of characteristics of a professional. Public Law 93-360 (Labor Management Relations Act, 1947 [amended, 1959, 1974]), which governs collective bargaining activities, defines the professional employee as follows:

> (a) any employee engaged in work (i) predominantly intellectual and varied in character as opposed to routine mental, manual, mechanical, or physical work; (ii) involving the consistent exercise of discretion and judgment in its performance; (iii) of such a character that the output produced or the result accomplished cannot be standardized in relation to a given period of time; (iv) requiring knowledge of an advanced type in a field of science or learning customarily acquired by a prolonged course of specialized intellectual instruction and study in an institution of higher learning or a hospital, as distinguished from a general

academic education or from an apprenticeship or from training in the performance of routine mental, manual, or physical processes; or

(b) any employee, who (i) has completed the courses of specialized intellectual instruction and study described in clause (iv) of paragraph (a), and (ii) is performing related work under the supervision of a professional person to qualify himself to become a professional employee as defined in paragraph (a).

The sociological and legal definitions are much more restrictive than the popular view of the term *professional*. One of the difficulties is the communication block that results from people using the term in different ways. When one person is using a restrictive, sociological definition and the other person responds from a standpoint of personal belief and feeling, agreement is almost impossible.

You can put this into better perspective if you know something about the historical development of the field of nursing.

Health Care in Ancient Cultures

The life of the primitive societies was necessarily a nomadic one. People wandered in search of food, warmth, and an environment compatible with life. Anthropologists believe that these primitive groups moved from Africa to spread across the world. The ice ages in northern latitudes drove these groups back to the warmer climate found around the Mediterranean Sea, in India, and in China where civilizations developed. The Mediterranean Sea was thought to occupy the center of the earth with all areas to its east known as "eastern" and those to the west known as "western" (Donahue, 1985). Located in the Near East were the countries of Egypt, Persia (Iran), Babylonia (Iraq), Assyria, and Palestine. The sophistication of health care practices varied considerably from one culture to another.

INDIA

Located in the southern part of the Far East, India was essentially isolated by mountains from other parts of the world. Excavations indicate that the first civilizations (3000–1500 BC) were highly developed with systems of sanitation, bathrooms and public baths, and other amenities. The Vedic age began in 1500 BC and the people worshiped the eternal spirit Brahma. Brahmanism (also known as Hinduism) was to become a major religion of the country. Sources of information about health practices come from the Vedas, a sacred book of Brahmanism dating back as far as 1600 BC and considered by some to be older than any other writings on earth. Medicine, as described in the books of *Ayur-Veda*, included major and minor surgery, children's diseases, materia medica, and diseases of the nervous and urinary systems (Nutting and Dock, 1935). Their surgery may have been the most highly developed of any ancient culture. Also developing out of this early religion was stratification of the society into four different castes. Later Buddhism was to emerge as the major religion of early India. During the Buddhist period, India is credited with an advanced understanding of disease prevention, hygiene and sanitation, medicine, and surgery. The importance of prenatal care to both mother and infant seemed well understood and practiced. In disregarding the caste system of the earlier religion, Buddhism made education and the right to peace possible for everyone. Public hospitals were constructed during this time, and some vital statistics were collected. The early hospitals were staffed with nurses whose qualifications were similar to those expected of today's practical nurse, except that the Indian nurses were all men. When Buddhism fell, the hospitals were abolished (Donahue, 1985).

CHINA

The ancient Chinese followed the teachings of Confucius, who sought to relieve the country's oppression by reviving ancient customs. Patriarchal rule dominated, and emphasis was placed on the value of the family as a unit. Ancestor worship attained great importance. Woman's role was seen as being vastly inferior to man's, her major value being determined by the number of sons she could produce. Early Chinese established the philosophy of the yang and the yin. The yang represented the active, positive, masculine force of the universe, and the yin represented the passive, negative, feminine force. These two forces were always contrasted to and complementary with each other. Health practices focused on prevention and good health resulted from a balance between the yang and the yin.

The Chinese also developed acupuncture skills that are still being practiced today. No faith was placed in the patient's history as a diagnostic tool, and diagnosis was made on the basis of a complicated pulse theory. The Chinese had elaborate materia medica, and many of the drugs they used, such as ephedrine, are used in modern medicine.

EGYPT

The oldest medical records so far discovered and deciphered are those from Egypt, dating back as far as 3000 BC. Early records were carved on stone or were written on papyrus. Ancient Egyptians, who settled along the Nile (while other cultures were settling along the Indus, Euphrates, and Tigris rivers), developed community planning that helped to avoid public health problems, especially those related to disease transmitted through water sources. Egypt is credited with being one of the healthiest of ancient countries, perhaps because of the progress it made in the fields of hygiene and sanitation. Strict rules were developed around such things as cleanliness, food, drink, exercise, and sexual relations. The Egyptians also established a "house of death," which was located at a site away from civilization, and they embalmed their dead. People in this early culture classified more than 700 drugs. Their skill in bandaging was carried over for history to observe in mummies. It is also believed that they were skilled in dentistry, often filling teeth with gold. The oldest known medical books come from this society. The books outline surgical techniques and methods of birth control, describe disease processes, and suggest remedies. Out of this culture came the first physician known to history, Imhotep (2900–2800 BC). He was recognized as a surgeon, an architect, a temple priest, a scribe, and a magician. Although women in ancient Egypt received more respect than in some other Eastern countries, it is not clear whether nurses existed as such. Most likely they served as "wet nurses" and as midwives.

PERSIA

One of the most extensive empires of the Near East was that of the Persians. Persia was located in the area of modern day Iran and, at one time, extended throughout the Fertile Crescent area. Their quest for territory and power resulted in their conquering much of that area. They believed in Zoroaster, a prophet who wrote the sacred books of Persia. His writing introduced the world to the concept of two creators—one good, one evil—and sacred elements of fire, earth, and water. The Persian society adopted many of the cultural practices of the lands they conquered, which included much of the medical and surgical practices of Egypt. They established early schools to prepare priest–physicians, from which evolved three types of physicians—those who healed by the knife, those who healed with herbs, and those who healed through exorcism.

BABYLONIA

Babylonia, like Egypt, was located in an area known as the Fertile Crescent and the Cradle of Civilization and from this country came the second oldest medical records (Nutting and Dock, 1935). Babylonia was located in the southern part of present-day Iraq, although its borders differed. The area was so named because of its well watered soil and warm climate, a combination that was favorable to the establishment of civilizations. The life-style of the Babylonians was entirely different from that of the Egyptians. Each city was a complete community in itself, governed by a divine ruler and a priest–king. Illness was believed to be the punishment for sinning and for displeasing the gods. A cure was brought about by purifying the body, usually by incantations and the use of herbs. Temples, in which the purification occurred, became centers of medical care.

The Babylonians were skilled mathematicians and astronomers. It is not surprising, therefore, that many of their beliefs were based on nature study and the potency of numbers and on observations of the movement of stars and planets. Horoscopes were cast in terms of a person's birth and the position of the planets on that occasion. The Babylonians found significance in the number seven, which we often hear referred to today as "the lucky number." From this culture developed the famous Code of Hammurabi (Hammurabi was then the king of Babylonia) in 1900 BC. The principal source of this code is a stone monument found in 1901 and preserved today in the Louvre in Paris. This code may represent the first sliding scale for fee payment by dividing the public into three classes. Those classified as "gentlemen" might expect to pay their surgeons in silver coins rather than in goods or services. A surgeon who bungled an operation on a "gentleman" carried heavy obligations; the surgeon might have his hands cut off if the surgery went poorly. This puts the malpractice rates absorbed by physicians today in a different light.

ASSYRIA

The Babylonians were succeeded as rulers in the Fertile Crescent by the Assyrians. This nation centered in the northern part of present-day Iraq and extended into what is now Syria and southern Iraq as they conquered other nations. Their laws were severe, with the death penalty frequently used. They believed in good and evil spirits, in magic, and in many gods, and that illness was punishment for sin and that a person's body could be occupied by evil spirits. Thus, the practice of medicine was developed around these religious beliefs.

PALESTINE

The Hebrews made their home in the area called Palestine, adjacent to Egypt. This area includes present-day Israel and some surrounding area. Primarily an agricultural society, the country was ruled by kings. The Hebrews are credited with more democratic sharing of knowledge than any of the other ancient civilizations. Through the leadership of Moses, the adopted son of the Egyptian pharaoh's daughter, the Hebrews developed the Mosaic Code, which represented an organized method of disease prevention. The code emphasized isolation of persons with communicable diseases, differentiated clean from unclean, and covered every detail of personal, family, and public or national hygiene. With regard to their treatment of women, Nutting and Dock (1935) write:

> All the stern and ungraciously sounding texts relating to the 'uncleanliness' of women, which when considered only in the abstract seem so needlessly humiliating, are in reality witnesses of the extreme care and solicitude of the Jews for the health of their women, and of the sanctity and beauty of their family life. These regulations secured to women the personal isolation and privacy, quiet, and consideration necessary on hygienic grounds, and especially made the time of childbirth a period of isolation and quiet, of cleanliness of body and clothing, and of rest for mind and body (pp 62–63).

Bible scriptures such as Leviticus 7:16–19 and 19:5–8, which forbade that meat be eaten past the third day after the animal was slaughtered, were no doubt written because of the warm climate and the lack of refrigeration. Similarly, the Mosaic and Talmudic regulation regarding the slaughtering of animals and the examination and inspection that checked for diseases of the internal organs were in keeping with their advanced sanitary ordinances. The duty to visit the sick also saw its origin in the early writings of Jewish rabbis even if the sick person was a Gentile. The Houses for the Sick during this early period were called Beth Holem.

The Hebrew culture recognized one god who had power over life and death. From this belief evolved the role of the priest as supervisor of medical practices relating to cleansing and purification. Priest–physicians took on the function of health inspectors.

GREECE

This culture occupied a peninsula that jutted out into the Mediterranean Sea from the southeastern part of Europe. The ancient Greek culture is remembered in part for its worship of gods and goddesses and for the emphasis that was placed on healthy bodies. (Remember that the Greeks started the Olympic games.) In Greek mythology, Asklepios (sometimes spelled Aesculapius or Asclepius), son of Apollo, was the chief healer. He is usually represented as carrying a staff, to show that he traveled from place to place, around which is entwined a serpent, representing wisdom and immortality. (Some persons believe that when the army medical services fashioned the caduceus, the symbol of the medical profession, the staff and serpent that were incorporated into the symbol came from this legend.)

Exquisite temples, located on beautiful sites, were built as shrines to Asklepios and became social and intellectual centers as well as places to obtain cures. The curative process usually began with animal sacrifice and continued through various purifying processes. In addition to these shrines, two other institutions offered care to the sick in ancient Greece. The xenodochium was an institution that first offered care to travelers and later cared for people who were sick and injured. This may have been the forerunner of the city or country hospital as we know it today. The iatrion was a facility offering ambulatory care and would correspond to our outpatient clinics.

It is rather surprising that from this Greek society, so heavily steeped in mythology, animal sacrifice, and faith in the power of the gods, was to come the Father of Modern Medicine. Hippocrates was born about 400 BC on the island of Cos. He stressed a natural cause for disease, treated the whole patient in a patient-centered approach to care, and introduced the scientific method of solving patient problems. He also taught the necessity of accurate observations and careful record keeping. Hippocrates did not attribute ill health to an infliction by the gods but rather believed that health depended on equilibrium existing between the mind and body and the environment. From this evolved the humoral theory of disease, which has lasted for centuries.

Many early physicians were also from Greece, although they often practiced their skills in Rome after Greece was conquered by the Roman Empire. Galen, Aesclepiades, and Pedanim Dioscorides were all Greek physicians who worked in Rome.

ROME

The medical advances of the ancient Romans fell short of those of the Greeks. Medical practices were often borrowed from the countries the Romans conquered, and the physicians from those countries were made slaves who provided medical services to the Romans. The Romans clung to gods, superstition, and herbs when faced with disease, although hygiene and sanitation were fairly well established. Many homes were equipped with baths, and cleanliness was valued. The role of women was considerably different from that in other ancient cultures. Women were allowed to own property, appear in public, and campaign publicly for causes they believed should be advanced, and they could entertain guests and sit with them at the table.

THE AMERICAS

No definite date can be assumed for the historical recording of civilization of the area that was to be known as the Americas. It is thought that early inhabitants probably came from Central Asia, gaining access across a land bridge in the Bering Strait into Alaska. Like other early tribes they were nomadic, seeking food and shelter. Several groups including the Incas and the Aztecs developed a high level of civilization. Medicine men were responsible for curing ills of both the body and the mind, and disease was believed to result from displeasing gods. The sun god was particularly important to these cultures. Rites, ceremonies, herbal treatment, charms, and, in some instances, human sacrifice contributed to healing practices. Little is known about the role of the nurse in these early civilizations, although the status enjoyed by women was good.

The writing about early health care makes little or no mention of nursing or nurses. Health practices varied depending on level of development of the society. Ritualistic ceremonies and worship of gods was common and the role of healer was assumed by various individuals within the culture. Each primitive society had its own curative agents, taboos, and practices, some more advanced than others. Absent from most cultures was a sound theory of disease.

Historical Perspectives of Nursing

Although the ancient cultures developed medicine as a science and profession, they showed little evidence of establishing a foundation for nursing. With the possible exceptions of the male attendants of the early Buddhist culture in India and the midwives, who had an established role in several cultures, nursing, as we think of it, did not exist. It was not until the early Christian period that nursing would emerge.

Muriel Uprichard identifies three heritages from the past that tend to inhibit the progress of nursing. They are "the folk image of the nurse brought forward from primitive times, the religious image of the nurse inherited from the medieval period, and the servant image of the nurse created by the Protestant-capitalist ethic of the 16th to 19th century" (Uprichard, 1973, p 24). Whether they impeded progress, certainly these concepts of the nurse have had an impact.

THE FOLK IMAGE OF THE NURSE

Since the time of the first mother, women have carried the major responsibility for the nourishing and the nurturing of children and for caring for elderly and aging members of the family. With this type of history, it is difficult to pinpoint a particular time or place for the beginnings of nursing as we know it. It is reasonable to assume that early tribes and civilizations had needs for health care. It is also reasonable to assume that within those tribes and civilizations, there would come forth people who demonstrated adeptness and special interests in meeting the needs of the sick, the injured, and child-bearing women. The education of these "nurses" was largely by trial and error, advancing those methods that appeared successful, and by the sharing of information with one another. Superstition and magic played a significant role in the treatment rendered; folklore abounded, and a close relationship existed between religion and the healing arts.

Nursing skills primarily evolved from intuition. For example, during the process of planning a diet for the family, the wise woman noticed that eating certain foods resulted in episodes of diarrhea and vomiting, whereas eating other herbs, roots, and leaves had a soothing effect on the body. Families developed recipes that were handed down from generation to generation; effective treatments and cures were recorded and shared.

THE RELIGIOUS IMAGE OF THE NURSE

The first continuity in the history of nursing began with Christianity. Christ's teachings admonished people to love and care for their neighbors. With the establishment of churches in the Christian era, groups were organized as orders whose primary concern was to care for the sick, the poor, orphans, widows, the aged, slaves, and prisoners, all done in the name of charity and Christian love. Christ's precepts placed women and men on a parity, and the early church made both men and women deacons, with equal rank. Unmarried women had opportunities for service that were never imagined earlier. Although these opportunities represented positive changes, as nursing developed an image closely tied to religion and religious orders, strict discipline was expected. Absolute attendance to the orders of persons in higher rank (priest or physicians) was demanded. This type of thinking was embedded in nursing for many years.

Of particular significance in the history of nursing are the deaconesses in the Eastern Christian churches. These women, who were required to be unmarried or widowed, were often widows or daughters of Roman officials, and thus had breeding, culture, wealth, and position. These dedicated young women practiced "works of mercy" that included feeding the hungry, clothing the naked, visiting the imprisoned, sheltering the homeless, caring for the sick, and burying the dead. The deaconesses were the early counterparts to the community health nurses of today. When they entered homes to distribute food and medicine they carried a basket, which would later become the visiting nurse bag of today. No discussion of nursing history would be complete without mentioning Phoebe, who is often referred to as the first deaconess and the first visiting nurse. She carried Paul's letters and cared for him and many others. In the Epistle to the Romans, dated about AD 58, reference is made to Phoebe and to her work.

Not clearly distinguished from the deaconesses were the widows and the virgins. The members of the *Order of Widows* had not necessarily been married. It seems that the title was used to designate respect for age. If married, a member was required to be widowed only once, and vows were taken never to remarry. The *Order of Virgins* emphasized virginity as essential to purity of life, and virgins ranked equal to the clergy. These three groups—deaconesses, widows, and virgins—shared many common characteristics and carried out similar responsibilities. Because these women often visited the sick in their homes, they are sometimes recognized as the earliest organized group of public health nurses. The movement peaked in Constantinople about AD 400, when a staff of 40 deaconesses lived and worked under the direction of Olympia, a powerful and deeply religious deaconess. The influence of the deaconess order diminished in the fifth and sixth centuries, when church decrees removed clerical duties and rank from the deaconess.

Although the position of deaconess originated in the Eastern Church, it spread west to Gaul and Ireland. In Rome, women who served in comparable positions were known as *matrons*. Active during the fourth and fifth centuries, these women held independent positions and had great wealth, which they contributed to charity and to nursing. Among these Christian converts were three women who contributed significantly to nursing.

St. Marcella

Saint Marcella established the first monastery for women in her own beautiful and palatial home in an exclusive area of Rome. This later became a center for Christian study and teaching. It was here that St. Jerome worked on translation of the Bible while teaching Christian principles. Marcella herself was regarded as an authority on difficult scriptural passages. During the sack of Rome, her home was invaded by warriors who expected to find valuables stored there. When they found little more than a bare building, they whipped Marcella, hoping that she would reveal the hiding places of riches. After the assault she is said to have fled to St. Paul's church, which was nearby where she died as a result of her injuries.

Fabiola

Fabiola is said to have studied at Marcella's home. She was reputably a beautiful woman from a great and wealthy Roman family; however, she was unhappy in her first marriage and so divorced her husband and remarried, again unhappily. Under the influence of Marcella, she converted to Christianity and, after the death of her second husband, began her career of charity. On becoming a Christian, Fabiola's new beliefs made marriage after divorce a sin. She publicly acknowledged this, committed her life to charitable work, and in AD 380 built the first public hospital in Rome described as a *nosocomium*. Here she cared for the sick and poor whom she gathered from the streets and highways, personally washing and treating wounds and sores that repulsed others. St. Jerome tells of some of her work and her attributes in his writings. She died about 399, and scores of Romans are said to have attended her funeral to show their respect for her.

St. Paula

Saint Paula was also a scholar of Marcella. Widowed, learned, and wealthy, she is said to have assisted St. Jerome, (whose lifetime exceeded that of all the women with whom he was associated), in the translation of the writings of the prophets. St. Paula traveled to Palestine and devoted a fortune to the estab-lishment of hospitals and inns for pilgrims traveling to Jerusalem. In Bethle-hem she organized a monastery, built hospitals for the sick, and developed hospices for pilgrims, where tired travelers and the ill were cared for. Some credit her with being the first to teach nursing as an art rather than as a service.

The Role of the Monastic Orders

The monastic orders also developed during this time. Through them young men and women were able to follow careers of their choice while living a Christian life. One of the earliest organizations for men in nursing, the Parabolani brotherhood, was established at this time. Responding to needs created by the Black Plague, this group reportedly organized a hospital and traveled throughout Rome caring for the sick. The order of Benedictines, which still exists, was founded during this period. Such famous monastic nurses as St. Brigid, St. Scholastica (a twin sister of St. Benedict), and St. Hilda were founding schools, tending to the sick and giving to the poor. The monasteries played a large role in the preservation of culture and learning as well as in offering refuge to the persecuted, care to the sick, and education to the uneducated. The learning of the classical period would have been lost when the empire fell were it not for the monks and monasteries. During this period (approximately AD 50 to 800), the first hospitals also were established. These hospitals, located outside the monastery walls, are still standing. There were more than 700 hospitals in England by the middle of the 16th century. The Hotel Dieu in Lyons was established in 542 and the Hotel Dieu in Paris, around 650. The Hotel Dieu in Paris was staffed by the first order specifically devoted to nursing, the Augustinian Sisters. The Santo Spirito Hospital in Rome, the largest medieval hospital, was established by papal order in 717.

The Crusades, which swept northern Europe, were to last for almost 200 years (1096–1291). The deaconess movement, suppressed by the Western churches, became all but extinct. Military nursing orders evolved as a result of the Crusades. The Knights Hospitallers of St. John was one such order. It was organized to staff two hospitals that were located in Jerusalem. The Knights, organized as a nursing order, at times were required to defend the hospital and its patients. For this reason they wore a suit of armor under their habits. On the habit was the Maltese cross. The same cross was to be used later on a badge designed for the Nightingale School. The badge became the forerunner of the nursing pin as we know it today. The symbolism of the pin will be dis-cussed later in this chapter. Orders of lay sisters called *consorores* developed to assist with the hospital work but were not granted the status of the Knights.

Secular orders of nurses also came into existence at this time in history. Operating much like the monastic orders, members of this group could termi-nate their vocations at any time and were not bound to the vows of monastic life. Examples of the secular orders include the Order of Antonines (1095);

the Beguines of Flanders, Belgium (1184); the Misericordia (1244); and the Alexian Brothers, founded during the bubonic plague epidemic of 1348. The only nursing education offered to these dedicated people was in the form of an apprenticeship; a newcomer to the organization would be assigned to a more experienced person and would learn from that person.

The inquiring student is encouraged to seek greater depth of knowledge about the orders, their purposes and goals, and the lives of those who devoted their energies to the care of the sick and the poor by consulting the nursing references given at the end of this chapter.

THE SERVANT IMAGE OF THE NURSE

The Middle Ages were followed by the Renaissance (occurring from the 14th through the 16th centuries) and the Reformation. During the Renaissance, also known as the Age of Discovery, a new impetus was given to education, but not to medical education, which was still caught up in the humoral theory of disease. Neither was it provided to nursing education, which was all but nonexistent.

The Reformation, a religious movement that started with the work of Martin Luther, began in Germany in 1517. It resulted in a revolt against the supremacy of the pope and the formation of Protestant churches across Europe. Monasteries were closed, religious orders were dissolved, and the work of women in these orders became almost extinct.

Also associated with the Reformation was a change in the role of women. The Protestant Church, which stood for freedom of religion and thought, did not grant much freedom to women. Once revered by the church and encouraged toward charitable activities, women of the Reformation were deemed subordinate to men. Their role was defined within the confines of the home; their duties were those of bearing children and caring for the home. Work in hospitals no longer appealed to women of high birth. Hospital care was relegated to "uncommon" women, a group comprising prisoners, prostitutes, and

Women faced with earning their own living were forced to work as domestic servants; and although nursing was considered a domestic service, it was not a desirable one. Pay was poor, the hours were long, and the work was strenuous. The nurse was considered the most menial of servants. Thus, began what may be called the "Dark Ages of Nursing."

The image of nurses and nursing during this time was described by Charles Dickens (1936) through the characters of Sairey Gamp and Betsy Prig in his book *Martin Chuzzlewit*:

> She was a fat old woman, this Mrs. Gamp, with a husky voice and a moist eye, which she had a remarkable power of turning up, and only showing the white of

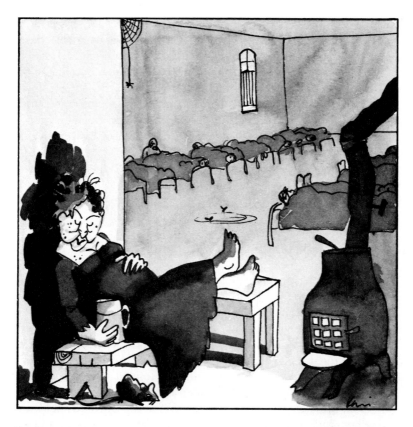

FIGURE 1–3 From the Middle Ages to the 19th century, nursing was often left to "uncommon women."

it. Having very little neck, it cost her some trouble to look over herself, if one may say so, at those to whom she talked. She wore a very rusty black gown, rather the worse for snuff, and a shawl and bonnet to correspond. . . . The face of Mrs. Gamp—the nose in particular—was somewhat red and swollen, and it was difficult to enjoy her society without becoming conscious of a smell of spirits. Like most persons who have attained to great eminence in their profession, she took to hers very kindly; insomuch, that setting aside her natural predilections as a woman, she went to a lying-in or a lying-out with equal zest and relish (p 318).

Mrs. Prig was of the Gamp build, but not so fat; and her voice was deeper and more like a man's. She had also a beard (p 417).

The 16th and 17th centuries found Europe devastated by famine, plague, filth, and horror. In England, for example, King Henry VIII had effectively eliminated organized monastic relief provided to orphans and other displaced persons. Throughout Europe vagrancy and begging abounded, and those caught begging were often severely punished by being branded, beaten, or chained in galleys where they served as oarsmen. Knowledge of hygiene was insufficient; the poor suffered the most. Social reform was inevitable. Several nursing groups were organized. These groups gave money, time, and service to the sick and the poor, visiting them in their homes and ministering to their needs. Such groups include the Order of the Visitation of Mary, St. Vincent de Paul, and in 1633, the Sisters of Charity. The last group became an outstanding secular nursing order. They developed an educational program for the intelligent young women they recruited that included experience in a hospital as well as visiting in the homes. Receiving help, counsel, and encouragement from St. Vincent de Paul, the Sisters expanded their services to include caring for abandoned children. In 1640, St. Vincent established the Hospital for Foundlings in Paris.

THE BEGINNING OF CHANGE

Countries in Europe remaining Roman Catholic escaped some of the disorganization caused by the Reformation. During the 1500s the Spanish and the Portuguese began traveling to the New World. In 1521, Cortes conquered the capital of the Aztec civilization in Mexico and renamed that capital Mexico City. Early colonists to the area included members of Catholic religious orders, who became the doctors, nurses, and teachers of the new land. In 1524, the first hospital on the American continent, the Hospital of Immaculate Conception, was built in Mexico City. Mission colleges were founded. The first medical school in America was founded in 1578 at the University of Mexico.

Farther north, Jacques Cartier sailed up the St. Lawrence River in 1535 and established French settlements in Nova Scotia. In 1639, three Augustinian nuns arrived in Quebec to staff the Hotel Dieu. Jeanne Mance, who had been educated at an Ursuline Convent, arrived in Montreal in 1641 to care for the Iroquois Indians and the colonists. The Ursuline Sisters of Quebec are credited with attempting to organize the first training for nurses on this continent. They taught the Indian women of the area to care for their sick.

The first hospital founded in what was to become the United States was started in Philadelphia in 1751, at the urging of Benjamin Franklin. Franklin believed that the public had a duty to provide care to the poor, friendless, sick, and insane. A bill, passed that year, authorized the establishment of the Pennsylvania Hospital (Kalisch and Kalisch, 1995).

In Europe, outstanding men of medicine began to make vital and valuable contributions to medical knowledge. William Harvey (1578–1657), who became known as the father of modern medicine, was the first to theorize about circulation of the blood. Anton van Leeuwenhoek (1632–1723) used a microscope to delineate bacteria and protozoa. Later, Rene Laennec (1781–1826) described the pathology of tuberculosis; Ignatz Semmelweis (1818–1865) explained the relationship between handwashing, or the lack of it, and puerperal fever; Louis Pasteur (1822–1895) discovered anaerobic bacteria and the process of pasteurization; and Joseph Lister (1827–1912) developed aseptic technique. In the United States Oliver Wendell Holmes (1809–1894) wrote the classic *The Contagiousness of Puerperal Fever*, published 5 years before the medical community became aware of the work of Semmelweis.

Among lay persons influencing social change during this time was a young minister in Kaiserwerth, Germany, Theodore Fliedner (1800–1864). With the assistance of his first wife, Friederike, Fliedner revived the deaconess movement by establishing a training institute for deaconesses at Kaiserwerth in 1836. During a fund-raising tour through Holland and England, Pastor Fliedner met Elizabeth Fry of England, who had brought about reform at New-gate Prison in England. Greatly impressed with Mrs. Fry's accomplishments, the Fliedners followed her example and first worked with women prisoners in Kaiserwerth. Later they opened a small hospital for the sick, and Gertrude Reichardt, the daughter of a physician, was recruited as their first deaconess. The endeavors at Kaiserwerth included care of the sick, visitations and parochial work, and teaching. A course in nursing was developed that included lectures by physicians. No small part was played by Friederike, who helped bring Theodore's visionary plans to fruition and who was herself much dedicated to the deaconess movement. While away from home promoting deaconess activities, she learned that one of her children had died. A second child died shortly after her return, and she herself died in 1842, after the birth of a premature infant. Pastor Fliedner was also assisted in his work by his second wife, Caroline Bertheau, who had some nursing experience before her marriage. In 1849 Pastor Fliedner journeyed to the United States, where he helped to establish the first Motherhouse of Kaiserwerth Deaconesses in Pittsburgh, Pennsylvania.

In England, at about the same time, Elizabeth Fry (1780–1845) organized the Institute of Nursing Sisters, often called the Fry Sisters, a secular group. To follow were the Sisters of Mercy, a Roman Catholic group formed by Catherine McAuley (1787–1841), and another Catholic group called the Irish Sisters of Charity, formed by Mary Aikenhead (1787–1858).

The Nightingale Influence

The three images discussed (the folk image, the servant image, and the religious image) all influenced the development of nursing, but in the latter half of the 18th century one woman changed the form and direction of nursing and succeeded in establishing it as a respected field of endeavor. This outstanding woman was Florence Nightingale.

Born May 12, 1820, the second daughter of a wealthy family, she was named after the city in which she was born, Florence, Italy. Because of her family's high social and economic standing, she was cultured, well traveled, and educated. At the age of 17 she had mastered several languages and mathematics and was extremely well read. Through the influential people she met, she was expected to select a desirable mate, marry, and assume her place in society. Florence Nightingale had other ideas. She wanted to become a nurse. To her family this was unthinkable. She continued to travel with her family and their friends. In her travels she met Mr. and Mrs. Sidney Herbert, who were becoming interested in hospital reform. Miss Nightingale began collecting information on public health and hospitals and soon became recognized as an important authority on the subject.

Through friends she learned about Pastor Fliedner's institute at Kaiserwerth. Because it was a religious institution under the auspices of the church, she could go there, although she could not go to English hospitals. In 1851 she spent 3 months studying at Kaiserwerth.

In 1853, she started working with a committee that supervised an "Establishment for Gentlewomen During Illness." She eventually was appointed superintendent of the establishment. As her knowledge of hospitals and nursing reform grew, she was consulted by both reformers and physicians who were beginning to see the need for "trained" nurses. Still her family objected to her activities.

When the Crimean War broke out, war correspondents wrote about the abominable manner in which the sick and wounded soldiers were cared for by the British Army. Florence Nightingale, by then a recognized authority on hospital care, wrote to her friend Sir Sidney Herbert, who was then Secretary of War, and offered to take a group of 38 nurses to the Crimea. At the same time he had written a letter requesting her assistance in resolving this national crisis. Their letters crossed in the mail. Her achievements in the Crimea were so outstanding, although they seriously affected her own health, that she was later recognized in 1907 by the Queen of England, who awarded her the Order of Merit.

In 1856 she returned to England, her health broken. Much has been written of her "illness," many suggesting it was, to a large degree, a neurosis. She retreated to her bedroom, and for the next 43 years conducted her business from her secluded apartment.

Throughout her lifetime Florence Nightingale wrote extensively about hospitals, sanitation, health and health statistics, and especially about nursing and nursing education. She crusaded for and brought about great reform in nursing education.

In 1860 she devoted her efforts to the creation of a school of nursing at St. Thomas' Hospital in London, financed by the Nightingale Fund. The basic principles on which Miss Nightingale established her school included:

> The nurses should be trained in teaching hospitals associated with medical schools and organized for that purpose.

The nurses would be carefully selected and should reside in nurses' houses that would be fit to form discipline and character.

The school matron would have final authority over the curriculum, living, and all other aspects of the school.

The curriculum would include both theoretical material and practical experience.

Teachers would be paid for their instruction.

Records would be kept on the students, who would be required to attend lectures, take quizzes, write papers, and keep diaries.

In many other ways Florence Nightingale advanced nursing as a profession. She believed that nurses should spend their time caring for patients, not cleaning; that nurses must continue learning throughout their lifetime and not become "stagnant"; that nurses should be intelligent and should use that intelligence to improve conditions for the patient; and that nursing leaders should have social standing. She had a vision of what nursing could and should be.

Florence Nightingale died in her sleep at the age of 90. The week during which she was born is now honored as National Hospital Week. The enthusiastic student is encouraged to learn more about this fascinating woman in Cecil Woodham-Smith's book *Florence Nightingale*.

Early Schools in the United States

After the establishment of the Nightingale School in England, nursing programs flourished, and the Nightingale system spread to other countries, including the United States. It was extended to America in 1849 when Pastor Fliedner arrived in Pittsburgh with four deaconesses. They assumed responsibility for the Pittsburgh Infirmary, which was the first Protestant hospital in the United States. The hospital is now called Passavant Hospital. Since that time, nursing education has grown in the United States.

The Civil War broke out in the United States in 1861. Although social reform was on its way, nursing was still in an embryonic, unorganized stage. Responding to the nursing needs created by the war, women volunteered to help, and after a brief training course, they performed nursing duties. Dorothea Dix, already well known for her concern for the mentally ill, was appointed superintendent of women nurses for the Union Army. Clara Barton, who served as a volunteer with the Sixth Massachusetts Regiment, was instrumental in founding the American Red Cross in 1882. Clara Barton's birthplace in Boston is maintained as a museum by the Unitarian Universalist Women's Federation, who also operate the Clara Barton Camp for Girls with diabetes, as a living memorial to this dedicated humanitarian. Lillian Wald created and developed the Visiting Nurse Service of New York and the Henry

Street Settlement House. Wald, a social activist, entered nursing at a time when nursing was not the first choice of well-to-do women (Backer, 1993).

African American nurses, such as Harriet Tubman, Susie Taylor, and Sojourner Truth carried out nursing duties for the Union army while supporting antislavery activities for the blacks. Mary Ann (Mother) Bickerdyke challenged the work of lazy, corrupt medical officers. Jane Stuart Woolsey and her sisters Georgeanna and Abby championed for standards of selection and training for nurses of the Union nurse corps. The Woolseys continued their efforts to establish sound nurse training schools after the Civil War. Students who want to learn more about the nurses of the Civil War should explore the writings of Walt Whitman, who was a nurse during this time, and Louisa May Alcott. Both wrote poignantly about nursing and war conditions of this period.

The conditions exposed during the Civil War coupled with the popularity of Florence Nightingale in England provided the impetus necessary to heighten the interest in nursing education in the United States. In 1869 the American Medical Association established a committee to study the issue. The New England Hospital for Women and Children established a 1-year program to train nurses in 1872, and by 1873 three additional schools were opened: the Bellevue Training School in New York City, the Connecticut Training School, and the Boston Training School. The evolution of nursing education in the United States is fully discussed in Chapter 2.

The Image of Nursing Today

During the late 1970s and early 1980s, a great deal of time and energy was invested in studying the image of nursing. Much of this work was done by Beatrice and Phillip Kalisch, who have written prolifically about the topic. Much of their writing deals with segments of an overall study of the image of the nurse in various forms of the mass media, including radio, movies, television, newspapers, magazines, and novels. They believe that popular attitudes and assumptions about nurses and what nurses contribute to the patient's welfare can influence the future of nursing to a large extent. It is their contention that since the 1970s, the popular image of the nurse has not only failed to reflect changing professional conditions but also assumed derogatory traits that have undermined public confidence in and respect for the professional nurse. Nurses should be concerned about negative or incorrect images because such images can influence the attitudes of patients, policy-makers, and politicians. Negative attitudes about nursing may also turn away many capable prospective nurses, who will choose another career that offers greater appeal in stature, status, and

In studying nurses on television (the single most important source of information in the country), Kalisch and Kalisch found that nurses often had no

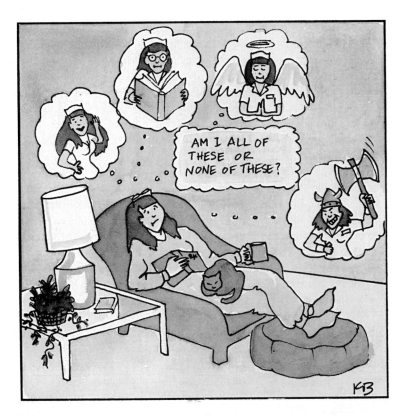

FIGURE 1–4 Nurses should be concerned about negative or incorrect images because these are sure to influence the attitudes of patients, policymakers, and politicians.

substantive role in the television stories. Often the nurse was part of the hospital background scenery for the physician characters, whose careers were viewed as more important and who scored high on such attributes as ambition, intelligence, rationality, aggression, self-confidence, and altruism. When nurses were singled out, most of the attention was directed toward solving the nurse's personal problems, as opposed to portraying her role as a nurse. The nurse frequently was portrayed as the "handmaiden" to the physician and scored high on such attributes as obedience, permissiveness, conformity, flexibility, and serenity. It is interesting to note that nurses ranked lower than physicians on such items as humanism, self-sacrifice, duty, and family concern, all of which are values traditionally ascribed to nurses (Kalisch and Kalisch, 1982a).

Kalisch and Kalisch found a rise and fall in the image of nurses in motion pictures, with the high point occurring during the war years of the 1940s and the low point occurring in the 1970s, when the nursing profession was denigrated and satirized in many films. This latter fact will have an impact on the attitudes of prospective nurses because the largest proportion of moviegoers each year are adolescents. The earlier, positive images of nurses usually came from films that were biographies of outstanding nurses such as Sister Kenny, who worked with polio patients, or Edith Cavell, a World War I heroine who was shot by the Germans for helping Allied soldiers escape from occupied Belgium. For a time the nurse–detective was a popular theme in films; such nurses were portrayed as being intelligent, perceptive, confident, sophisticated, composed, tough, and assertive. During the 1970s, however, nurses in films often were portrayed as being malevolent and sadistic (eg, the roles of Nurse Ratched in *One Flew Over the Cuckoo's Nest* and Nurse Diesel in *High Anxiety*). This was the lowest point in the history of films for the nurse figure with regard to such values as duty, self-sacrifice, achievement, integrity, virtue, intelligence, rationality, and kindness. Few films centered on the individual achievement or personal autonomy of the nurse. When compared with the physician's role, nursing was seen as less important (Kalisch and Kalisch, 1982b).

In studying the image of nursing in novels, Kalisch and Kalisch analyzed 207 books. As was true of the review of films and television, they found that the nurse in the novel was almost always female, usually single, childless, white, and younger than the age of 35.

Because nurses almost always have been depicted in novels as women, emphasis has also been on traditional female roles (ie, wife, mistress, mother). Three nurse stereotypes have resulted: 1) the nurse as man's companion; 2) the nurse as man's destroyer; and 3) the nurse as man's mother or the mother of his children. The man of the novel was often a physician. Novelists of the 1970s and 1980s have, as was seen in movies, often maligned their nurse characters, ignoring the nurses' professional motivations and health care perspectives (Kalisch and Kalisch, 1982c).

Muff (1982) has analyzed feminine myths and stereotypes and has elaborated on nursing stereotypes. In looking at books about nurses written for school-aged children (eg, Cherry Ames, Sue Barton, Kathy Martin, and Penny Scott), she has made the following conclusions. Nursing is described as glamorous; medicine and nursing are imbued with a sense of mystery and elitism; nursing is simplistic; nurses move from job to job; and nurses are subservient and deferential, following orders, running errands, and idolizing the physicians for whom they work. All of the nurses in these books were educated in hospital-based diploma programs in which the hard-earned "R.N." was finally won after hours of hospital service, although the Martin and Scott series were both written in the 1960s.

Muff (1982) has also examined the role of the nurse as it is captured in the romance novel. In many instances appearances (eg, color and condition of the hair) were most important, and the nurse was portrayed as a "pure" girl, dressed in white, whose main aim was to get a man, usually the doctor. Those women who were not looking for husbands were in nursing for altruistic reasons, and duty and self-sacrifice were glamorized. Muff also found that the image of the nurse as found in the novel generally could be classified into one of the following categories: ministering angels, handmaidens, battle-axes, fools, and whores. She also stated that the stereotypes of nursing presented by television and films usually would fit one of these categories. When reviewing the nurse image on get-well cards, she had to add a new category, that of "token torturer."

Only newspapers and news magazines tended toward realism rather than fantasy. News articles tended to cover information about the nursing shortage, including some reasons for it, for example, working conditions, salaries, benefits, and hardships. Articles also provided information about new nursing roles, or special features, such as nurses in Vietnam (Muff, 1982). With the outbreak of war in the Middle East in 1991, nurses received positive recognition by the various media. Nurses serving in reserve status with branches of the military were among the first called up when the conflict began. Although some might argue that nursing has better things to do than worry about how the nurse is revealed in the media, a consistently misrepresented image can negatively affect the way the public thinks about nurses. Therefore, nurses have responded to television advertisements or programs that portray nurses and nursing in a negative light with letters and telephone calls. In instances in which a product was involved, a boycott on the purchase of that item has proved to be a fairly effective way to bring about a change. Actions such as these were responsible for the discontinuance of a television show title "The Nightingales" that cast nursing in an inaccurate and demeaning image.

Various nursing organizations have waged campaigns to enhance the image of nursing. In 1981, the National League for Nursing (NLN) took an active role in developing media that portrayed nursing in a positive light. The National Commission on Nursing Implementation Project was responsible for initiating an advertising campaign over television and radio that emphasized nursing as a prestigious, desirable, and respected career. Some hospital associations, such as the Texas Hospital Association, also launched recruitment operations that focused on the desirability of nursing as a career.

Studies for and About Nursing

As schools of nursing grew in number, the quality of many of the schools and their graduates often suffered, and many of Florence Nightingale's admonitions regarding nursing education were forgotten. Nurses, doctors, friends, and critics of nursing became concerned about the inadequate preparation being offered. Before the problem could be corrected, it was necessary to learn more about the programs, how nurses were being used in the employment market, and the problems that resulted. To accomplish this, studies about nursing and nurses were initiated.

We recognize that many students in nursing are not excited by studies, especially those conducted years ago. However, the development of nursing as a profession has been affected by them, and it seems important that the significant studies be discussed. We think you will recognize some recurring themes that remain current today.

Although the first studies were not begun until the early 1900s, the number of studies since the 1950s is voluminous. It is impossible to pick up any professional publication and not find mention of some new study in progress. In an effort to classify and catalog references to these studies, Virginia Henderson has prepared A *Nursing Studies Index.* In 1952, a group of nurses, under the sponsorship of the Association of Collegiate Schools of Nursing, launched a new journal called *Nursing Research,* which was designed to disseminate information about nursing research.

EARLY STUDIES

One of the earliest studies was carried out under the guidance of M. Adelaide Nutting in 1912. Published by the U.S. Bureau of Education, it was entitled "The Educational Status of Nursing." The study investigated what and how students were being taught at the time and under what conditions students were living. Although it did not receive the attention it probably deserved, it began to establish nursing as a profession and led the way to later studies.

The Winslow-Goldmark Report, sometimes simply called the Goldmark Report, followed in 1923. This was also referred to as "The Study of Nursing and Nursing Education in the United States" (Winslow-Goldmark Report, 1923). The report focused on the preparation of public health nurses, teachers, administrators, clinical learning experiences of students, and the financing of schools. Subsequently, the Yale University School of Nursing was established.

A three-part study, sponsored by the Committee on the Grading of Nursing Schools, was conducted in the years 1928 to 1934. The first part, which was socioeconomic in nature and entitled "Nurses, Patients, and Pocketbooks," attempted to determine if there was a shortage of nurses in the United States; the second part, an "Activity Analysis of Nursing," looked at nurses' activities that could be used as a basis for improving the curricula in nursing schools; part three, "Nursing Schools Today and Tomorrow," described the schools of the period and made recommendations for professional schools.

The last of the early studies that we mention was not really a study but often is referred to as one because of its far-reaching effects. A *Curriculum Guide for Schools of Nursing,* published in 1937, was a revised version of earlier publications. It outlined the curricula for a 3-year course, emphasizing sound educational teaching procedures. It was read and followed by many schools that were operating programs at that time.

MIDCENTURY STUDIES

By the 1950s studies about nurses and nursing were numerous and dealt with many aspects of the profession. Only a few of those studies are mentioned here.

Of particular significance was a study published in 1948 entitled "Nursing for the Future." Conducted by Esther Lucille Brown, the study is also known as the Brown report. Funded by the Carnegie Foundation, the study was done to determine society's need for nursing, and recommendations were made for higher education for nurses. It prompted serious examination of professional education and pointed out weaknesses in the existing educational programs. The investigators recommended that basic schools of nursing be placed in universities and colleges and encouraged the recruitment of large numbers of men and members of minority groups into nursing schools. This report set the stage for studies of nursing education that followed in the 1950s and 1960s and for recommendations that were to continue into the 1990s.

The Ginzberg report was published the same year. This study reviewed problems centering around the current and prospective shortage of nurses. The conclusions and recommendations were published in the book entitled *A Program for the Nursing Profession*. The study recommended that nursing teams consisting of 4-year professional nurses, 2-year registered nurses, and 1-year practical nurses be developed. Some of these conclusions are not far from where we are now.

In 1958, a study entitled "Twenty Thousand Nurses Tell Their Story" was published. It was part of a 5-year research project that was conceived by the ANA and financially supported by nurses throughout the country. The report was prepared by Everett C. Hughes, a professor of sociology at the University of Chicago. The study looked at nurses, what they were doing, their attitudes toward their jobs, and their job satisfaction. As a result, nurses learned a great deal about themselves.

Another significant study was initiated by Mildred Montag in 1952. This study on "Community College Education for Nursing" resulted in the creation of associate degree nursing education (see Chapter 2).

SIGNIFICANT STUDIES OF THE 1960s AND 1970s

In 1961, the Surgeon General of the U.S. Public Health Service appointed a 25-member panel called the Consultant Group of Nursing. This group was to advise him on nursing needs and identify the role of the federal government in assessing nursing services to the nation. In 1963, this group presented a report entitled "Toward Quality in Nursing," which recommended a national investigation of nursing education that would place emphasis on the criteria for high-quality patient care. After publication of this report, the ANA and the NLN appropriated funds and established a joint committee to study ways to conduct and finance such a national inquiry. It was decided that the study would expand to consider probable requirements in professional nursing to occur over several decades to come as well as examine changing practice and educational patterns of the present time. W. Allen Wallis, president of the University of Rochester, headed the study. Financing was obtained from the American Nurses Foundation, the Kellogg Foundation, the Avalon Foundation, and an anonymous benefactor. The National Commission for the Study of Nursing and Nursing Education was set up as an independent agency and functioned as a self-directing group. The 12 commissioners were chosen for their broad knowledge of nursing, for their skills in related disciplines, or for their competencies in relevant fields, with no commissioner representing a particular interest group or position. In August 1967, at the first meeting of the commission, Jerome P. Lysaught was appointed director to conduct the planning and operation of the inquiry.

The study focused on the supply and demand for nurses, nursing roles and functions, nursing education, and nursing as a career. The commission found it necessary not only to examine these key concerns but also to relate these issues to the social system that provides care to the public.

The final report of the commission, entitled "An Abstract for Action," was published in 1970. It included 58 specific recommendations and concluded with four central recommendations. It also listed three basic priorities: 1) increased research in both the practice and education of nurses; 2) enhanced educational systems and curricula based on research; and 3) increased financial support for nurses and for nursing.

The four general recommendations were as follows:

1. That the Federal Division of Nursing, the National Center for Health Services Research and Development, other governmental agencies, and private foundations appropriate grant funds or research contracts to investigate the impact of nursing practice on the quality, effectiveness, and economy of health care

2. That the same agencies and foundations appropriate research funds and research contracts for basic and applied research into the nursing curriculum, articulation of educational systems, instructional methodologies, and facilities design so that the most functional, effective, and economic approaches are taken in the education and development of future nurses

3. That each state have, or create, a master planning committee that will take nursing education under its purview, with such committees to include representatives of nursing, education, other health care professions, and the public, to recommend specific guidelines, means for implementation, and deadlines to ensure that nursing education is positioned in the mainstream of American educational patterns

4. That federal, regional, state, and local governments adopt measures for the increased support of nursing research and education. Priority should be given to construction grants, institutional grants, advanced traineeships, and research grants and contracts. It was further recommended that private funds and foundations support nursing research and educational innovations where such activities are not publicly aided. It was recommended that funds come from the federal government, and public and private agencies (National Commission for the Study of Nursing and Nursing Education, 1970).

In 1973, a progress report from the National Commission for the Study of Nursing and Nursing Education concerning the status of the implementation of the recommendations of the original report was published under the title "From Abstract into Action." The commission believed that it was imperative that nursing achieve the goals established in the recommendations so that nursing could emerge as a full profession and in the interest of optimal health care for this country.

STUDIES OF THE 1980s AND EARLY 1990s

One of the major studies of nursing conducted in the 1980s was that of the National Commission on Nursing. This group was composed of a forum of 30 commissioners from disciplines such as nursing, hospital management, business, government, education, and medicine, all of whom were concerned about the current nursing-related problems in the health care system, especially the apparent shortage of nurses. The commission was sponsored by the American Hospital Association, Hospital Research and Educational Trust, and the American Hospital Supply Corporation. Its chairman was H. Robert Cathcart. The group began its work in September 1980 and focused on areas that dealt primarily with the environment in which nurses work, the relationship between nursing education and nursing practice, nursing issues, and the status of nursing as a profession (National Commission on Nursing, 1981).

The commission began systematically to examine and evaluate data sources. Journal articles, state studies, and policy documents were reviewed. A series of public hearings held in six major cities across the nation provided the opportunity for input about nursing issues from each region of the country. Two open forums also were held. After the hearings the commission conducted an Inventory of Innovative Programs and Projects.

The highlights of these findings, along with the commission's recommendations and future action plans, were published in the initial report of the group in September 1981. The final recommendations were published in 1983. Although the findings and recommendations are too lengthy to be included in this chapter in their entirety, it is important to mention the five major categories of issues identified by the study (National Commission on Nursing, 1981, p 5):

1. The status and image of nursing, which includes changes in the nursing role
2. The interface of nursing education and practice, including models for education to prepare for practice
3. The effective management of the nursing resource, including such factors as job satisfaction, recruitment, and retention
4. The relationship among nursing, medical staff, and hospital administration, including nursing's participation in decision-making
5. The maturing of nursing as a self-determining profession, including defining and determining the nature and scope of practice, the role of nursing leadership, increasing decision-making in nursing practice, and the need for unity in the nursing profession.

A series of publications that explore the work of the National Commission on Nursing is available from the Hospital Research and Educational Trust, 840 North Lake Drive, Chicago, IL 60611 (telephone: 312-280-6620). The publication *New Directions in Nursing* deals with nursing practice, credentialing, licensure, accreditation, and education.

Many of these issues are discussed in other sections of this book. A number of the issues are not new to nursing; most of them will not be completely resolved in the next decade. As a new graduate, you will have the opportunity to influence the outcome.

Many of the commission's findings were no surprise to people who are involved with nursing. Included was information that indicated that physicians and health care administrators often did not understand the role of nurses in patient care and that traditional and outdated images of nurses (including Victorian stereotypes and traditional male–female relationships) impeded acceptance of current roles. Some physicians and administrators perceived nurses as being overeducated, and they did not support an increase in the nurse's authority to make decisions concerning health care.

The findings that individuals and nursing groups are not unified in defining fundamental, professional goals for nursing, and that nursing, as a profession, lacks cohesiveness and a clear understanding of its role and direction were no revelations to many seasoned nurses. These same people were also not astonished to learn of the numerous and diverse associations that represent nursing but lack any arrangement to determine common goals for nursing education, practice, and credentialing. The disagreement and confusion about educational preparation for nurses and the controversy about entry into practice were identified as further blocks to the advancement of the profession. Clearly there is a need for a system of nursing education that promotes realistic expectations, provides appropriate support for practice and advancement, and includes educational mobility in nursing.

Following in the footsteps of the National Commission of Nursing was the National Commission on Nursing Implementation Project, which began in 1985. Funded by the W. K. Kellogg Foundation for 3 years, the project was cosponsored by the NLN, the ANA, the American Organization of Nurse Executives, and the American Association of Colleges of Nursing. Administered by the American Nurses' Foundation, it had as its purpose to provide leadership in seeking consensus about the appropriate education and credentialing for basic nursing practice, effective models for the delivery of nursing care, and the means for developing and testing nursing knowledge. The focus of this project was to lay the groundwork and take action wherever possible to support effective, high-quality nursing care delivery in the immediate and long-range future.

The results of another study of nursing were released in January 1983. This 2-year study, mandated under the 1979 Nurse Training Amendments, was conducted by the Institute of Medicine Committee on Nursing and Nursing Education and was funded by the Department of Health and Human Services at a cost of $1.6 million. The objectives of the study included providing advice regarding federal support for nursing education, to gain more information about nurses such as why they do not seek employment in medically underserved areas and why they leave the profession, and to make recommendations regarding measures to improve the supply and use of nursing resources (Institute of Medicine, 1983).

The Institute of Medicine study made 21 specific recommendations to Congress. The study found that the shortage of nurses of the 1960s and 1970s had largely disappeared and that federal support of nursing education should focus on graduate study. The first recommendation of the study was that the federal government discontinue efforts to increase the supply of "generalist nurses."

The fallacies in these findings were soon realized. Across the nation nursing enrollments plummeted in the late 1980s. When combined with the expanded roles being assumed by nurses and the increased need for nurses in the delivery of health care throughout the nation, this soon resulted in a serious national shortage of nurses. These shortages are of a critical nature in specific areas such as certain geographic regions and in services to certain groups such as geriatric and economically disadvantaged patients.

Responding to the increasing need for nurses, many of the studies of the early 1990s focused on the roles of nurses in the delivery of health care and on educational patterns that would encourage capable individuals to choose nursing as a career and programs that would facilitate educational mobility. Issues related to nurses' image and the nursing shortage merged. A new Commission on the National Nursing Shortage replaced the Federal Commission on Nursing, and $275,000 was budgeted to assist in its function. This commission had as its role developing strategies to decrease the nursing shortage, which included areas related to recruitment, retention, restructuring of nursing services for most effective utilization of nursing personnel, and gathering data about nursing and the information systems used in nursing.

Traditions in Nursing

Over the years nursing has, because of its history, developed a number of traditions. Some of these traditions are being challenged, primarily because they are simply not practical in today's workplace (eg, the wearing of a nursing cap). It is worthwhile, however, to reflect just a little on the development of these traditions and to discuss their relationship to nursing.

THE NURSING PIN

The nursing pin may date back to the time of the Crusades when Crusaders, marching to Jerusalem to recover the Holy Land, wore crosses on their heads or chest as symbols of good fortune. Following the capture of Jerusalem in 1099, some of the Crusaders noted the excellent nursing care provided by the Hospital of Saint John and decided to join the nursing group. A uniform was drawn up for the group that included a black robe with a white Maltese cross on the chest. The Maltese cross is an eight-pointed cross formed by four arrowheads joining at their points. When the Knights Templars and the Knights of the Teutonic Order were formed in 1118 and 1190, respectively, this symbol was carried forward.

The actual symbolism of the pin relates to customs established in the 16th century when the privilege of wearing a coat of arms was limited to noblemen who served their kings with distinction. As centuries passed, the privilege was extended to schools and to craft guilds, and the symbols of wisdom, strength, courage, and faith appeared on buttons, badges, and shields. It was probably this concept that Florence Nightingale was capturing when she also chose the Maltese cross as a symbol when selecting a badge for the graduates of her first nursing school.

As nursing developed as a profession, each school chose a unique and different pin, awarded on completion of the program, and as a symbol to the public of work well done. Many of the early schools, particularly those associated with hospitals supported by religious groups, have incorporated the cross into their pin. On graduation from the program, a "pinning" ceremony would be held and new graduates would be awarded their nursing pin. This tradition continues in numerous schools today although some students are electing not to purchase a school pin.

THE NURSING CAP

The history of the nursing cap is a little less clear. It would seem reasonably to have evolved out of the period of time when nursing was greatly influenced by religion. The white cap of the deaconesses of the early Christian era and the nun's veil of the Middle Ages have been said to be the forerunners of the nursing cap as we know it today (Mangum, 1994). It was considered proper for women to keep their heads covered at that time. The veil was modified to become a cap and was associated with provided service to others. The cap worn by students at Kaiserwerth when Florence Nightingale was a student was hood shaped, had a ruffle around the face, and tied under the chin. In addition, short hair cuts were not acceptable for women and the use of a head covering helped to control the hair.

As women's hair styles changed and hair was worn shorter, the head covering became smaller and lost its scarf or veil attachment in the United States and Canada. (The hair covering aspect remained a part of the cap in many areas of England and Europe.) As hospitals developed nursing education programs, they each created their own cap and nursing pin as a symbol of that particular hospital and nursing school. Some of these were rather "frilly" and were fashioned after the ether cone through which ether was dropped. A "capping" ceremony was part of the ritual of the nursing student. Often held in a nearby church, the students who had successfully completed their probationary period or perhaps the first year of study, were "capped" among much pomp and circumstance. (See Chapter 2 for more detail regarding nursing education.)

As the role of nurses changed and as high technology became a significant part of the hospital work environment, nurses found that caps were bothersome as they tried to carry out their duties. They were knocked askew by curtains, equipment, and tubing. By the 1980s, many hospitals were no longer requiring the cap as a part of the uniform. Nursing programs responded by dropping the cap as a required article of dress. If students wished to have a cap, it was purchased from a local uniform store and had no particular identification with the program.

THE NURSING UNIFORM

Like the nursing cap, which is actually a part of the early uniform, the requirement for special dress came from the religious and military history of nursing and has always been significant in nursing. This is due in part to the fact that dress provides a strong nonverbal message about one's image. The nurse attired in a white uniform, at least in the 1950s and 1960s, communicated an impression of confidence, competence, professionalism, authority, role identity, and accountability. As nurses have adopted more casual dress, some of this identity has been lost and hospital committees, nursing programs, and nurses have spent considerable time discussing appropriate attire.

Early uniforms were long, usually stiffly starched, and had detachable collars and cuffs. A full uniform often included a long cape that would cover the uniform. By the 1900s, the uniform became more functional and the hemline was raised. By the mid-1960s, pantsuits became accepted and nurses in certain settings, particularly psychiatric and pediatric units, were challenging the appropriateness of uniforms, especially if the clothing were all white. By 1970, significant changes were occurring in the uniforms with the acceptance of styles that "made the nurse more approachable." In psychiatric settings, "no uniform" became the standard of the day. Today athletic shoes have become acceptable in many institutions and "scrubs" have become so accepted that they are featured in pamphlets advertising uniforms. In 1987, the Springhouse Corporation conducted a survey of nurses throughout the United States and found that most nurses prefer scrubs or lab coats worn over street clothes. The result of this change has been that nurses today are no longer identifiable by uniform. The stethoscope worn around the neck provides the consumer some orientation to a person's position (ie, that they are a health care worker rather than a maintenance person), and hospital identification badges provide further information but may not include the person's full name.

Today there is controversy over the appropriate attire for nurses. Mangum and associates (1991) recommend that nurses wear clothing that clearly distinguishes them as professional nurses. Although not suggesting a cap, they have advocated for the more traditional white dress or pantsuit. Others argue that it matters less what nurses wear, but rather it is what they know that is critical. Perhaps compromise is necessary.

Key Concepts

- ⇨ Two major factors will shape the direction of nursing: education and research. Education for nursing has moved progressively into postsecondary settings and away from vocational apprenticeship-type preparation. The move has been toward more research in nursing as a theoretical foundation for nursing education and practice.
- ⇨ In its development as a profession, nursing has struggled with its definition, its image, and its role in the health care delivery system.
- ⇨ Its history has had an influence on the way the profession is recognized by the public.
- ⇨ Nursing's history included three significant images: the folk image of the nurse, the religious image of the nurse, and the servant image of the nurse.
- ⇨ During the Reformation, nursing fell into a period known as "The Dark Ages in Nursing," when only those individuals who could not find other employment cared for the ill.
- ⇨ Florence Nightingale had a significant impact on nursing, changing the form and direction of nursing and establishing it as a respected field of endeavor. Many of her precepts are still a part of nursing.
- ⇨ A number of studies about nursing have been conducted since the 1950s. These relate to nursing as a profession, nursing education, the

image of nursing, the environment in which nurses work, and nurses themselves.

⇨ Nursing, as a profession, has many traditions, some of which are being challenged today. Among the traditions are the pin, the cap, and the uniform.

CRITICAL THINKING ACTIVITIES

1. If you had the power to change one single event in the history of nursing what would it be? Why would you make that change? How do you think that would have effected nursing today?
2. How do you think the changes in health care reform will affect the image of nursing today? Provide a rationale for your answers.
3. What areas of nursing currently need the most study? Why? How would nursing benefit if those studies were completed?
4. If you were to set the standard of dress for nurses in a 200-bed community hospital, what would you require. Provide your rationale for this decision. If you had the responsibility for enforcing the dress code, how would you go about it?

References

Abdellah FG. Patient-Centered Approaches to Nursing. New York: Macmillan, 1960

American Nurses Association. Nursing: A Social Policy Statement. Kansas City, MO: American Journal of Nursing Co, 1980

American Nurses Association. First Position on Education for Nursing. Am J Nurs 65(12): 106–111, 1965

Backer BA. Lillian Wald: Connecting caring with activism. Nurs Health Care 14(3):122–129, 1993

Benner P. From Novice to Expert: Excellence and Power in Clinical Nursing Practice. Menlo Park, CA: Addison-Wesley, 1984

Bixler GK, Bixler RW. The professional status of nursing. Am J Nurs 45(9):730, 1945

Dickens C. Martin Chuzzlewit. In The Works of Charles Dickens, vol II. New York: Books Inc, 1936

Donahue MP. Nursing: The Finest Art. St Louis: CV Mosby, 1985

Flexner A. In Bernard LA, Walsh M: Leadership: The Key to the Professionalization of Nursing. New York: John Wiley & Sons, 1981

Henderson V. The Nature of a Science of Nursing. New York: Macmillan, 1966

I.O.M. study sees need for funds in graduate, specialty areas. Am J Nurs 83(3):343, 344, 454, 1983.

Johnson D. The behavioral system model for nursing. In Riehl JP, Roy C: Conceptual Models for Nursing Practice, 2nd ed. East Norwalk, CT: Appleton-Century-Crofts, 1980:207–216

Kalisch PA, Kalisch BJ. The Advance of American Nursing, 3rd ed. Philadelphia: J.B. Lippincott Co., 1995

Kalisch PA, Kalisch BJ. Nurses on prime-time television. Am J Nurs 82(2):264, 1982a

Kalisch PA, Kalisch BJ. The image of the nurse in motion pictures. Am J Nurs 82(4):605, 1982b

Kalisch PA, Kalisch BJ. The image of nurses in novels. Am J Nurs 82(8):1220, 1982c

King IM. A Theory for Nursing: Systems, Concepts, Process. New York: John Wiley & Sons, 1981

Labor Management Relations Act (1947) as amended by Public Laws 86-257 (1959) and 93-360 (1974), Section 2

Mangum, S. Uniforms and caps: Do we need them? In Strickland OL, Fishman DJ: Nursing Issues in the 1990s. Albany, NY: Delmar Publishers, 1994:46–66

Mangum S, Garrison C, Lind C, Thackerary R, Wyatt M. Perception of nurses' uniforms. Image: The Journal of Nursing Scholarship 23:127–130, 1991

Muff J. Handmaiden, battle ax, whore. In Muff J: Socialization, Sexism and Stereotyping. Prospect Heights, IL: Waveland Press, Inc. 1988:113–156

National Commission for the Study of Nursing and Nursing Education: Summary, report and recommendations. Am J Nurs 70(2):279, 1970

National Commission on Nursing. Initial Report and Preliminary Recommendations. Chicago: Hospital Research and Educational Trust, 1981

Neuman B. The Neuman System Model: Application to Nursing Education and Practice. East Norwalk, CT: Appleton-Century-Crofts, 1982

Newman MA. Professionalism: Myth or reality. In Chaska NL: The Nursing Profession: Turning Points. St Louis: CV Mosby, 1990:49–52

Nightingale F. Notes on Nursing: What It Is, and What It Is Not. (An unabridged republication of the first American edition, as published by D. Appleton and Company in 1860.) New York: Dover Publications, 1954

Nutting MA, Dock LL. A History of Nursing. New York: GP Putnam's Sons, 1935

Orem D. Nursing: Concepts of Practice, 2nd ed. New York: McGraw-Hill, 1980

Orlando IJ. The Discipline and Teaching of Nursing Process. New York: GP Putnam's Sons, 1972

Pavalko RM. Sociology of Occupations and Professions. Itasca, IL: Peacock Publishers, 1971

Pavelka M. Definition of nursing practice. Issues 3(Summer):3, 1982

Peplau HE. Interpersonal Relations in Nursing. New York: GP Putnam's Sons, 1952

Rogers ME. Science of Unitary Human Beings: A Paradigm for Nursing. Paper presented before the International Nurse Theorist Conference, Edmonton, Alberta, May 1984

Roy C. Introduction to Nursing: An Adaptation Model, 2nd ed. Englewood Cliffs, NJ: Prentice-Hall, 1984

Schlotfeldt RM. Resolution of issues: An imperative for creating nursing's future. J Prof Nurs 3:136–142, 1987

Strauss A. The structure and ideology of American nursing: An interpretation. In Davis J: The Nursing Profession. New York: John Wiley & Sons, 1966:60–108

Uprichard M. Ferment in nursing. In Auld E, Birum LH: The Challenge of Nursing. St Louis: CV Mosby, 1973:24–31

Wiedenbach E. Clinical Nursing, A Helping Art. New York: Springer Publishing Co, 1964

Winslow-Goldmark Report. The Study of Nursing and Nursing Education in the United States. New York: Macmillan, 1923

Further Readings

Aaronson LS. A challenge for nursing: Reviewing a historic competition. Nurs Outlook 37(6): 274–279, 1989

Bunting S, Campbell JC. Feminism and nursing. Adv Nurs Sci 12(4): ll–24, 1990

Bullough VL, et al. The Emergence of Modern Nursing. New York: Macmillan, 1969

Christy T. Equal rights for women: Voices from the past. Am J Nurs 2(2):288–293, 1971

Christy T. First fifty years. Am J Nurs 9(9):1778–1784, 1971

Christy T. Portrait of a leader: Lavinia Lloyd Dock. Nurs Outlook 17(6):72–75, 1969

Christy T. Portrait of a leader: M. Adelaide Nutting. Nurs Outlook 17(1):20–24, 1969

Christy T. Portrait of a leader: Isabel Hampton Robb. Nurs Outlook 17(3):26–29, 1969

Christy T. Portrait of a leader: Isabel Maitland Stewart. Nurs Outlook 17(10):44–48, 1969

Dolan JA. Nursing in Society: A Historical Perspective, 14th ed. Philadelphia: WB Saunders, 1978

Gamer M. The ideology of professionalism. Nurs Outlook 27(2):108–111, 1979

Griffin GJ, Griffin JK. Jensen's History and Trends of Professional Nursing, 7th ed. St Louis: CV Mosby, 1973

Hanson KS. The emergence of liberal education in nursing education, 1893–1923. J Prof Nurs 5(2):83–91, 1989

Kalisch BJ, Kalisch PA. Heroine out of focus: Media images of Florence Nightingale: I. Popular biographies and stage productions. Nurs Health Care 4(4):181–187, 1983

Kalisch BJ, Kalisch PA. The nurse–detective in American movies. Nurs Health Care 3(3): 146–153, 1982

Kalisch BJ, Kalisch PA, Scobey M. Reflections on a television image. Nurs Health Care 5(5): 248–255, 1981

Larisey MM. Attic treasures: A look at nursing history. Nurs Forum 25(1):20–24, 1990

Melosh B. Not merely a profession: Nurses and resistance to professionalization. Am Behav Scientist 32(6):668–679, 1989

Parsons M. The profession in a class by itself. Nurs Outlook 34(6):270–275, 1985

Roberts MM. American Nursing: History and Interpretation. New York: Macmillan, 1954

Sleeper R, et al. Issues in Health Care: The Edna A. Fagan Health Care Lecture Series. Publication No. 14-1599. New York: National League for Nursing, 1976

Woodham-Smith C. Florence Nightingale. New York: McGraw-Hill, 1951

2 | Educational Preparation for Nursing

Objectives

After completing this chapter, you should be able to

1. Describe the educational preparation and role of the nursing assistant.
2. Describe the educational preparation and role of the licensed practical nurse.
3. Discuss the educational preparation provided by a hospital-based diploma program of nursing.
4. Discuss the educational preparation provided by a baccalaureate degree program of nursing.
5. Discuss the educational preparation provided by an associate degree program of nursing.
6. Identify the purposes of other forms of nursing education: the external degree, registered nurse baccalaureate programs, master's preparation, doctoral studies, and nondegree programs.
7. Discuss the concept of articulated programs.
8. Define the continuing education unit and discuss its purpose.
9. Compare and contrast the major points supporting mandatory continuing education and the major points supporting voluntary continuing education.

Ellis JR, Hartley CL: NURSING IN TODAY'S WORLD:
CHALLENGES, ISSUES, AND TRENDS, 5th ed.
© 1995 J.B. Lippincott Company

Unlike many other professions that provide a single route of educational preparation, the development of nursing as a profession has resulted in three major educational routes that prepare graduates to write the National Council Licensure Examination (NCLEX) for registered nursing. This circumstance has offered various alternatives and opportunities to the prospective student, and at the same time, has resulted in much confusion. The health care consumer often finds it difficult to interpret the vast array of initials (eg, RN, RNCS, CRN, MN, or DNS) that can now follow a nurse's name. Some of these credentials represent legal titles, some are earned by education, and others are acquired by demonstrating expertise through examination (certification). The employer has difficulty differentiating among the three major types of registered nurse graduates who, at least initially, enter the work environment with similar behaviors. The educator is charged with the responsibility of graduating a "safe" practitioner but may lack clear direction as to how the professional preparation provided by the various educational routes should differ in purpose, structure, and outcomes. This situation has also provided a springboard for much discussion, debate, and, in some instances, dissension among nurses, educators, and interested lay persons regarding aspects of each program as they relate to professional nursing practice.

The three avenues preparing men and women for registered nursing are the hospital-based diploma programs, the baccalaureate programs located in 4-year colleges and universities, and the 2-year associate degree programs primarily found in junior and community colleges. It is also possible for students to begin their nursing education in programs that culminate in a master's degree, and at least one program exists in which a student can earn a doctorate before being eligible to write the state licensing examination for registered nursing. You can better comprehend much of the politics of nursing today if you have an understanding of the history and development of the educational preparation of nurses.

At least two other groups of caregivers are identified with nursing: the nursing assistant who is certified and the practical (vocational) nurse, who is licensed through a separate examination from that taken by the registered nurse. We will briefly discuss the education of each of these groups.

The Nursing Assistant

For years care has been provided to patients in hospitals and long-term care facilities by individuals we called nursing aides or assistants. These caregivers were hired without formal preparation for their responsibilities and were provided "on-the-job training" once their work began.

In 1987, Congress passed the Omnibus Budget Reconciliation Act (OBRA), which regulates the education and certification of nurse aides. This act stipulated that by October 1, 1990, all persons working as nurse assistants in long-term care facilities were required to complete a competency evaluation program or approved course (Hegner and Caldwell, 1995; Sorrentino, 1992). The certification falls under state jurisdiction but is guided by federal regulations. These regulations require that an individual who wishes to be certified complete a minimum of 75 hours of theory and practice and pass both a theory and clinical examination. In many states the hours of preparation exceed the 75 hours established in the law. Following the federal legislation, the National Council of State Boards of Nursing Inc., developed the Nurse Aide Competency Evaluation Program (NACEP), which identifies the minimum skills to be attained and can be used as a guide by programs registering or certifying nursing aides. The state agency bearing the responsibility for certifying and maintaining the listing of nursing assistants varies from state to state. Most commonly it is done by the Board of Nursing of the state or by the Department of Health and Human Services.

The certified nursing assistant (CNA) functions under the direction of the registered nurse or the licensed practical (vocational) nurse. Each state identifies the skills that may be performed by the nursing assistant. Typically these include basic nursing skills, especially in the area of communication, personal hygiene and grooming, assisting patients with nutritional and elimination needs, and helping with mobility. The preparation emphasizes the importance of a safe environment and includes instruction in the use of side rails and restraints. Some states also require a designated number of hours per year of continuing education. The training occurs in a variety of settings including high schools, long-term care facilities, hospitals, community colleges, regional occupational programs, and privately operated programs. Some persons consider this preparation as the first rung on the ladder of nursing education and, in some states, the nursing assistant may be exempt from certain classes required in licensed practical (vocational) nursing programs.

Practical Nurse Education

The practical nurse is no newcomer to the health care delivery system. In the past, the practical nurse was the family friend or community citizen who was called to the home in emergencies. This person, usually self-taught, learned by experience which things were effective and which were not. She would perform basic care procedures such as bathing and also would cook for the family and do light housekeeping duties. Although the controls on licensing of practical nurses and on the accreditation of curriculum have been slower in evolving than those regulating professional nursing, states gradually began enacting licensure laws governing the practice of practical nursing. By 1945, 19 states and one territory had licensure laws but in only one state was licensure of the practical nurse mandatory (Kalisch and Kalisch, 1995). When states began adopting mandatory licensure laws governing the practice of practical nursing, a large number of individuals who had been functioning in this capacity were granted a license by waiver, thus never really having any formal training (see Chapter 4 on credentialing). However, most of these people have now retired from nursing practice.

It is a little uncertain when the first program to offer formal preparation for practical nursing began. Some suggest training programs were started in 1897 (Kalisch and Kalisch, 1995). More popular is the belief that the first programs were initiated through the YWCA in Brooklyn, New York, around 1892. The school started through the YWCA was known as the Ballard School, after Lucinda Ballard, who provided the funding to operate the school. The course of study was approximately 3 months long. The students, called "attendants," were trained to care for invalids, the elderly, and children in a home setting.

Although the YWCA may seem to many of us to be a strange place for a practical nurse program, we must remember that in the late 1890s and early 1900s, young women traveled from their homes to large cities seeking new careers and a better life. Many of these women found inexpensive housing at YWCAs. Because most of them were untrained and had no marketable skills, the YWCA provided a natural site for a school.

Other early practical nursing programs included the Thompson School, founded in Brattleboro, Vermont, in 1907; the American Red Cross Program, begun in 1908; and the Household Nursing Association School of Attendant Nursing, begun in Boston in 1918.

Although by 1930 only 11 schools were in existence, the number of programs expanded rapidly during the 1940s. During World War I and especially during World War II the need for people who had some skills, but, more importantly, who could be prepared quickly, became crucial. As this need became more and more critical, the practical nurse, who until this time was primarily found in the home, moved out into the world.

In 1941, the Association of Practical Nurse Schools was founded; in 1942 membership was opened to practical nurses and the name was changed to the National Association of Practical Nurse Education and Service (NAP-NES). The first planned curriculum for practical nursing was developed in 1942, and in 1945, NAPNES established an accrediting service for schools of practical nursing. The National Federation of Licensed Practical Nurses (NFLPN) was organized in 1949. In 1957, this group, working with the American Nurses Association (ANA), attempted to clarify the role and function of the practical nurse, just as various groups throughout the nation have worked at delineating the roles of other nursing program graduates. The Council on Practical Nursing was established by the National League for Nursing (NLN) in 1957. In 1966, the Chicago Public School Program became the first practical nurse program to be accredited by the NLN.

The general curriculum, which requires 9 months to a year to complete, varies considerably from state to state and even from school to school. In many instances the education is weighed in clock hours instead of credit hours as used in the professional programs. Most of today's practical nurse educational programs stress clinical experiences, primarily in structured care settings such as hospitals and nursing homes. Basic therapeutic knowledge and introductory content from biologic and behavioral sciences correlate with clinical practice. Usually about one third of the time is spent in the classroom and two thirds in the clinical areas.

The setting in which the educational preparation of the practical nurse occurs may vary tremendously. A program may be offered by a high school, trade or technical school, hospital, junior or community college, university, or independent agency. There has been a movement to incorporate practical nurse education and associate degree programs in the community college. All students are grouped together for "core" courses during the first academic year. At the end of this time, the student has the option of stopping the educational program and seeking licensure as a licensed practical nurse or continuing for an additional year and seeking licensure as a registered nurse. Many students opt to do both. Graduates of these core programs in practical nursing usually possess a broader and more in-depth understanding of the biologic sciences and, in some instances, the social sciences also because these are part of the core curriculum and may be college-level courses that are transferable to a 4-year institution. As issues related to educational mobility and "articulation" between programs have received much attention (see Chapter 3), the combined programs have been popular in areas where they exist.

Graduates of practical nurse programs take the NCLEX-PN and if successful use the title licensed practical nurse (LPN) or, in California and Texas, the title licensed vocational nurse (LVN). The scope of their practice focuses on meeting the health needs of patients/clients in hospitals, long-term care facilities, and the home. LPNs or LVNs work with patients/clients whose conditions are considered stable. Their work is supervised by a registered nurse or a licensed physician.

Like the associate degree and the hospital-based diploma programs for registered nursing, the educational preparation and the future of practical nursing has received much discussion. Some would advocate two levels of nursing with one being the practical nurse. Others would eliminate practical nursing altogether. In 1987, North Dakota became the first state (and to date the only state) to require all candidates taking the licensure examination for practical nursing to have completed an associate degree in practical nursing. With the "graying" of America and the increasing need for more nurses in home health and long-term care facilities, practical nurses play a significant role in health care delivery.

Diploma Education

The earliest type of nursing education in the United States occurred in diploma programs administered by hospitals. The first hospital with a nurse training school was the New England Hospital for Women, which accepted five probationers on September 1, 1872 (Kalisch and Kalisch, 1995). Linda Richards generally is recognized as the first nurse graduated in the United States. Diploma, or hospital, schools of nursing flourished during the late 1800s and early 1900s. These training schools provided free or inexpensive staffing for the hospitals offering the educational program. Until 1888, when the first school for males opened as the Mills School of Nursing at Bellevue Hospital, the students were all female. The first African American nursing school graduate was Mary Eliza Mahoney, who graduated from the program at the New England Hospital for Women and Children in 1879 (Kalisch and Kalisch, 1995).

Initially the education was largely an apprenticeship and resulted in students providing much of the work force of hospitals. Although some formal theory classes were conducted, learning was achieved primarily by "doing." There was no standardization of curriculum and no accreditation. Programs were developed to meet the service needs of the hospital rather than the educational needs of the students, and programs varied considerably from hospital to hospital.

In the early schools the responsibility for administration of the educational program frequently was vested in the director of nursing service, who also had the role and title of director of nursing education. Many of the instructors were graduates of the program who undoubtedly possessed nursing skills but knew little of teaching or learning theories, teaching skills and techniques, curriculum design and development, or evaluation processes. In many instances the teacher was also a head nurse on one of the units in the hospital. Formal lectures often were delivered by members of the medical staff.

The curriculum generally was laid out in blocks of study that included medical nursing, surgical nursing, psychiatric nursing, obstetrics, pediatrics, operating and emergency department experience, as well as support courses in anatomy, physiology, nutrition, pharmacology, history of nursing, and often a course titled "professional adjustments." If a hospital was unable to provide certain learning opportunities, for example, psychiatric experience, students were sent on "affiliation" to a hospital where they could receive that education. The hospital dietitian may have been involved in teaching the nutrition course, and nurses usually provided the remainder of the education, including instruction in biologic sciences. The students usually were assigned to the hospital units during the early and late hours of the day (when the staffing needs were the greatest), working what were known as "split shifts." Lectures were given between 1 and 3 o'clock in the afternoon. Most days were at least 12 hours long.

Almost all the students were single young women who started the program immediately on completion of high school. They entered the school as "probies" (short for probationer) for a 6-week to 6-month probationary period. This was a testing time for both the student and the school, a time for the student to seriously look at nursing as a career and a time for the school to examine the student's aptitude for nursing. Although not exactly comparable to the experience of freshmen entering some private colleges, this situation had a few similarities. The probie often could be identified by dress; for example, the apron might be worn without a bib during this period. There was no real hazing at this time; however, the probie might be sent on errands that capitalized on her lack of knowledge and that might result in embarrassment later. (A typical assignment would be to send the probie to the central service area of the hospital for a supply of fallopian tubes.)

The students were housed in dormitories attached to the hospital. The dorms generally had a housemother, and codes of behavior were strict and well enforced. For example, students who failed to adhere to 9:30 PM curfews, who were caught smoking in their rooms, or who committed other acts of indiscretion were at risk of expulsion from the school. Usually marriage was not

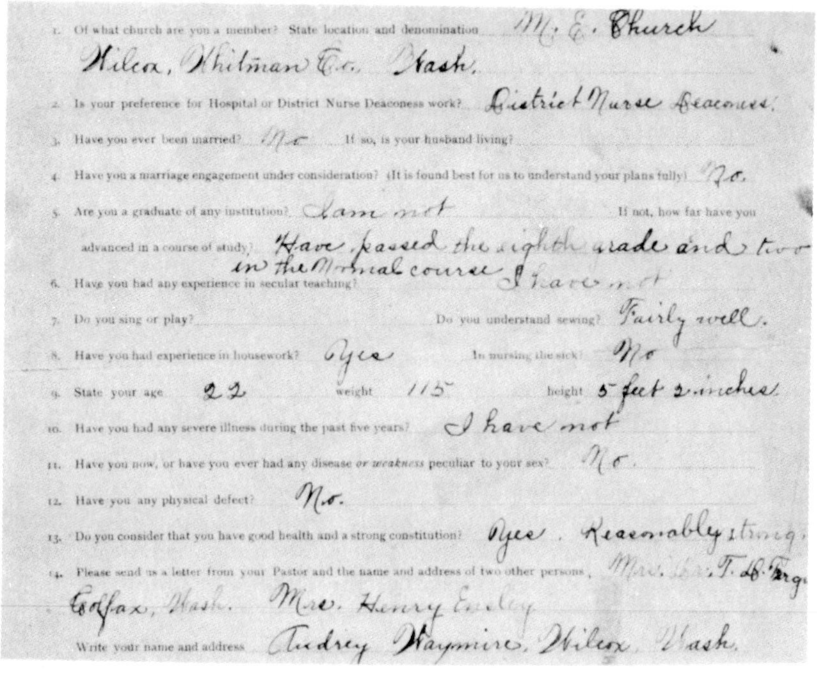

FIGURE 2–1 Typical application for admission to nursing school.

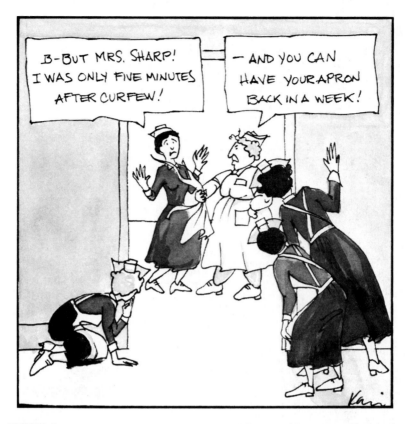

FIGURE 2–2 A student who had committed a minor infraction of the rules might have forfeited an article of apparel.

permitted during the time the students were in training. Because the students literally lived with one another, a type of socialization and identification occurred and students had a built-in support system through one another. Dress codes were rigid, and students who committed minor infractions of social behavior were reprimanded in a number of ways. The following is a quote from a special publication developed on closure of a diploma school:

In 1921, a nurse was discharged for "cigarette habit." Skirts of nurses' uniforms were getting shorter but there was periodic measurement to be sure some were not too short.

The year 1924 would see Deaconess' first student protest. Student nurses were required to wear their hair long in those days. A number of them though made arrangements with a barber in the Victoria Hotel to stay open late one evening and they all went down and had their hair bobbed in the latest style. They were deprived of their caps for several weeks and ordered to wear switches

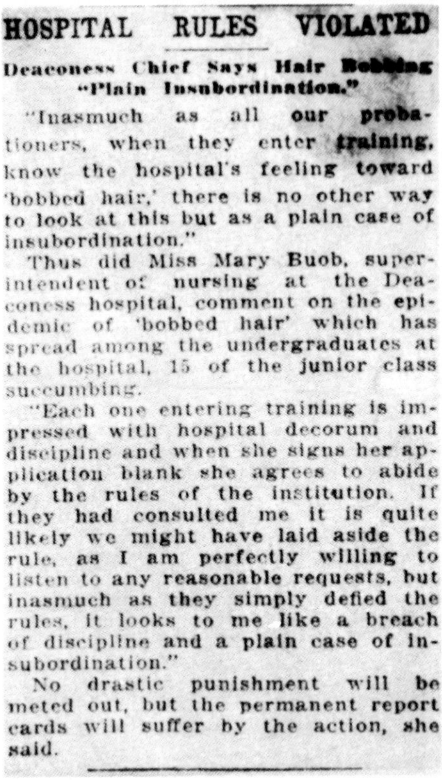

HOSPITAL RULES VIOLATED

Deaconess Chief Says Hair Bobbing "Plain Insubordination."

"Inasmuch as all our probationers, when they enter training, know the hospital's feeling toward 'bobbed hair,' there is no other way to look at this but as a plain case of insubordination."

Thus did Miss Mary Buob, superintendent of nursing at the Deaconess hospital, comment on the epidemic of 'bobbed hair' which has spread among the undergraduates at the hospital, 15 of the junior class succumbing.

"Each one entering training is impressed with hospital decorum and discipline and when she signs her application blank she agrees to abide by the rules of the institution. If they had consulted me it is quite likely we might have laid aside the rule, as I am perfectly willing to listen to any reasonable requests, but inasmuch as they simply defied the rules, it looks to me like a breach of discipline and a plain case of insubordination."

No drastic punishment will be meted out, but the permanent report cards will suffer by the action, she said.

FIGURE 2-3 A newspaper clipping from 1924.

and what-nots, their punishment comparatively slight, since "banks and other business regularly dismissed employees for social offense" (Deaconess Hospital School of Nursing, 1980, p 10).

Students surviving the probationary period finished the remainder of the year as freshmen. They then became juniors for a year, and completed the final year of the 3-year program as seniors. During the senior year the student often had responsibility for supervising the units of the hospital, with perhaps a month spent on each of the work shifts—days, evenings, nights. At the completion of the 3 years, the students were awarded a diploma, which was not recognized as an academic degree because hospitals legally were not chartered as educational institutions. If graduates wanted to continue their education toward a baccalaureate degree they often encountered problems because the 3 years spent preparing for nursing was not recognized with academic credit.

Symbolism and ceremony were an important part of these programs. Each school had its own identifiable uniform, cap, and pin. The traditional "capping" ceremony at which the student received a nursing cap after a given period of study (usually 3 months to 1 year) was a high point in the educational program. Parents and loved ones attended these ceremonies, which were often conducted in churches, particularly if the nursing program was sponsored by a hospital supported by a religious group. Today many programs have eliminated the cap, conforming to nursing as it is practiced in hospitals. Many view the cap as interfering with the ability of the nurse to work in confined or congested quarters and around much technical equipment.

Of even greater significance was the pinning ceremony that heralded completion of the program. Among much pomp and circumstance family and friends gathered to observe as the nursing director ceremoniously "pinned" each new graduate. Graduates often recited, in unison, the Nightingale Pledge (see accompanying display), written in 1893 by Lystra E. Gretter, superintendent of Harper Hospital school in Detroit (Calhoun, 1993). This ritual if often repeated in pinning ceremonies today. As nursing education has moved into institutions of higher education, some of the traditional ceremonies have been discontinued. Some argue that the ceremony recognizing program completion in the collegiate environment is the college commencement and that "special" celebrations for students of particular areas of study are not appropriate. In other cases, the tradition is continued.

Although the education described above may seem archaic by today's standards, a word must be said in defense of such programs. As a result of the many hours spent in hospital service, the students usually emerged from such programs skilled in "nursing arts" and were able to assume positions as staff or charge nurses without orientation. Although they may have shown weaknesses in knowing why something was done, they were certainly able to "do it." The graduate usually had a fairly good concept of her role as a nurse and was capable of functioning competently in that role, although some nurses today might not agree with some aspects of that role. One often hears older

The Nightingale Pledge

I solemnly pledge myself before God and in the presence of this assembly:
    To pass my life in purity and to practice my profession faithfully;
    I will abstain from whatever is deleterious and mischievous and will not take or knowingly administer any harmful drug; I will do all in my power to maintain and elevate the standard of my profession, and will hold in confidence all personal matters committed to my keeping and all family affairs coming to my knowledge in the practice of my calling;
    With loyalty will I endeavor to aid the physician in his work, and devote myself to the welfare of those committed to my care.

Gretter, 1893

nurses, hospital administrators, and physicians extol the virtues of the "good ol' days" when schools produced graduates "who could do something." Certainly, for more than a century, the diploma schools carried the major responsibility for producing graduates who could meet the health care needs of the nation.

By the late 1940s and early 1950s, many diploma schools had affiliated with nearby colleges and universities, and general education requirements such as anatomy, physiology, sociology, and psychology were offered. At this time also the National League of Nursing Education (later to become the NLN) was assuming an active role in curriculum guidance and accreditation. Programs gained a stronger educational foundation because they were required to align themselves more closely with other types of postsecondary education.

Most diploma schools in operation today have sound educational programs that meet the criteria necessary for accreditation, qualified faculty, and clinical learning experiences that meet the student's learning needs rather than hospital's service needs. Graduates have been provided a foundation of study in the biologic and social sciences and may have some courses in the humanities. The programs may be affiliated with a college or university so that postsecondary credit can be formally awarded. There is a strong emphasis in diploma programs on patient/client experiences, and the course of study also includes experience in nursing management (ie, being in charge of a nursing unit). Graduates work in acute, long-term, and ambulatory health care facilities.

During the mid-1960s, there was a significant decline in enrollments in diploma schools. As the push to move nursing education into institutions of higher education reached new heights (see Chapter 3), many hospital-based schools elected to discontinue their programs. Others merged with local community colleges or universities that assumed the administrative responsibility for managing the program of education and awarded an associate or baccalaureate degree when graduation requirements were satisfied. Elimination of hospital-based programs is particularly true in the western part of the United States where only one or two programs remain in existence.

Baccalaureate Education

The first school of nursing to be established in a university setting was started at the University of Minnesota in 1909. The program existed as a quasi-autonomous branch of the university's school of medicine. Close inspection of the curriculum would reveal a program little different from the 3-year hospital program; nothing was required in the way of higher general education, and graduates were prepared for the registered nurse certificate only. Education was predominantly apprenticeship in nature, and students provided service to hospitals in exchange for education. However, it did result in nursing education existing as part of an academic organization and by 1916 programs were reported at 16 colleges and universities.

Most of the early programs offering a baccalaureate degree in nursing extended over a 5-year period. This allowed for the 3 years of nursing school curriculum similar to that of the hospital programs, and for the additional 2 years of liberal arts. In 1924, the Yale School of Nursing became the first to be established as a separate department within a university; Annie W. Goodrich was its dean. However, the growth of these schools was not rapid. Although the development of baccalaureate education for nurses may not seem like a major step to young people of today, you need to remember that it was not until 1920 that the 19th Amendment to the Constitution of the United States granted women the right to vote. Many individuals considered nursing to be a less than desirable occupation, vocational in its orientation, overshadowed by militaristic and technical aspects, and confined to women. A liberal education, scholarship, and knowledge were thought to be incompatible with the female personality and possibly posed problems for marriage later. The nursing curriculum, with its emphasis on performance of skills rather than the philosophical and theoretical approaches used in the humanities, was not well accepted by universities. Opposition to collegiate education for nurses also came from physicians who argued that nurses would be "overtrained." They were not certain that a sound knowledge base was as important as the acquisition of technical skills and manual dexterity that could be acquired with brief training at the bedside. Physicians also argued that baccalaureate education for nurses would result in their services being too costly.

Many nursing leaders have advocated for baccalaureate education as the minimum educational preparation for supervisory and administrative nursing roles. Baccalaureate education further provides the background needed for public health positions, including school nursing and the educational base for entry into graduate education in nursing. In 1965, the ANA recommended baccalaureate preparation in nursing as the minimum educational preparation for entry into professional nursing practice (see Chapter 3). The American Nurses' Credentialing Center, which offers certification in 24 specialty areas, requires a baccalaureate degree for initial basic certification in a nursing specialty and requires a master's degree for initial certification as a clinical specialist or nurse practitioner. Those certified before these new requirements took effect are permitted to maintain their certification. Some of the other nursing specialty organizations that provide certification do not require a baccalaureate degree for certification.

CHARACTERISTICS OF BACCALAUREATE EDUCATION

Baccalaureate nursing programs are located in 4-year colleges and universities. When the program of studies includes an upper division (junior and senior years), baccalaureate nursing major that is built on 2 years of liberal arts and science courses taken during the freshman and sophomore years, it is known as a *basic* or *generic* baccalaureate program.

Applicants to such programs must meet the entrance (and graduation) requirements established by the university and those of the nursing school. The admission requirements usually specify academic preparation at the high school (or preadmission) level, which includes courses in foreign language, higher-level study of mathematics and science, and a high cumulative grade point average. Relatively high scores on college admission tests may also be necessary.

During the freshman and sophomore years of study, students who pursue a nursing education take liberal arts and biologic and physical science courses with college students who are preparing for other majors. In some schools these courses may be completed on a part-time basis; but if this occurs, the entire course of study covers more than a 4-year span. The number of required liberal arts and science courses may vary from program to program but usually constitutes about one half the total number of credits specified for graduation from the college or university. Students usually begin their study of nursing content in their junior year, thus the term "upper-division major" in nursing. Nursing theory can be taught that builds on an understanding of the physical and biologic sciences and liberal arts studied the previous 2 years.

Recently, there has been some tendency for schools offering baccalaureate nursing education to introduce nursing content at some point in the sophomore year of study. These courses, if offered at this point, often include an overview of the nursing profession and some of the fundamental nursing skills.

Students in baccalaureate nursing programs learn basic nursing skills. They also learn concepts of health maintenance and promotion, disease prevention, and supervisory and leadership techniques and practices and are provided with an introduction to research. Clinical course work includes experience in community health settings and practice as leaders on a nursing team within the acute care hospital as well as basic care procedures. Emphasis is placed on developing skills in critical decision-making, on exercising independent nursing judgments that call for broad background knowledge, and on working in complex nursing situations in which the outcomes are often not predictable. Acting as a patient/client advocate, the graduate of a baccalaureate nursing program collaborates with other members of the health care team in structured and unstructured settings and supervises those with lesser preparation. The baccalaureate graduates often work with groups as well as with individuals.

In 1986, the NLN Council of Baccalaureate and Higher Degree Programs revised a statement originally developed in 1979 on the "Characteristics of Baccalaureate Education in Nursing." This statement concludes with the following list of activities that the graduate of the baccalaureate programs in nursing should be capable of performing.

- Provide professional nursing care, which includes health promotion and maintenance, illness care, restoration, rehabilitation, health counseling, and education based on knowledge derived from theory and research.
- Synthesize theoretical and empirical knowledge from nursing, scientific, and humanistic disciplines with practice.
- Use the nursing process to provide nursing care for individuals, families, groups, and communities.
- Accept responsibility and accountability for the evaluation of the effectiveness of their own nursing practice.
- Enhance the quality of nursing and health practices within practice settings through the use of leadership skills and a knowledge of the political system.
- Evaluate research for the applicability of its findings to nursing practice.
- Participate with other health care providers and members of the general public in promoting the health and well-being of people.
- Incorporate professional values as well as ethical, moral, and legal aspects of nursing into nursing practice.
- Participate in the implementation of nursing roles designed to meet emerging health needs of the general public in a changing society (National League for Nursing, 1987).

CHANGES IN BACCALAUREATE EDUCATION

In recent years the nature of baccalaureate education has changed. Some schools, seeking to add an advanced component, have added courses that permit a degree of specialization at the baccalaureate level (eg, additional courses in coronary or intensive care nursing). Other schools are providing more grounding in research, either as preparation for graduate school or for a more varied role in nursing. Another interesting variation occurs in California. In that state the rules and regulations for schools of nursing stipulate that all courses required by the Board of Nursing for licensure as a registered nurse be offered within the first 36 months of full-time training, the first six academic semesters, or the first nine academic quarters, whichever is shortest (California Board of Registered Nursing, 1992). In essence this means that all educational preparation required for application for licensure of students enrolled in baccalaureate programs in that state must be completed by the end of the junior year. This leaves the senior year to be filled with specialty experience, preceptorships, or whatever the school might deem appropriate education. This change in the licensure law has also caused some problems. Some students complete their junior year and successfully pass the licensing examination. They then elect to drop out of school and work as a registered nurse.

Although they are licensed in the state of California, these students have no degree from any school, which creates problems if they seek licensure in another state.

Associate Degree Education

The movement for associate degree education began in 1952. It has the distinction of being the first and, to date, the only type of nursing education established on the basis of planned research and experimentation. Three events undoubtedly influenced its beginning. First, it followed in the wake of the community college movement across the United States, which saw the organization and growth of 2-year community colleges that not only offered the first 2 years of a traditional 4-year college program but also brought to the community many vocational and adult education programs. The goal of the community college was to make some form of college education available to all who would desire it. Second, the cadet nurse program was created during World War II and demonstrated that qualified students could be adequately educated in less than the traditional 3 years. Lastly, the development of associate degree education was influenced by the studies conducted about nursing education in the United States, as discussed Chapter 1.

CHARACTERISTICS OF ASSOCIATE DEGREE EDUCATION

Associate degree education, which had its birth in the Cooperative Research Project in Junior and Community College Education for Nursing at Teachers College, Columbia University, was directed by Mildred Montag. The original project included seven junior and community colleges and one hospital school, located in six regions of the United States. This type of nursing education has expanded from only two schools in 1952 to more than 800 in 1995.

The four basic characteristics of associate degree education include 1) encompassing the nursing program as an integral part of the college that controls and finances the program; 2) ensuring the members of the nursing faculty the same privileges and responsibilities granted to other faculty; 3) organizing the curriculum for completion in 2 years with a clearly stated philosophy, rationale, and conceptual framework; and 4) ensuring that students are treated as are other community college students with regard to admission, progression, and graduation requirements (National League for Nursing, 1973). The programs are designed to award an associate degree on completion and graduates are eligible to write the state licensing examination for registered nursing.

The curriculum required approximately half of the credits needed for the associate degree to be fulfilled with general education requirements such as

English, anatomy, physiology, speech, psychology, sociology, and similar courses and that the other half be comprised of nursing courses. Clinical learning experiences were carefully selected to correspond with content being delivered in classroom lectures. The pre- and post-conference was used to help reinforce the relationship between the two.

COMPETENCIES OF THE ASSOCIATE DEGREE GRADUATE

In 1990, the Council of Associate Degree Programs of the NLN revised and retitled a document published in 1978 that described the abilities of the associate degree graduate. Retitled "Educational Outcomes of Associate Degree Nursing Programs: Roles and Competencies," this document condensed what was earlier described as five roles into three. These are Role as Provider of Care, Role as Manager of Care, and Role as Member within the Discipline of Nursing. The competencies are focused around these three roles and describe the behaviors the associate degree graduate demonstrates on graduation as well as the competencies the graduate would be expected to demonstrate 6 months following graduation. These last competencies are identified as "anticipated competencies" (National League for Nursing, 1990).

The advent of associate degree education in nursing has brought with it greater diversity in the students who enroll. Nursing students were traditionally a homogeneous group consisting of mostly single white women ranging in age from 18 to 35 who were usually scholastically in the upper third of their high school class. Associate degree programs (although sometimes adding selective admission policies to the "open door" philosophy of the community colleges) attract older people, married women, minorities, men, and students with a wider range of educational experiences and intellectual abilities. People who already possess baccalaureate or higher degrees in other fields also seek admission to associate degree programs, often because it can be completed in a shorter period of time than would be needed to earn another baccalaureate degree.

CONCERNS FACING ASSOCIATE DEGREE EDUCATION

Over the years associate degree education, as with all educational programs, has experienced change. There is a growing tendency to place more emphasis and time on nursing courses than on general education courses. Faculty, prepared with master's degrees in nursing, have difficulty defining *essential content*. They often respond to suggestions from advisory committees that ask for graduates with greater knowledge particularly as it relates to some specialty areas (eg, coronary care). The 1990 changes in the described role of the graduate necessitated some inclusion in the curriculum of management principles and skills. In some instances, changes in the basic requirements of the college for completion of associate degrees have increased the number of credits nursing students must complete. The concept of "core course" taken by all who graduate from the college has been popular. More content and greater credit hours have resulted in programs that can take up to 3 years to complete.

Criteria for accreditation of these programs established by the accredited schools that are members of the Council of Associate Degree Programs of the NLN have set 108 quarter hours or 72 semester credits as the maximum number of credits for any program (National League for Nursing, 1991). Many schools have difficulty meeting this criterion. Where the structure of the program would allow completion in 2 years, the selective admission criteria developed by faculty to deal with burgeoning numbers of applicants may not. When enrollments in nursing programs dropped throughout the nation in 1986, associate degree programs were the least affected. Today most programs receive many more applications for admission than positions available in beginning nursing classes. This has resulted in the need to develop some method for selecting students. In some instances this has been a "waiting list," which honors the concept of "first come—first served." Other schools have used systems similar to a lottery. Also popular are "factoring" systems built around the concept of awarding points for courses completed, past work experience, cumulative grade point average, and similar criteria. These factoring systems often result in the student spending at least a year in college before starting nursing courses to secure a position in the beginning nursing class.

An increasing number of graduates are seeking additional education beyond the associate degree, and the "ladder" concept in nursing education is growing. Registered nurse baccalaureate and "two-on-two" programs are increasing as these graduates demand easier matriculation into 4-year institutions of learning. In some states legislation has been passed strongly encouraging, and in some instances mandating, articulation plans allowing graduates to move from one level of nursing education to another with minimum loss of credit. These issues are discussed later in the chapter.

Although initially associate degree education was poorly understood by the employer, the public, and to some extent, nursing educators in general, this route to nursing education is now firmly established as credible preparation for a nursing career. Over the years, the controversy regarding "entry into practice" and the preparation needed for "professional" nursing has lost much of its passion and controversy. This is due to several factors. First of all a national nursing shortage occurring in the late 1980s and early 1990s placed a premium on all registered nurses. Along with this shortage and rising hospital costs was a serious movement to introduce into the health care work force individuals with varying titles (such as registered care technician) who had lesser educational preparation but for whom the nurse would be responsible. This brought nursing factions together in a common cause and has undoubtedly helped to push the nursing profession to greater articulation between the existing routes of educational preparation. Some efforts have been made to differentiate the practice of graduates with different types of educational preparation, and some hospitals recognize baccalaureate preparation with a pay differential. But all in all, the discord and dissonance regarding entry into practice that pervaded nursing in the 1970s and 1980s has been significantly decreased. Questions regarding what to title the associate degree graduate, how to license that graduate, and use of the term "technical" nurse may become part of nursing history.

Master's and Doctoral Programs That Prepare for Licensure

In concluding our discussion of the various educational programs that prepare the graduate to write the state licensing examination for registered nursing, we need to mention the generic master's programs.

The history of such programs goes back a number of years, to programs at Yale and several other schools of nursing where students were admitted with a baccalaureate degree in another area. They were granted a master's degree in nursing after completing an established program of study of approximately 2 years that prepared the graduate for registered nurse licensure. In addition, there is one program, located at Case Western Reserve University, in which the student earns a doctorate in nursing before being eligible to write the licensing examination.

Interest in this type of educational preparation for nursing is increasing. It reflects, in part, the thinking of some nurse leaders that the minimum preparation for professional nursing should be the master's degree. It also provides a higher degree to those persons who possess basic baccalaureate preparation in another area of study and are making a career change. With increasing emphasis being placed on the need for a baccalaureate degree for professional practice, making this type of program an option is certainly credible. When programs offering this option are not available, many students who have degrees in other disciplines have chosen to pursue a 2-year associate degree in nursing. Despite availability, some persons with degrees in other disciplines opt for the 2-year degree because of time and expense.

Similarities Among Programs

Currently there appear to be as many similarities in the various avenues to nursing education as there are variances. These similarities may be grouped into several broad classifications that include academic standards, administrative concerns, and areas relating to students.

ACADEMIC SIMILARITIES

In the academic realm, three similarities stand out:

1. All graduates write the NCLEX for registered nursing in their state. All writers must meet the same minimum cutoff score to pass the test and become licensed.
2. All schools must meet the criteria established for state board approval and (in many instances on a voluntary basis) the criteria developed for national accreditation.
3. All faculty are pushed to develop curricula responsive to the needs of today's health care delivery system that demands greater efficiency, an ability to work in a highly technological environment, knowledge of new protocols, and greater responsibility and accountability.
4. The recruitment of faculty possessing master's and doctoral degrees in an ongoing effort. Salaries in education have lagged behind those in practice. The graduate with a master's degree can find many challenging roles in hospitals, clinics, and even private practice and earn more at the same time.
5. Members of the faculty are pushed to meet the increasing demands of education, clinical excellence, tenure, and possibly vocational certification. Workloads and the time invested in the performance of professional responsibilities often are disparate with that of instructors from other areas of the campus, even though they are considered colleagues in the educational setting.

ADMINISTRATIVE SIMILARITIES

From an administrative perspective, two similarities are noted:

1. Adequate financial support is a major concern. All programs are relatively expensive to operate in comparison to other forms of education provided in colleges and universities. Federal and state agencies, as well as colleges and universities, are tightening the reins on funding and are demanding greater accountability. In tough economic times, the nursing program may be identified as one to be phased out. Less financial assistance is available to students in the form of scholarships and loans than in the past. Tuition costs are rising.
2. Finding appropriate learning experiences is a challenge. Most programs find themselves searching and competing with other schools for learning experiences in clinical agencies. To some extent this competition is related to changes in societal values and the health care delivery system. Families are electing to have fewer children and, more recently in some societies, to deliver these children at home. The result has been fewer patients in the obstetric units of hospitals.

Pediatric patients are managed on an outpatient basis as much as possible, and hospitalization, when required, is kept to a minimum. The management of the client with psychiatric disturbances is moving from institutions to community mental health centers whenever feasible. Finally, the increase in the number and size of schools in urban areas creates high demand for clinical facilities in those areas.

SIMILARITIES RELATING TO STUDENTS

In the area relating to students, three similarities are noted:

1. Selection of students is a major task. All schools must develop sound educational programs while balancing student enrollments against faculty recruitment and retention factors. In many instances the number of applications exceed the positions available in beginning classes. This has resulted in the development of selective admission policies that have been carefully scrutinized by school officials and then reviewed by the school's attorney for correct legal form and for legal ramifications before being accepted by the school's policy-making group.
2. Legal concerns are demanding increased time and attention. Programs are caught up in more legal concerns than in the past because applicants and students seek their "rights as individuals" and challenge admission and dismissal policies. The National Student Nursing Association Student Bill of Rights and Responsibilities is widely accepted by schools of nursing throughout the country. This bill sets forth the students' basic rights and establishes grievance procedures if a student believes that these rights have been violated (see Chapter 13, Fig. 13–5). Another legal concern relates to malpractice coverage for students. Some collegiate programs, now removed from the umbrella coverage of the hospital, ask that students purchase malpractice insurance to provide protection against financial losses that could occur as the result of suits that could be based on errors committed in the learning process.
3. There is greater diversity in the student body. All programs are experiencing a wider diversity in the characteristics of applicants seeking admission to the programs. Programs are receiving more applications from men, minorities, older adults, and persons who possess degrees in other fields of study. Students with English as a second language are presenting new challenges to nursing faculty in all types of programs.

One usually finds nursing educators united in their efforts to create quality programs that will graduate students who can function satisfactorily in a changing and challenging health care delivery system (Table 2–1).

(*text continues on page 70*)

TABLE 2–1 Educational Opportunities for Registered Nursing: A Comparison

	Diploma	Associate Degree	Baccalaureate
Location	Is usually conducted by and based in a hospital	Most often conducted in junior or community colleges, occasionally in senior colleges and universities	Located in senior colleges and universities
Length of Study	Requires generally 24–30 months but may require 3 academic years	Requires usually 2 academic or sometimes 2 calendar years	Requires 4 academic years
Requirements for Admission	Requires graduation from high school or its equivalent, satisfactory general academic achievement, and successful completion of certain prerequisite courses.	Requires that applicants meet entrance requirements of college as well as of program	Requires that applicants meet entrance requirements of the college or university as well as those of program
Program of Learning	Includes courses in theory and practice of nursing and in biologic, physical, and behavioral sciences	Combines a balance of nursing courses and college courses in the basic natural and social sciences with courses in general education and the humanities	Frequently concentrates on courses in the theory and practice of nursing in the junior and senior years
	May require that certain courses in the physical and social sciences be taken at a local college or university		Provides education in the theory and practice of nursing and courses in the liberal arts as well as the behavioral and physical sciences
Clinical Component	Provides early and substantial clinical learning experiences in the hospital and a variety of community agencies; these focus on an understanding of the hospital environment and the interrelationship of other health disciplines	Requires as a significant part of the program supervised clinical instruction in hospitals and other community health agencies	Provides clinical laboratory courses in a variety of settings where health and nursing care are given

Opportunity for Educational Advancement	Little or no transferability of courses unless affiliated with a community college or university	Is structured so that some credits may be applied to baccalaureate degree	Provides the basic academic preparation for advancement to higher positions in nursing and to master's degree
Competency on Graduation	Graduate is prepared to plan for the care of patients with other members of the health care team, to develop and carry out plans for the care of individuals or groups of patients, and to direct selected members of the nursing team. Has an understanding of the hospital climate and the community health resources necessary for the extended care of patients	Graduate is prepared to plan and give direct patient care in hospitals, nursing homes, or similar health care agencies and to participate with other members of the health care team, such as licensed practical nurses, nurses aides, physicians, and other registered nurses in rendering care to patients	Graduate is prepared to plan and give direct care to individuals and families, whether sick or well, to assume responsibility for directing other members of the health care team, and to take on beginning leadership positions. Practices in a variety of settings and emphasizes comprehensive health care, including preventive and rehabilitative services, health counseling and education, and care in acute and long-term illnesses Has necessary education for graduate study toward a master's degree and may move rapidly to specialized leadership positions in nursing as teacher, administrator, clinical specialist, nurse practitioner, and nurse researcher
Licensure	Must successfully complete state licensing examination	Must successfully complete state licensing examination	Must successfully complete state licensing examination

Other Forms of Nursing Education

Educational offerings in nursing have grown tremendously since the 1960s. This is due in part to the changing role of the nurse in health care delivery and to the need for more adequate education to meet the preparation requirements of that role. Another contributing factor is the continuing push to make nursing truly professional. The result is the need for practitioners, with master's and doctoral degrees, who are interested and competent in research techniques and skills. A third significant reason for advancing nursing education relates to requirements placed on the profession for leadership in nursing administration and education. Nurse educators, joining the ranks of other professionals in the academic environment, are required to possess equivalent educational background. Nurses who assume roles in nursing administration have found the need for a solid understanding of management and finance principles acquired by study at the master's and doctoral level.

REGISTERED NURSE BACCALAUREATE PROGRAMS

Recent years have seen an increase in the number of registered nurse baccalaureate (RNB) programs. These programs are designed for registered nurses with either a diploma or an associate degree who wish to return to school to complete a baccalaureate degree in nursing. Another variation are programs that admit registered nurses with an associate degree who can graduate 3 years later with a master's degree in nursing. A baccalaureate degree is awarded part way through the program. Some schools have also added programs designed to admit the licensed practical (vocational) nurse who will emerge with a baccalaureate degree in nursing. These programs carry various names in different parts of the country, including baccalaureate registered nurse (BRN) programs, two-on-two, and, in the Midwest, capstone programs.

There are several reasons for the increase in this form of nursing education. Employers are requiring greater preparation for supervisory roles. Highly qualified young men and women are entering associate degree programs because of cost and time factors and are then planning more education several years after completing the original program. Nursing as a profession is pushing toward increasing the number of nurses prepared with baccalaureate and higher degrees.

The RNB programs vary greatly throughout the United States. In some instances they exist in universities that already offer the generic baccalaureate program. The students may be integrated with generic baccalaureate students, partially separated, or totally separated. Another form of RNB preparation is the two-on-two approach, in which registered nurse students transfer into the college or university with junior standing and complete an additional 2 years of upper-division nursing classes. In some instances, this is the only program in nursing offered by that college or university; that is, the college does not offer a basic program that prepares a graduate for licensure. Some schools offer nurse practitioner preparation in conjunction with the baccalaureate degree, although the growing tendency is to place this at the master's level.

The general trend is to allow the transfer of credits in basic education courses such as psychology, sociology, and in the natural and biologic sciences earned at junior and community colleges. Often some transfer credit is given for nursing (eg, 45 quarter credits), or the courses may be challenged. Distribution requirements of the particular college or university must be satisfied, and upper-division nursing courses must be completed in such areas as physiologic nursing, community health, and supervision. A minimum of 2 years usually is required for completion of the program, although the time may be longer, depending on the number of requirements satisfied at the time of entry.

When the programs offering baccalaureate education to registered nurses were first launched, they were criticized by some nurse educators. The criticism seemed to revolve around three central themes. The first was based on the fact that the ladder concept in nursing education was slow to develop. Based on the original planning for associate degree programs, many nurse educators perceived associate degree education as terminal and did not accept it as a stepping stone to baccalaureate education.

The second concern related to the problems associated with evaluating previous learning and granting credit for that learning. How should one equate nursing process that was taught at the freshman level in the community college with nursing process that was taught at the junior level in the senior university?

The third difficult area was that of determining what and how additional courses in nursing should be offered. A serious question existed as to whether the standards, program objectives, and educational structures that had been developed for the generic student were appropriate for the registered nurse. What learning experience could be included that would help to "socialize" the student for the role of a baccalaureate graduate? What additional nursing courses were needed to form the upper-division major in nursing that would provide a basis for graduate education?

Because the skills of the various graduates were not clearly delineated, it was difficult to develop a curriculum that would enable the RNB graduate to demonstrate specific terminal behaviors. When attempts were made to develop such programs, baccalaureate educators found themselves confronted with another concern: they were working with adult students. This required them to rethink teaching–learning principles to provide effective education. Students were seeking a learning program that allowed for part-time study, provided more evening and weekend classes, and permitted part- or full-time employment while pursuing more education. They wanted the education brought to them rather than going to the educational setting.

Recently, RNB education and two-on-two educational programs have gained more acceptance. In some instances, schools operating both basic and

RNB programs report graduating more RNB students than basic graduates. At least three factors are responsible for the change in attitude toward RNB education. First, the ANA Commission on Nursing Education has provided a push to increase the availability of baccalaureate programs for registered nurses. Nursing educators are challenged to create and accept more innovative educational strategies.

The second factor comes from pressure within each state itself. A number of states have enacted legislation, sometimes in response to the nursing shortage, that requires the development of a statewide plan for articulation between various types of nursing education programs. In most instances the legislation establishes a date by which the plan will be implemented.

The last push for increased development of educational mobility has come from organizations in the health care arena. The American Medical Association (AMA) House of Delegates has suggested career mobility as one way to alleviate the nurse shortage. Members of the NLN passed a resolution at the convention held in 1989 requiring that the NLN drop entry issue activities and take steps that would increase educational mobility.

Some of the RNB programs currently in operation provide for part-time study or for studies completed through evening courses. The desirability of such an approach for nurses who must work to support their education is obvious. Other innovative RNB programs provide baccalaureate education to people living in areas geographically remote from colleges or universities. These programs have used new technologies available for the electronic transmission of information.

THE EXTERNAL DEGREE

The concept of an external degree is not new. Universities in Australia, the Soviet Union, and England have long recognized independent study validated by examination. The University of London has awarded college degrees earned in this fashion since 1836. The major difference between the external degree and the traditional educational experience is that students awarded an external degree are not required to attend classes or follow any prescribed methods of learning. (They may choose to take some classes.) Learning is assessed through highly standardized and validated examinations. This approach to education had not been developed in the United States until about the mid-1950s and then in only selected areas. Schools in the United States that were first to recognize the value of this self-directed learning were New York's Empire State College and the University Without Walls consortium.

The New York Regents External Degree (REX) Program of the University of the State of New York has become part of this movement. The New York Board of Regents established the College Proficiency Examination Program in 1961. Similar to the College-Level Examination Program tests developed by the Educational Testing Service, the examinations allow students to gain credit and meet the regents' external degree requirements without attending classes.

In 1971, the New York Board of Regents authorized an external associate degree program in nursing; the external baccalaureate degree in nursing was to follow in April 1976 with the first baccalaureate degrees awarded in 1979. The W. K. Kellogg Foundation provided funds to support the initiation of the program. The programs have grown in popularity, and both the associate degree program and the baccalaureate program are accredited by the NLN programs.

The nursing program, like other external degree programs in arts, science, and business, uses an assessment approach and is primarily—although not exclusively—designed for those with some experience in nursing. It is philosophically based on principles of the adult learner, which advocate flexible and learner-oriented education. Specifically, the responsibility for demonstrating that learning has occurred is placed on the student, and the responsibility for identifying the content to be learned and objectively assessing that this has occurred rests with the faculty. The nursing major is divided into cognitive and performance components. The cognitive learning is documented through nationally standardized and psychometrically valid written examinations. Clinical skills are evaluated through four criteria-referenced performance examinations at regional performance assessment centers throughout the country. Because performance examinations are quite different from typical evaluation procedures, the people who administer the examinations must complete a training program to prepare them to perform the evaluations. The major thrust of the training sessions is to exchange teaching–helping behaviors with those of the neutral observer whose role is to determine that criteria have been met.

Collaborative relationships have been established with academic institutions that want to assist REX candidates who live in their area. The local colleges advertise the program to area nurses and offer courses designed to assist the student who is preparing for examination. Close collaboration occurs between REX faculty and the local college faculty. Students who want to learn more about this program are encouraged to write to the University of the State of New York, Regents External Degree Program, Cultural Education Center, Albany, NY 12230.

Despite objections, alternative and nontraditional avenues to nursing education continue to grow and appeal to the learner. Nursing education, like nursing care, should be tailored to the consumer's needs.

Nursing Education at the Graduate Level

The critical need for nurses who have had additional preparation to function in educational settings, in supervisory roles, and as clinical specialists and to fulfill the expanded role of the nurse has resulted in the increase of programs at the graduate level.

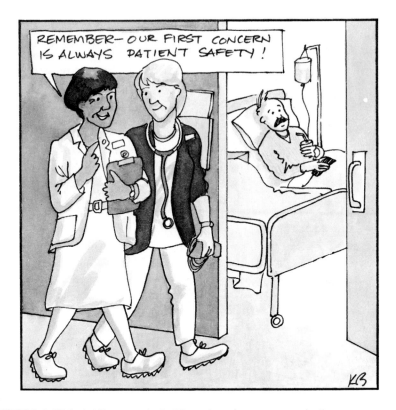

FIGURE 2–4 Clinical skills are evaluated through performance examinations.

MASTER'S PREPARATION

A variety of models of master's preparation in nursing exist. Most could be classified as traditional in approach, but a study of master's programs found that 36% used nontraditional options (Forni, 1987). Some less traditional approaches include outreach programs; summers-only programs; RN-to-MSN tracks that provide a direct route to master's degrees for registered nurses who have graduated from diploma or associate degree programs; programs for groups with special needs, such as registered nurses with non-nursing baccalaureate degrees or those seeking preparation as technical nurse educators; and programs that admit non-nurses and foreign graduates. Some schools offer off-campus classes, perhaps rotating sites, and some use telecommunication systems to deliver core content by way of television. In at least one school all classes are on Fridays. Several unique programs (eg, those at Yale University, Pace University, and the University of Tennessee at Knoxville) offer a master's degree in nursing after completion of a baccalaureate degree in another field. Such programs, called generic master's degree programs, were discussed earlier in the chapter.

Most programs require at least a full year for completion; many have been expanded to 2 years. Master's programs in nursing are often found in senior colleges and universities that have baccalaureate programs in nursing. They have the option of seeking voluntary accreditation from the NLN.

Persons seeking information about master's degree programs in nursing should be aware of the NLN publication, *Master's Education: Route to Opportunities in Contemporary Nursing*.

DOCTORAL STUDIES

The number of requests for admission to doctoral study in nursing has greatly increased since the early 1980s. The impetus for this movement stems from the need for advanced study for academic advancement or tenure in the educational setting and reflects the need in nursing research for the advancement of the profession as a whole.

Before doctorates in nursing were offered, doctoral study in other fields allowed nursing into the mainstream of education in the United States. A doctorate outside the area of nursing was often the only doctorate available to the person seeking further education; doctorates in nursing are relatively new to the educational milieu, as opposed to such degrees in psychology, sociology, anthropology, or physiology. Certainly nursing can and has benefited from other disciplines.

Doctoral programs in nursing offer various degrees such as the doctor of nursing science (DNSc), the doctor of science in nursing (DSN), the doctor of nursing education (DNEd), or the doctor of philosophy (PhD) in nursing. Other types of doctorates are also available to nurses, such as the doctor of education (EdD) or the doctor of public health (DPH).

The difference in preparation and function of graduates possessing these various degrees is confusing, but for the most part nurses with doctorates provide leadership roles in education, often serving as a dean or director of nursing programs. They may also chose to be involved in the research and development of a body of nursing knowledge.

Although assuming no role in the accreditation of doctoral programs, the NLN has published a pamphlet entitled "Doctoral Programs in Nursing" that provides information about various programs of doctoral study in nursing.

Directly Articulated Programs

Another recent innovation in nursing education is a program that provides direct articulation between lower-level and higher-level programs. Many of the legislative mandates are encouraging this type of education. The purpose

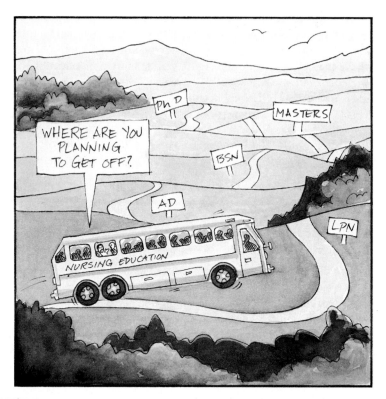

FIGURE 2–5 Among innovations occurring in nursing education over the past decade are programs that provide direct articulation between lower-level and higher-level programs.

of such a program is to facilitate opportunities for students to start nursing education, stop when some goal (such as practical nurse licensure) is achieved, or keep moving up the educational ladder.

The plan, which is especially attractive to practical (vocational) nurse and associate degree students, allows them to move up the career ladder from practical nurse to associate degree nurse to the nurse with a baccalaureate degree. Students in an articulated licensed practical nurse/associate degree program would spend a year preparing to be an LP(V)N and another year completing the associate degree. If they want to continue after this 2-year period, they can earn a baccalaureate degree at another institution after 2 more years of study. From that point a student could continue work toward a master's degree.

Such programs usually involve planning between two or more institutions, but, depending on start and stop points, they may occur within a single institution. Of concern to nurse educators today is whether nursing assistants should be included in this ladder approach and, if so, how they can be accommodated. Some state boards of nursing have already stipulated that a mechanism be established to recognize in some way, the previous knowledge acquired by the nursing assistant.

These multiple entry, multiple exit programs are not without problems. Initially they are difficult to develop because of the tremendous amount of joint planning needed. Leveling of content in nursing as well as in the supporting areas of natural and behavioral sciences is critical. Understanding what has been taught and determining how to evaluate current knowledge is also important. Educators need to speak the same language and develop mutual respect.

Nondegree Programs

Specialized programs have been developed to help to prepare individuals for roles of increased breadth and scope. Some of these programs are incorporated into the preparation leading to a particular degree; others exist as part of a school's continuing education program.

The registered nurse anesthesia and the midwifery programs both award a certificate after completion of a standardized and rigorous course of study lasting from 18 months to 2 years. Each program stipulates its own admission requirements, some requiring licensure only, others requiring a baccalaureate degree.

Programs that have been introduced more recently include nurse practitioner and nursing specialist preparation in areas of nursing practice such as pediatrics, gerontology, family health, genetics, and women's health care. The recent health care reform has resulted in an increased emphasis on the role of advanced nursing practice in health care delivery and more demand for educational programs to prepare these practitioners. Advanced skills in clinical decision-making and coordinating care from the hospital to the community and to the home are essential parts of this preparation (Lipman and Deatrick, 1994). Programs that prepare nurse practitioners concentrate study in specific areas over a period of time lasting from several months to a year or more. Requirements for admission vary tremendously. Some require licensure for admission, others stipulate the baccalaureate degree, and still others require that the education occur at the post-master's degree level. (The American Nurses' Credentialing Center requires the master's degree for all those seeking initial nurse practitioner certification.)

The proliferation of such programs has been so great that a complete listing is impossible. A student interested in pursuing such preparation is encouraged to write to the college or university of choice for information about available programs.

Internships and Residencies for the New Graduate

When nursing education moved from hospital-based diploma programs into higher education, a new problem was created. Employers of the new graduates, who expected these graduates to function as experienced and qualified professionals on the day after graduation, complained that they were not prepared to assume staff nurse positions within their institutions.

The changes that had occurred in nursing education, including changes in diploma education, had resulted in shortened clinical experience. Many graduates of diploma schools of the 1950s would have as much as 4000 clock hours of clinical experience, albeit more as an apprenticeship and a service to the hospital than as a learning experience. Graduates of associate degree programs, with integrated curricula and objective-based learning experiences, emerged into the work world with clinical learning time of 800 or fewer clock hours. Baccalaureate and hospital-based programs also had decreased their clinical hours as curricula were reorganized.

Critics in nursing service were distressed by a new type of graduate who could think, analyze, and synthesize but who was inexperienced in "doing." Most graduates needed an orientation to the work facility and to their new role in that organization and time to become efficient in the administration of their newly learned skills. Although few would question the need for internships and residencies for the new physician, the need for a similar experience for new nursing graduates was viewed as appalling. The new graduates, unable to live up to the expectations placed on them, became frustrated and discouraged and often opted for a less stressful situation, sometimes even outside nursing. Nursing educators, in defending the education provided, cited other professions, such as law and engineering, in which graduates needed a period of time to adapt to the world of work.

By the 1970s, it was apparent that something must be done. Although the cost was a problem, orientation programs, internships, and residencies for new graduates were instituted by hospitals. The programs were intended to ease the transition from the role of student to that of staff by providing the opportunity to increase clinical skills and knowledge as well as self-confidence. Programs can last from several weeks to a year and are designed for graduates of all nursing programs—associate degree, diploma, and baccalaureate. They often include rotations to various units within the hospital, including specialty areas, and they accommodate different shifts. Usually some formal classwork is associated with the experience, but the majority of the time is spent in direct patient care, often under the supervision of a preceptor.

Some direct benefits to institutions, other than a better prepared new employee who remains in employment, have resulted from such programs. Inadequacies in policy and procedure books have been uncovered and, as a result, these books have been rewritten. Performance evaluation tools that are more objective in format have emerged. Nursing practice throughout an agency may have become more standardized. Job satisfaction has increased. It is no longer unusual for hospitals to advertise planned orientation and internships as benefits offered to the new graduate who would seek employment at their institution.

Continuing Education

Continuing education programs are widely publicized in today's nursing literature. They are frequently presented just prior to and as part of major nursing conventions. Some professional meetings carry continuing education credit. Other continuing education programs exist as an extension of nursing program at a college or university.

Continuing education in nursing is defined as "planned learning experiences beyond a basic nursing educational program. The learning experiences are designed to promote the development of knowledge, skills, and attitudes for the enhancement of nursing practice, thus improving health care to the public" (American Nurses Association, 1974).

Like so many other areas of nursing, this is not new. In an article entitled "Nursing the Sick," written around 1882, Florence Nightingale wrote:

> Nursing is, above all, a progressive calling. Year by year nurses have to learn new and improved methods, as medicine and surgery and hygiene improve. Year by year nurses are called upon to do more and better than they have done. It is felt to be impossible to have a public register of nurses that is not a delusion (Nightingale, as cited in Seymer, 1954, p 349).

The first continuing education courses for nurses probably would be considered postgraduate instruction today. In 1899, Teachers College at Columbia University instituted a course for qualified graduate nurses in hospital economics. Nursing institutes and conferences were first offered to nurses in the 1920s. Often these were given to make up for deficiencies in basic nursing curricula of the time. Hospital in-service or staff development programs were also beginning to be discussed in nursing literature around this time. Today most hospitals employ someone who is responsible for the staff education program. By 1959, federal funds became available for short-term courses, giving much thrust to continuing education. In 1967, the ANA published "Avenues for Continued Learning," its first definitive statement on continuing education; and in 1973, the ANA Council on Continuing Education was established. The Council, which is responsible to the ANA Commission on Education, is concerned about standards of continuing education, accreditation of the programs, transferability of credit from state to state, and development of guidelines for recognition systems within states. In 1974, "Standards for Continuing Education in Nursing" was published by the ANA, and the federal government altered the Nurse Traineeship Act of 1972 to include an option that would provide continuing education as an alternative to taking increasing numbers of students into programs receiving federal capitation dollars.

By the 1970s, almost all nursing publications had something to say about continuing education for nurses. Practically all states were organizing or planning to organize some method by which the nurse could receive recognition for continued education. These systems were called continuing education approval and recognition programs, or continuing education recognition programs, and most state systems followed the guidelines and criteria prepared by the ANA.

The continuing education unit (CEU) became a rather uniform system of measuring, recording, reporting, accumulating, transferring, and recognizing participation in nonacademic credit offerings. The definition of a CEU was developed by the National Task Force on the Continuing Education Unit, which represented 34 educational groups. Although nursing was not one of the groups, the definition has been accepted by the profession. Ten hours of participation in an organized continuing education experience under responsible sponsorship, capable direction, and qualified instruction is equal to one CEU.

Today colleges, universities, hospitals, voluntary agencies, and private proprietary groups are all offering continuing education courses to registered nurses. Cost of that education varies tremendously. Nurses attending meetings and conferences may earn a CEU, or part of one, for merely being in the meeting. No attempt is made to assess whether learning has occurred. Professional journals are including sections on programmed instruction that can be completed in the comfort of one's living room. These have an evaluation mechanism. Telecourses are offered by television. Workshops, institutes, conferences, short courses, and evening courses abound. Yet some nurses do not feel the need to keep up with these current offerings.

A system for accreditation and approval of continuing education in nursing was developed and implemented by the ANA in 1975. Accreditation was awarded for a period of 4 years and assured the public that the continuing education offerings provided consistent quality. A new system, put into operation August 1, 1987, allows organizations that offer continuing education to seek accreditation as either a provider or an approver. A provider is any organization that is responsible for the development, implementation, and evaluation of courses. An approver could be the state nurses' association, a specialty organization, or a federal nursing service that has been designated to approve the continuing education process. Organizations can be both approvers and providers. This program made the system more accessible to groups seeking approval of courses or classes by bringing the process closer to the membership and to those offering the programs.

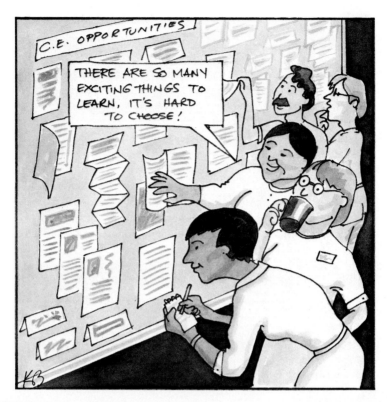

FIGURE 2–6 Today colleges, universities, hospitals, voluntary agencies, and private proprietary groups are all offering continuing education courses to registered nurses.

An issue today is whether continuing education should be mandatory or voluntary. Mandatory continuing education affects licensure, that is, any nurse renewing a license in a state requiring (mandating) continuing education will have to meet that state's regulations for completing CEUs. Voluntary continuing education is not related to relicensure. Government agencies and state legislatures are exerting pressure on nurses, as they have on physicians, attorneys, dietitians, dentists, pharmacists, and other professionals, to provide evidence of updated knowledge before renewal of license.

A position supporting mandatory continuing education raises some other issues. How shall the learning be measured? Who should accredit the programs? How can quality be ensured? By whom and where shall records be retained? Who should bear the cost? What should be the time frame for continuing education? How many hours, courses, and credits should be required?

You can write directly to a state board of nursing for information on specific requirements (see Appendix A for addresses).

Key Concepts

▷ Three major avenues to preparation for licensure as a registered nurse exist in the United States: the hospital-based diploma, the university-based baccalaureate degree and the associate degree offered most commonly in community colleges. Many similarities exist among these programs. In addition, various other nontraditional approaches to nursing education have evolved.

▷ Educational programs prepare nursing assistants and licensed practical (vocational) nurses for roles in the health care delivery system.

▷ The increasing need for nurses has resulted in decreased dissension regarding educational preparation for nursing and greater creativity in educational approaches.

▷ Master's and doctoral programs that prepare nurses for leaderships positions within the profession continue to grow. The actual doctoral degree awarded is varied.

▷ One of the most rapidly growing areas is that of advanced practice, accelerated by health care reform.

▷ Continuing education, whether it is represented by further education that results in a higher degree or whether it takes the form of classes, seminars, or workshops that update and increase expertise, is being encouraged by more and more organizations. Staying current in practice is critical to safe patient care.

CRITICAL THINKING ACTIVITIES

1. Imagine that you could restructure nursing education for the ideal world. How would you do so? How many levels would you provide for? Would each be terminal or articulated with others? How would you see the graduate of each program functioning in health care delivery?

2. If nursing education had not had its beginnings in the hospital, where do you think it would have started? Where do you think it would be now?

3. If nurse practitioners are to work in a collaborative way with physicians and as primary care providers, what type and level of education do you believe should be required? How would you go about ensuring that this would occur?

4. Given the situation we have today with three routes to preparation for registered nursing, what would you do about differentiating the skills of the graduate of each program? How should that influence nursing practice? How might it be accomplished?

5. Do you believe continuing education should be a mandatory requirement for renewal of one's license? Why or why not? How would you go about the record-keeping aspects if your answer is yes? How would you go about ensuring competence if your answer is no?

References

American Nurses Association. Standards for Continuing Education for Nursing. Kansas City, MO: American Nurses Association, 1974

Calhoun J. The Nightingale Pledge: A commitment that survives the passage of time. Nurs Health Care 14(3):130–136, 1993

California Board of Registered Nursing. Laws Relating to Nursing Education Licensure: Practice with Rules and Regulations. Sacramento: California Board of Registered Nursing, 1992

Deaconess Hospital School of Nursing. Eighty-One Years of Nursing: 1989–1980. Spokane, WA: Deaconess Hospital, 1980

Forni PR. Nursing's diverse master's programs: The state of the art. Nurs Health Care 8(2):770–775, 1987

Hegner BR, Caldwell E. Nursing Assistant: A Nursing Process Approach, 6th ed. Albany, NY: Delmar Publishers, 1995

Kalisch PA, Kalisch BJ. The Advance of American Nursing, 3rd ed. Philadelphia: JB Lippincott, 1995

Lipman TH, Deatrick JA. Enhancing specialist preparation for the next century. J Nurs Educ 33(2):53–58, 1994

National League for Nursing. Criteria and Guidelines for Accreditation of Associate Degree Program, 7th ed. Publication No. 23-2439, Council of Associate Degree Programs. New York: National League for Nursing, 1991

National League for Nursing.: Educational Outcomes of Associate Degree Nursing Programs: Roles and Competencies. Publication No. 23-2348, Council of Associate Degree Programs. New York: National League for Nursing, 1990

National League for Nursing. Characteristics of Baccalaureate Education in Nursing. Publication No. 15-1758, Council of Baccalaureate and Higher Degrees. New York: National League for Nursing, 1987

National League for Nursing. Characteristics of Associate Degree Education in Nursing. Publication No. 23-1500, Council of Associate Degree Programs. New York: National League for Nursing, 1973

Nightingale F. Nursing the sick. In Seymer LR. Selected Writings of Florence Nightingale. New York: Macmillan, 1954

Sorrentino, SA. Textbook for Nursing Assistants, 3rd ed. St. Louis: Mosby-Year Book, 1992

Further Readings

Allen VO, Sutton C. Associate degree nursing education: Past, present, and future. Nurs Health Care 2(9):496–497, 1981

American Association of Colleges of Nursing. Guidelines for Baccalaureate Education in Nursing for Registered Nurse Students in Colleges and Universities. Publication Series 79, No. 3. Washington, DC: American Association of Colleges of Nursing, 1980

American Nurses Association. A Case for Baccalaureate Preparation in Nursing, ANA publication No. NE-6 15M. Kansas City, MO: American Nurses Association, 1979

Battista-Calderone A. Designing interactive video instruction: An educator's perspective. Nurs Health Care 10(9):504–510, 1989

Bramble K. Nurse practitioner education: Enhancing performance through the use of the objective structured clinical assessment. J Nurs Educ 33(2):59–65, 1994

Brubaker BH. A faculty learns to make self-pacing work. Nurs Health Care 11(2):74–77, 1990

Coleman E. On redefining the baccalaureate degree. Nurs Health Care 7(4):193–196, 1986

Craver DM, Sullivan PP. Investigation of an internship program. J Contin Educ Nurs 16(4):114–118, 1985

Davids SL, Laeger E. Developing a BSN program across two institutions: Arizona State University West Campus/Glendale Community College—the adjuvant model. Nurs Health Care 11(2):84–87, 1990

Frik SM, Pollack SE. Preparation for advanced nursing practice. Nurs Health Care 14(4):190–195, 1993

Feldman HR, Jordet C. On the fast track. Nurs Health Care 10(9):490–493, 1989

Kasprisin CA, Young WB. Nurse internship program reduces turnover, raises commitment. Nurs Health Care 6(3):137–140, 1985

Kurzen CR. Contemporary Practical/Vocational Nursing. Philadelphia: JB Lippincott, 1989

Lambert C, Lambert VA. Relationships among faculty practice involvement, perception of role stress, and psychological hardiness of nurse educators. J Nurs Educ 33(4):171–179, 1993

Mead ME, Berger S, Nicksic E. Contracts for continuing education. J Contin Educ Nurs 16(4):121–126, 1985

Montag ML. Community College Education for Nursing. New York: McGraw-Hill, 1959

Parkinson CF, Parkinson SB. A comparative study between interactive television and traditional lecture offerings for nursing students. Nurs Health Care 10(9):498–502, 1989

Schwartz MD. An introduction to interactive video systems. Computers Nurs 2(1):8–13, 1984

Seymer LR. The Nightingale training school: One hundred years ago. Am J Nurs 60(5):658–661, 1960

Smith PL. Non-nurse college graduates in a specialty master's program: A success story. Nurs Health Care 10(9):494–497, 1989

Tanner CA, Hartshorn J, Rosenfeld P. Critical care nursing in baccalaureate programs. Nurs Health Care 10(9):482–488, 1989

Woolley AS. Defining the product of baccalaureate education. Nurs Health Care 7(4):199–201, 1986

3

Perspectives on Nursing Education

Objectives

After completing this chapter, you should be able to

1. Discuss the impact of the Brown report.

2. Explain factors that prompted improvements in nursing education in the 1950s and 1960s.

3. Discuss the development and effect of the ANA position paper on nursing education and on nursing organizations.

4. Outline the arguments against the ANA position on entry from the viewpoint of associate degree and hospital-based schools.

5. Explain what is meant by a "grandfather" clause and the effect of such a clause on responses to proposed changes in nursing licensure.

6. Analyze the problems created for nursing mobility by changes in individual state licensure laws.

7. Discuss the concept of differentiated practice and provide a rationale for its development.

8. Explain how the nursing shortage, computers in health care, and changes to community-based practice have had an impact on nursing education.

9. Discuss the impact of reduced federal funding on nursing education.

10. Explain why nursing theories are important to the profession.

11. Identify one theory that you believe describes nursing as it should be practiced and give your rationale for selecting this theory.

In our discussion of nursing and nursing education thus far, we have provided a background for understanding the development of nursing as a profession and a discussion of the various educational paths that will prepare you for the practice of that profession. Nursing education, because it prepares the graduates of tomorrow, must be responsive to change. Social, technical, political, and financial factors will affect the way that nursing is practiced and the manner in which students will be educated for the profession in the future.

Major Factors of the 1950s and 1960s That Influenced Nursing Education

During the 1950s and 1960s society was undergoing numerous changes. At the same time several major events occurred that had an enormous impact on the direction of nursing education. The effects of these events are still apparent in nursing education of today.

THE BROWN REPORT

Throughout the years perhaps no aspect of nursing has been more studied than the educational preparation of nurses (see Chapter 1). When you realize the efforts made to establish nursing as a profession, you can understand why nursing education has been so scrutinized. In American society, education has been the key for opening the doors of power, prestige, and economic security. Nursing and nurses have been seeking all of these.

One of the important early studies about nursing was conducted in 1948 by Esther Lucille Brown, who was not a nurse. She was concerned that young women were not choosing nursing as a profession and believed as a result of her study that the majority of schools were not providing a professional education. In her report "Nursing for the Future," Brown (1948) recommended that nursing education move away from the system of apprenticeship that predominated at the time and into a planned program of education similar to that offered by other professions. She recommended that the schools be operated by universities or colleges, hospitals affiliated with institutions of higher learning, medical colleges, or independently. She also recommended that programs be periodically examined or reviewed and that a list of accredited schools be published and distributed.

The Brown report attracted the attention of many nursing leaders who shared her concerns about recruiting qualified women into nursing. This study also followed on the footsteps of World War II. Nurses who had been involved in the military gained a new sense of autonomy and independence that they were not willing to leave behind. Committees were formed to respond to the suggestions put forth in the Brown study, particularly those related to accreditation of programs. A classification of schools evolved with schools being ranked by overall excellence. At the same time the National League for Nursing Education (NLNE, later to become the National League for Nursing [NLN]) was recommending that hospital schools of nursing consider transferring control and administration of their programs to educational institutions. The NLNE also urged that federal grants be provided to nursing schools to allow for their improvement.

DEVELOPMENT OF THE STATE BOARD
TEST POOL EXAMINATION

Along with this push for the improvement of nursing education, licensing authorities were pressured to establish a uniform licensing examination. The NLNE offered to assist states develop and adopt machine-scored examination questions that would ensure greater uniformity in testing. Originally only six states participated in the testing developed by the NLNE, but by 1949, 41 states were using this "State Board Test Pool Examination." In 1951, all licensing jurisdictions adopted a standard passing score (350). The development of the State Board Test Pool Examination helped all schools to focus on common goals. (See Chapter 4 for more information on the development of the licensing examination.)

NATIONAL ACCREDITATION OF NURSING PROGRAMS

By 1952, the NLN had a temporary accreditation program in place and was helping schools find ways to improve their programs of instruction. The accreditation program had a noticeable effect on standards of nursing education. As a result of accreditation activities, schools were forced to look at the educational preparation of faculty, the workload of faculty and students, the structure of clinical teaching, withdrawal rates, and state board examination scores. As schools began to look beyond their local community to national standards, the quality of education was enhanced. Schools that had achieved national accreditation were recognized and their graduates had added opportunities in regard to advanced education or certain types of employment.

CHANGES IN NURSING SERVICE

While changes were occurring in the education of nurses, equally significant changes were taking place in the activities for which nurses were responsible in the workplace. With the advent of antibiotics and other major advances in medical treatment, the public was seeking care in hospitals as opposed to home treatment. Infants previously born at home were now being born in hospitals. Increased hospitalization practices drove the need for qualified nurses to a new high. Hospitals were often desperate to find nurses to fill the needed positions, which represented half of all hospital personnel.

The role of the nurse was also changing. Nursing staff were assuming responsibilities formerly associated with the role of the physician. Unfortunately, they were also assuming responsibilities that could have been done by housekeeping, dietary, laboratory, and pharmacy departments. Nurses began spending more time managing personnel, delegating responsibilities, and carrying out other administrative activities. These changes in practice required nurses prepared with higher levels of education (ie, baccalaureate and master's degrees).

As attempts were made to increase the number of nursing personnel prepared as registered nurses, the 2-year associate degree programs came into existence (see Chapter 2). These programs, housed in community and junior colleges, prepared a graduate educated in 2 years and skilled in bedside nursing. The number of associate degree nursing programs grew rapidly during the 1960s. These programs appealed to men, minorities, and older students who had not traditionally sought educational preparation for nursing. The number of baccalaureate programs also increased during this time.

THE REPORT OF THE SURGEON GENERAL'S CONSULTANT GROUP

In 1961, the surgeon general of the United States Public Health Service appointed a group that would advise him on the federal government's role in providing adequate nursing services to the country. This group was known as the Surgeon General's Consultant Group on Nursing. A report of this group was published in 1963.

This report emphasized the need for more nurses and pointed to the lack of adequate financial resources for nursing education as a major problem. The report also identified several other concerns, among them the facts that too few schools were providing adequate nursing education, that too few college-bound young people were being recruited into the profession, and that more nursing schools were needed in colleges and universities. Graduation from a program offering a baccalaureate degree in nursing was recommended as the minimum educational preparation for nurses assuming leadership roles (U.S. Public Health Service, 1963).

The Surgeon General's Consultant Group on Nursing also made recommendations that federally funded low-cost loans and scholarships be made to students in both professional and practical nursing programs. It advocated the use of federal funds to construct additional nursing school facilities and to ex-

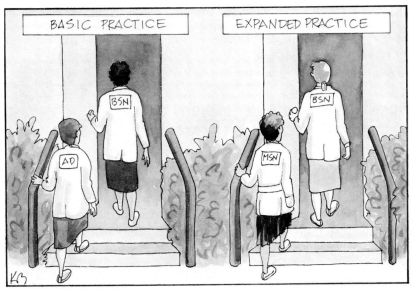

FIGURE 3–1 Basic practice and expanded practice require different educational backgrounds.

pand educational programs. The Nurse Training Act of 1964 was an outgrowth of these recommendations (see Chapter 11).

THE PUSH BY THE ANA FOR EDUCATIONAL CHANGE

In the early 1960s, the issue of educational preparation of nurses became a major concern of the American Nurses Association (ANA). The ANA believed that improvement of nursing practice depended on the advancement of nursing education. In 1962, a committee on education was appointed by the ANA Board of Directors to pursue the promotion of the baccalaureate degree as the basic educational foundation for professional nursing. For 2 years the Committee on Education studied the major changes and trends in and around nursing, especially as the trends affected patient care. This activity culminated in the development and publication in 1965 of "A Position Paper on Educational Preparation for Nurse Practitioners and Assistants to Nurses."

The paper took four major positions:

1. The education for all those who are licensed to practice nursing should take place in institutions of higher education.
2. Minimum preparation for beginning professional nursing practice at the present time should be baccalaureate degree education in nursing.
3. Minimum preparation for beginning technical nursing practice at the present time should be associate degree education in nursing.

4. Education for assistants in the health service occupations would be short, intensive preservice programs in vocational education institutions rather than on-the-job training programs (American Nurses Association, 1965, p 107).

Responses to the ANA Position Paper

No other single action or position would so affect nursing as did this position paper. For almost 40 years the profession has been divided over the issues it brought forth. Among the more perplexing of the problems associated with the position paper was the lack of definitive statements on the competencies of the graduates of each of the programs. The roles, functions, and responsibilities that each would assume within the health care delivery system were not clear. Although the position paper was fairly specific in describing the educational expectations of "professional" and "technical" nursing practice, most graduates of programs preparing for registered nurse licensure were employed by acute care hospitals. All beginning nurses, whether prepared with associate degrees, baccalaureate degrees, or in hospital-based programs, performed similar activities. This situation still exists to a large extent today.

RESPONSES OF ASSOCIATE DEGREE NURSING EDUCATION

Associate degree nursing, housed in institutions of higher education, was in its "toddler" stage when activity regarding the position paper began gathering momentum. Already attractive to many potential nurses and responsive to the older student, men and minority groups, advocates of associate degree education found the position of the ANA unacceptable. In particular, they did not want to see their graduates designated "licensed practical nurses." As discussion increased and positions became more demarcated, many nurses associated with associate degree education dropped their membership in ANA because they could not support this position.

RESPONSES OF HOSPITAL-BASED NURSING EDUCATION

Persons who were supportive of hospital-based nursing education were no more enchanted with the position than were their associate degree counterparts. Throughout the evolution of nursing in the United States, hospital-based programs had been the mainstay of nursing education. The majority of working nurses had received their basic education in these programs. They viewed themselves and their graduates as "professionals" and anything less was unacceptable. In addition, the heavy emphasis on clinical experience that was the backbone of the diploma programs, resulted in graduates who were ready, without additional orientation, to move into the workplace on the day of graduation. The programs included "leadership" components, and graduates saw themselves functioning in that role, at least in acute care hospitals.

Although many nurses objected to the position taken by the ANA, a steady push for implementation of the position paper continued throughout the 1970s. By the mid-1980s, the controversy was probably at its height.

ACTIVITIES OF THE STATE ASSOCIATIONS

In 1974, the New York Nurses' Association became the first state nurses' association to adopt a resolution regarding the entry-into-practice issue. They recommended that by 1985 all applicants for registered nurse licensure in New York State have the minimum of a baccalaureate degree, with an upper-division major in nursing. The proposed legislation was also designed to change the educational requirement for the licensed practical nurse to an associate degree. Although the resolution did not move far in terms of legislation, it started movements in other states and became the springboard for vigorous debate in the entire health care field regarding the appropriate educational preparation required of a professional nurse.

Other states were soon to follow with position statements. By August 1986, at least 48 state nurses' associations had taken positions supporting a change in the educational requirements for entry into nursing practice. The change most commonly recommended was to stipulate the baccalaureate degree in nursing as the requirement for licensure at the professional level and the associate degree in nursing as the requirement for licensure at the technical level. This would mean that there would be one entry point for each level of licensure. Boards of nursing would need to redefine the legal scope of practice for each level (Edge, 1986). Some states had settled on titles to be used by nurses prepared at the two levels; few had developed a competency statement for the categories.

In January 1986, North Dakota published and put into effect administrative rules that required nursing programs to develop specific curricula leading to the associate degree for practical nurse programs and the baccalaureate degree for registered nurse programs to be approved by the North Dakota Board of Nursing. This requirement became effective January 1, 1987. The North Dakota legislature was not involved in this change because educational requirements for licensure were not a part of the act itself. (They were stipulated in the rules and regulations that do not require legislative activity for change.) They were adopted by the board on January 16, 1986 (North Dakota Rule, 1986).

Other states with nurse practice acts that would allow for the changing of educational requirements for licensure through the rules process carefully watched the activities occurring in North Dakota. Some states had organized groups dedicated to protecting the role of the associate degree graduate. Oregon became the first state to have a bill passed in the state legislature that would bar the state board of nursing from making any change in entry-level requirements without legislative approval. Utah and Pennsylvania were to follow (ADNs, Community College, 1985; Pennsylvania Legislature, 1987).

OTHER NURSING ORGANIZATIONS AND THE ENTRY ISSUE

Gradually, other nursing specialty groups and associations endorsed the baccalaureate degree as minimum preparation for entry into professional nursing practice. Among the first organizations to support the position was the National Student Nurses' Association (NSNA), which voted in favor of this at its convention in 1976.

In 1979, several associations indicated support of the baccalaureate degree as the minimum educational level for future entry into professional practice. These were the Association of Operating Room Nurses (AORN), the Emergency Department Nurses' Association, the Association of Rehabilitation Nurses, the American Association of Occupational Health Nurses, and the Executive Board of the Nurses' Association of the American College of Obstetricians and Gynecologists (now called the Association of Women's Health, Obstetric, and Neonatal Nursing [AWHONN]). Many of these organizations had stipulations or qualifications on their position that related to regional planning, career mobility, and clarification of concepts of levels of practice. Eventually most of the major nursing organizations supported the position, at least conceptually.

The NLN has perhaps struggled with its position as much as has any nursing organization. Historically, because the composition of the memberships of the NLN includes educational councils representing practical, diploma, associate degree, and baccalaureate and higher-degree nursing programs, the organization voiced its support for all types of programs. Although in 1982 NLN issued a controversial position paper supporting the baccalaureate degree as minimum preparation for "professional" practice, it has taken a more neutral stance. At the 1987 biennial convention, the membership "postponed indefinitely" resolutions addressing this issue and in 1989 instructed the NLN to put its energies into activities that would promote upward mobility in nursing.

Discussion of the entry issue would not be complete without including decisions made by two other organizations. One of those organizations is the National Council of State Boards of Nursing. At an August 1986 meeting, representatives of the state boards voted without debate and opposition to

take a "formal position of neutrality on changes in nursing education requirements for entry" (Hartung, 1986, p 124).

The final group we will consider is the National Federation of Licensed
Practical Nurses (NFLPN). During the 1980s, this organization was faced
with hospital layoffs of large numbers of practical nurses in favor of hiring
more highly educated registered nurses. In August 1984, the membership
passed a resolution that would support increasing the period of study of the
practical nurse program to 18 months and the awarding of an associate degree
at the completion of the program of study. It was the intent of the resolution
that much of the additional time would be spent in perfecting clinical expertise, and the written rationale for the recommendation was openly one of job
security. The title of licensed practical nurse would be retained for graduates of
such programs who had passed the National Council Licensure Examination
for practical nursing (NCLEX-PN) (NFLPN, 1984). Seven years later only
one state had moved toward implementation, but the NFLPN continues to
support this position. Because a large number of practical nurse programs exist
in vocational–technical schools, the recommendation of the ANA to place
all nursing education in institutions of higher education remains unacceptable to the practical nurse group. They emphasize the critical need for practical nurses in long-term care facilities.

Problems Associated With Changes in Licensure Requirements

A number of problems are associated with making any changes in licensure
requirements. Four major issues are related to titling, scope of practice, grandfathering, and interstate endorsement.

TITLING

One of the most controversial problems associated with changing requirements for licensure is that of the use of titles. Although the position statement
calls for two levels of nursing practice, the titles to be used by persons working
at each level have not been specified by many states. Some state associations
have incorporated titles into their position statements, generally using the
title "RN" for the baccalaureate graduate and "LPN" for the 2-year associate
degree graduate. This has caused widespread dissatisfaction among the ranks
of associate degree graduates, students, and educators who believe that this
denigrates the associate degree graduate, who currently may use the RN title if
successful on state licensing examinations. The use of these titles is also up-
setting to graduates of current diploma schools, from which no degree is
granted. It would seem that neither title could be used by those graduates.

Following the decision of the ANA to title the associate degree graduate "associate nurse" and the NLN's suggestion to designate the title "registered associate nurse" to the 2-year graduate, some states recommended the use of those titles. Staunch supporters of associate degree education were not willing to make this compromise, arguing that since the beginning of the associate degree movement in the 1950s, the graduates have held the title "registered nurse." In supporting their stand on titling they pointed to the past success of the associate degree graduates on the NCLEX-RN.

SCOPE OF PRACTICE

Of equal concern to the issue of titling is that relating to the description and delineation of the scope of practice for the two levels of caregivers. The scope of practice, as discussed in Chapter 4, is that section of the Nurse Practice Act that outlines the activities a person with that license may legally do. As states have moved toward plans for implementing two levels of practice, the process of making nursing diagnoses and developing nursing care plans has been included in the scope of practice of the professional nurse only. Associate degree educators have been adamant in their contention that unless the scope of practice for the 2-year graduate also includes these behaviors, that graduate will be unemployable and able to do less than the licensed practical nurse of today (Illinois RNs, 1986).

THE GRANDFATHER CLAUSE

Historically, the licensing of professions and occupations has been within the realm of the police power of each individual state. Police power exists to safeguard the health and welfare of citizens. When a state licensure law is enacted, or if a current law is repealed and a new law enacted, the grandfather clause has been a standard feature that allows persons to continue to practice their profession or occupation after new qualifications that they might not meet have been enacted into law. The legal basis for the process is found in the 14th Amendment to the U.S. Constitution, which says that no state may deprive any person of life, liberty, or property without due process of law. The Supreme Court has ruled that the license to practice is a property right.

The use of the grandfather clause in nursing is by no means a new process. For example, it was not until the mid-1950s that theoretical and practical experience in psychiatric nursing was required in all nursing curricula and that psychiatric content was included in state licensing examinations. When laws changed to make this a requirement, hundreds of practicing nurses had never had a formal course in psychiatric nursing and had not been required to write a psychiatric examination to qualify for licensure. The right of these nurses to continue to be licensed, and thus to practice their profession, was protected by a grandfather clause. (Most of these nurses are now retired from the active practice of nursing.)

When applied to the entry-into-practice issue, the grandfather clause would guarantee that registered nurses who had been educated in associate degree or diploma programs before a specified date would have the right to continue their licensure as registered nurses as long as they met all other conditions for licensure renewal. As an example of the application of this process, let us assume that changes in a state's licensure laws to require a baccalaureate degree as the minimum educational preparation for registered nurse licensure became effective July 1, 1998. After July 1, 1998, diploma and associate degree graduates would be licensed as technical nurses. All associate degree and diploma graduates licensed before July 1, 1998 would be considered registered nurses, as protected by the grandfather clause. Some people believe that the entry-into-practice resolutions would not have passed in state conventions without the assurance of a grandfather clause. Some voting delegates seemed more concerned "how will this affect me, personally" than about the impact of the resolution on nursing as a whole.

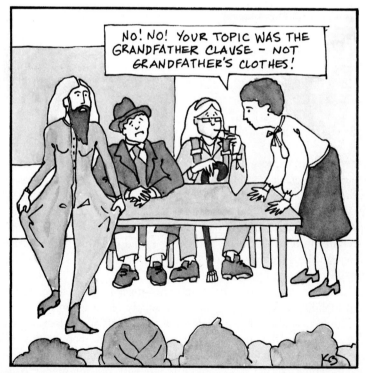

FIGURE 3–2 When a state licensure law is enacted or if a current law is repealed, the grandfather clause has been a standard feature that allows persons to continue to practice their profession.

The grandfather clause is limited to the protection of a nurse's license. Additional qualifications can be established by employers for certain jobs for registered nurses. For example, some employers now require that unit managers and supervisors have a baccalaureate degree, whereas others do not. Employers may require a master's degree for a position as a clinical nurse specialist or a director of nursing. In the public health arena, it has long been the practice to require a baccalaureate degree in nursing because other types of nursing programs do not provide a background in public health nursing. In some areas of the country, changes have occurred in the educational requirements of school nurses. Similar actions have already occurred with regard to qualifications for teachers in nursing schools. Accreditation standards for the Council of Associate Degree Programs now stipulate that nurse educators possess a master's degree in nursing, and the doctoral degree is being recommended for educators in baccalaureate programs.

Some nurses believe that the grandfather clause should be conditional. If it were conditional, persons licensed before the changes in the licensure law would continue to use their current title for a stipulated period, for example, 10 years. At the end of that period, if they had not completed the education mandated in the changes (or any other conditions that might have been added), they would have to use the title stipulated in the new law for persons with their educational preparation. This condition would require that there be access to the required education for those needing it. Because of the complexity and the questionable status of the issue, there is little likelihood that conditional "grandfathering" will occur.

INTERSTATE ENDORSEMENT

Another concern expressed over licensure changes is related to interstate endorsement of licensure among states. Nursing is one of the few professions to have developed a process by which national examinations with standardized scores are administered in each state or jurisdiction. This allows a nurse who has passed the licensing examination in one state to move to another state and seek licensure in that state, without the need to retake and pass another examination. Because nurses have been highly mobile, this has been a great advantage.

Changes in one state without similar changes in other states will affect nursing mobility. It would also affect the supply of nurses in an individual state. Throughout the nursing shortage of the late 1980s, this was a serious concern. Although that nursing shortage has resolved, many policy-makers believe that there will continue to be a need for nurses in the future and are reluctant to support action that would interfere with nursing supply. As states move toward making changes in their practice acts, it is hoped that similar changes will be considered across the nation so that interstate endorsement can be maintained without requiring reexamination.

Distinguishing Differences

Toward the beginning of the 1990s, some nursing leaders began to reassess the entry-into-practice issue. Although this reevaluation may have been encouraged by the nursing shortage of the late 1980s and the push toward cost cutting typical of the 1990s, it may also reflect new thinking regarding the role of nurses and nursing. Many nursing leaders encouraged recognition of the need for different types of practitioners prepared with different types of education and urged respect for all. Other nursing leaders began to advocate for the master's as the minimum requirement for professional practice, a concept reinforced in new requirements for nurses in advanced specialty practice.

COMPETENCY EXPECTATIONS
AND DIFFERENTIATED PRACTICE

The task of describing and differentiating the competencies and the scope of practice of nurses graduating from the various types of nursing education programs is one of the major challenges facing nursing today. It represents a problem the nursing profession faces without changes imposed by the position paper. At the present time, graduates of baccalaureate nursing programs and graduates of 2-year associate degree programs write the same licensing examination for practice as a registered nurse. Logically this would seem to make little sense. This approach fails to recognize the broad range of functions in nursing and the potential for improving the quality of care that can be given to those needing that care if different roles and responsibilities could be identified. Because the licensing examinations measure standards for minimum safe practice, some have suggested that the current licensing examinations are not testing those skills that are developed in a baccalaureate program. Also, in the work environment of the acute and long-term care facility, little differentiation exists in beginning staff nurse positions filled by graduates of associate degree or baccalaureate programs.

Realistic statements regarding competencies of each level or category of nursing are necessary so that each category can be used effectively and efficiently within the health care delivery system. Validated competencies will also provide a basis for the development of curriculum patterns that will ensure adequate preparation of each category of caregiver without running the risk of overeducation or undereducation at any one level. They can also serve as a foundation for the development of educational mobility patterns within the profession.

Some work has been done toward describing the competencies of graduates of the different programs in nursing. In 1990, the Council of Associate Degree Programs of the NLN, published "Educational Outcomes of Associate Degree Nursing Programs: Roles and Competencies," a revision of an earlier competency statement. Associate degree programs seeking NLN accreditation are encouraged to establish programs that support these competencies.

The "Characteristics of Baccalaureate Education in Nursing," revised by the Council of Baccalaureate and Higher Degrees of NLN in 1987, accomplishes a similar purpose for baccalaureate education. Two projects sponsored by the Midwest Alliance in Nursing have focused on defining competencies. One, entitled "Defining and Differentiating ADN and BSN Competencies and Facilitating ADN Competency Development" was funded by the W. K. Kellogg Foundation. The second, entitled "Continuing Education for Consensus on Entry Skills," was funded by a grant from the Division of Nursing of the Department of Health and Human Services. The goal of these studies was to achieve a regional consensus among nursing service persons and educators from both types of programs on differentiated statements of scope of practice for each level of graduate.

Since 1986, the National Council of State Boards of Nursing has conducted several studies aimed at role delineation and job analysis of entry-level registered nurses. The purpose of these studies was to validate the NCLEX-RN. Please refer to Chapter 4 for more discussion of the studies conducted by the National Council.

Although it seems appropriate for nurse educators to come to terms with the competencies of the various graduates, in some instances nursing service has seized the issue and is developing programs within institutions that recognize various types of educational preparation in job descriptions. *Differentiated nursing practice* refers to "practice expectations that are consistent with expected competencies of graduates from different kinds of education programs" (Harkness, Miller, and Hill, 1992 p 26). When this can be implemented in practice, every nurse can be used to that person's maximum capacity. In instances where differentiated practice has been set in motion, three levels of care provider have been identified: the patient care manager, the clinical nurse, and the patient care technician. The patient care manager manages care for patients in the caseload on a 24-hour basis, develops care plans, and generally directs the activities surrounding patient care needs. The clinical nurse provides care on a shift basis, adds to the care plan, and generally provides or delegates care. The patient care technician assists in care delivery and performs or assists with specified tasks. This would be similar to the approach described by Newman in which "One nurse plans and coordinates on a continuing long-term basis; another nurse organizes and coordinates the care in immediate short-term settings; and another nurse provides the day-to-day direct care in both institutional and home settings" (Newman, 1994, p 51). Newman further stipulates that these three roles require different types of expertise and different educational preparation.

Despite slow movement in the area, there continues to be a push to realistically define the competencies of the graduates of the various programs. Once identified, differentiated roles can be implemented in the practice setting that will allow graduates to practice as educated.

CERTIFICATION AS RECOGNITION

Another aspect of this issue is how differentiated practice should be recognized. In Maine, a regulation was passed that would have required the development of an additional licensing examination to be given to the baccalaureate graduate. That has been placed on hold for a variety of reasons, one being that the state is considering legislation that would change all health occupations licensure.

The ANA has consistently supported the belief that the law should regulate minimum safe practice and that advanced accomplishment should be recognized by certification awarded by the profession. This is the case in medicine. Currently the American Nurses Credentialing Center and some specialty nursing organizations offer specialty certification to nurses. Most of these speciality certifications require a baccalaureate degree and some require a master's degree. This is discussed more completely in Chapter 4.

Forces for Change in Nursing Education

Three decades have passed since the ANA first began activities to require the baccalaureate degree for entry into professional nursing. During the 40 years that nurses have been debating educational preparation for nursing, a number of other issues have emerged and a number of changes have occurred. As nursing advances as a profession, nursing education must remain responsive to the many changes that have occurred and are occurring in the profession.

THE NURSING SUPPLY

In the early 1990s, discussions and debates related to educational preparation were quickly dropped. The United States found itself with a serious nurse shortage. Hospitals that at one time sought to employ only graduates with baccalaureate degrees once again offered positions to associate degree graduates, and those hiring only registered nurses again offered jobs to licensed practical (vocational) nurses.

Two factors were largely responsible for this nurse shortage. The first was an increasing demand for nurses in the expanding health care delivery system and the second was the drop in nursing school enrollments in the late 1980s. Like many things in nursing, this was soon to change. As this book goes to print, new graduates again find themselves in the position of searching for positions and often accepting the one that was second or third choice. Shortages are occurring in the areas of advanced practice, in teaching, and other areas in nursing that require experience and additional education. Emphasis is being placed on increasing the opportunities for nurses to enter programs preparing for advanced practice.

EDUCATIONAL MOBILITY

One of the approaches to changes in nursing supply has been an increased emphasis on educational mobility in nursing. Rather than debate which is the appropriate educational preparation, educational mobility recognizes the unique contribution of nurses educated at all levels and facilitates advancement from one level to another with minimal repeat of course work. This movement has received impetus in some states from legislative mandates that stipulate that plans for articulation from one type of nursing program to another must be developed and implemented within a given period of time. In other instances, such activity has occurred without legislative action. Many states are beginning to establish statewide plans that will facilitate the enrollment of the practical nurse in associate degree programs or the advancement of the associate degree graduate to registered nurse baccalaureate programs.

INCREASED EMPHASIS ON COMPUTER LITERACY

Computers and computerized equipment have become common in today's health care settings. Health care facilities have long used computers for business operations, but they have been slower to move into computerization in patient care situations. That is now changing drastically. The federal government is mandating the use of computerized systems for some aspects of records for those covered by Medicare and Medicaid. Collecting clinical data such as vital signs and hemodynamic values of critically ill patients, computer voice-activated charting at the bedside, central main frames, and computerized nursing care plans and Kardexes are but a few of the examples of the computer applications being instituted.

This new technology places yet another challenge before nursing education, that of preparing the graduate for a highly technological work environment. It adds another dimension to the content that must be part of the nursing program. This comes at a time when the average age of the nursing student is higher than it has ever been. Unlike the new high school graduate, older students often have had little experience with computers. Despite the growing use of personal computers, many students have no computer skills; some instructors also have no computer knowledge. This makes selecting computer programs and assisting the student difficult. In some instances, continuing education must occur before instruction can begin.

The situation is further complicated by the cost of equipment to teach these skills. Nursing education, like other forms of higher education, has encountered serious budgetary constraints and cuts. Computer equipment is expensive and quickly outdated as new programs are developed before the equipment that was ordered can be installed.

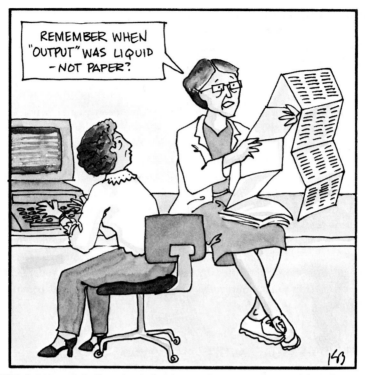

FIGURE 3–3 As hospitals, like other industries, put the computer to work in their agencies, the new graduate will be forced to have a beginning understanding of computer language and the operation of the machines.

The answer may be found in collaborative efforts between nursing service and education. Application of computer learning, like clinical learning, may occur in the hospital setting, after basic orientation on campus.

THE USE OF TECHNOLOGY IN NURSING EDUCATION

As computers and computer technology become common in the health care setting, they represent one of the major advances seen in nursing education. The computer age has reached the nursing classroom. The traditional nursing lecture is now being augmented or replaced with computer-assisted instruction. Interactive programs will permit students to practice decision-making skills in a safe environment. These programs allow students to select the best alternative for care without placing the patient in any jeopardy. The development of computer software in nursing education exceeds one's ability to know all the alternatives for instruction. Again, the cost of purchasing the equipment and the software for this instruction is significant. Some organizations, such as the Helen Fuld Trust Foundation, have made monies available to nursing education for this innovation and change.

Some of the technological advances used in nursing education facilitate the process of making nursing education more geographically accessible to the student. Outreach programs, which take the educational program to the student rather than requiring the student to come to the college, have been started in many parts of the country. These have been particularly useful in helping to meet the needs of the registered nurse seeking baccalaureate preparation. Cable television and video instruction have extended the perimeter of the classroom.

The use of videotaping and television in the classroom and in the practice laboratory has already proved to be an effective and efficient method to extend the ability of one instructor to assist many students. Videotaped demonstrations eliminate the need for tedious repetitions of basic procedures for small groups. Students can view videotapes at their own convenience and can use videotaped playbacks to assess their own skills, freeing the instructor for other instructional activities. Interactive classrooms allow students at distant learning sites to communicate with an instructor and a class on a university campus.

COMMUNITY-BASED PRACTICE

Another significant change in nursing practice is the trend toward community-based practice. Most nursing programs, especially hospital-based and associate degree programs, are strongly oriented toward the hospital as the primary clinical teaching environment. "Community," as it was historically used in nursing education, was associated with public health nursing and was to be found in baccalaureate education only.

Today we find even home health aids working in community settings. Nursing educators are being challenged to define what part of their nursing curriculum should be taught in a community setting. Many believe the time the students have on hospital clinical units to be inadequate and are not willing to shorten it. Others are uncertain how the experience should be provided if the hours are found for the instruction. In many instances, the students have little more than an observational experience. Some have none. The next few years will see change in this area.

THE ADULT LEARNER

Nursing educators are also revising programs of study to address the needs of the adult learner, rather than fashion all educational patterns toward the recent high school graduate. Programs that permit part-time study, and thus allow the student to work while attending school, have also been developed. Classes traditionally conducted during peak morning hours are being moved to late afternoon hours or to weekends to appeal to and meet the needs of the working student. Programs designed to accommodate to varying learning rates through self-paced modules respond to individual learning needs. Remedial classes in basic mathematics, grammar, study skills, or English as a second language have been made available to students who may not have had the same educational opportunities as others.

LEARNING ABOUT POLITICAL POWER

Nurses are increasingly recognizing the need to become more political to effect the changes they see as necessary in the health care delivery system. This means that courses will need to be developed that will provide nurses the knowledge needed to function comfortably and effectively in this new political role. Politics requires learning about power, a term some nurses want to reject as being incompatible with the aims of the profession. Kalisch and Kalisch (1982, pp 1–2) have defined power as "the ability to affect something or to be affected by something. Power means the capacity to alter behavior." Because they offer critically needed services, nurses possess much potential power, but they need a basic understanding of how to use that potential to create desired changes. As nurses assume a stronger patient advocacy role, they must possess better understanding of the social system, policy formation and implementation, the legislative process, lobbying, and political mobilization. Many programs have made a step in this direction by including content in assertive behavior in their nursing curricula, but this is only a beginning.

Some nurses see themselves functioning as independent practitioners or in joint practices. This role requires additional understanding of business management and economics and a knowledge of advanced clinical skills. Alternative health care providers will find themselves in a competitive system. Escalating medical costs may mean that as a nation, we need to modify our concept of health care delivery so that it responds to the needs of persons of all ages and in all economic strata.

CONCERNS ABOUT FUNDING

One of the gravest problems facing nursing education today is that of funding. In 1964, through the Nurse Training Act, $238 million was authorized for the advancement of nursing education, and $4.6 million was authorized to administer the programs. The programs, five in all, included construction of nursing facilities, improvement of teaching, continuation of traineeship programs that reimbursed students for advancing their nursing education, provision of loans to nursing students, and monies specifically set aside to improve instruction in hospital-based schools. This act was responsive to the recognized shortage of trained health personnel. In 1963, the Consultant Group on Nursing in their final report, "Toward Quality in Nursing," estimated that we would need 130,000 more nurses in 1970 than were available in 1960. This would mean that nursing schools would need to increase their numbers of graduates by 75%. The consultants also urged an increase in the number of nurses with graduate degrees and baccalaureate degrees and an increase in the number of licensed practical nurses.

In the years immediately following the passage of the Nurse Training Act, many schools and students were to benefit from these funds. When the Nurse Training Act expired in 1969, the Health Manpower Act continued most of Nurse Training Act programs. The 1971 Nurse Training Act, which followed, authorized the largest expenditure of funds for nursing in the history of the country—$855 million. After that period, the federal funding for nursing constantly decreased. The $160 million appropriated in 1973 dropped to $145 million in 1974. Presidents of the United States, both Republican and Democrat, believed that the nurse shortage had ended. They also contended that nursing students could apply for the federal aid made available to students in general (eg, basic educational grants). All thought that the amount of money allocated to nursing education was "excessive."

Since 1979, the funds allocated to nursing education have been consistently cut. As funding was reduced, the purposes for which the funds were made available also changed. Fewer dollars were made available for the basic education of nursing students. Emphasis was placed on funding advanced training for nurses and the preparation of nurse practitioners. Funds were also available for nursing research. Student loans were continued, but the total amount was reduced and "forgiveness clauses," which required students to repay only part of the loan if they became actively involved in nursing on graduation, were eliminated. At the same time, tuition costs sharply increased. Capitation funding, which provided money to schools based on student enrollment, was eliminated.

We are feeling the impact of the loss of these dollars and the effect on the nursing profession. Students are having to find other means for funding their education. Greater numbers of students are attending school part-time to allow time for employment while attending school.

Nursing education has suffered from the same reduction in state and local funding that has burdened other programs in higher education. Budget requests must often be reduced and needs set aside. Most critical to nursing are the dollars allocated to faculty salaries. As the salaries for nurses working in the health care delivery system have reached new highs, it is becoming increasingly difficult to attract well qualified and highly motivated persons to teaching positions in nursing education programs. Nurses with the education and expertise to be good teachers and positive role models for students can command much higher salaries outside the educational environment.

THE INCREASED EMPHASIS ON NURSING THEORIES

As nursing continues to grow as a profession, one of the areas receiving increased emphasis is nursing theory. This will undoubtedly continue. As nursing education keeps pace with the advancement of nursing knowledge, there has been a push to develop curricular patterns that also respond to the work of nursing theorists. During the late 1970s and the 1980s, criteria for accreditation of nursing programs as established by the educational councils of the NLN placed importance on the need for a conceptual framework around which a program of learning is developed. Many programs selected the approach of a particular nursing theorist and structured the program of learning around that theorist's work. Although this curricular design may be receiving some decreased emphasis today, the program of learning for the nursing program in which you are enrolled may be based on concepts outlined by a particular nursing theorist. Perhaps one of the hospitals to which you are assigned for clinical experience also uses the principles of a nursing theory to structure the delivery of care.

A theory is a "scientifically acceptable general principle which governs practice or is proposed to explain observed facts" (Riehl and Roy, 1974, p 3). Because nursing as a developing profession is seriously involved in research on which to build a sound body of nursing knowledge, theories are valuable to us. They provide the bases for hypotheses about nursing practice. They make it possible for us to derive a sound rationale for the actions we take. If the theories are testable, they will then allow us to build our knowledge base and to guide and improve nursing practice. This is explained in the words of Barbara Stevens (1984, p 1):

> A nursing theory . . . attempts to describe or explain the phenomenon called nursing. A theory is always a shorthand way to understand or characterize a phenomenon. It points out those components or characteristics that give the phenomenon its identity. It pulls out the salient parts of a phenomenon so that one can separate the critical and necessary factors . . . from the accidental and unessential factors.

She goes on to describe a theory as a map whose purpose is "to give one a handle on the phenomenon with which it deals." Today there are many published nursing theories. In an attempt to structure and organize those theories, various authors have categorized or classified them. Not all are classified similarly. Included are general classifications such as the art and science of humanistic nursing, interpersonal relationships, systems, and energy fields. Others include groupings that categorize growth and development theories, systems theories, stress adaptation theories, and rhythm theories.

Some examples of growth and development theories with which you are probably familiar are those of Maslow, Erikson, Kohlberg, Piaget, and Freud. Most basic nursing texts incorporate a discussion of the concepts developed by these theorists. The theories are so named because they focus on the developing person. They have the common characteristic of arranging this development in terms of stages through which a person must pass to reach a particular level of development. From a nursing standpoint they allow us to monitor the progress through the various stages and evaluate the appropriateness of that progress. You will recognize Maslow for his approach to self-actualization, Erikson for his psychosocial development, Kohlberg for his theories of moral reasoning, Piaget for his approach to cognitive development, and Freud for psychosexual theories on which medicine later based the school of psychoanalysis. These theories are not truly theories of nursing, however, because they were not developed for the purpose of explaining, testing, and changing the practice of nursing. They represent some of the "borrowed" knowledge around which we build our profession.

Most nursing theories are developed around a combination of concepts. Among those concepts, four subject areas usually are included: 1) an approach to the total person; 2) an approach to health–illness; 3) an approach to the environment (or society); and 4) an approach to nursing. Nursing theories may also be classified with regard to the structure or approach around which they are developed.

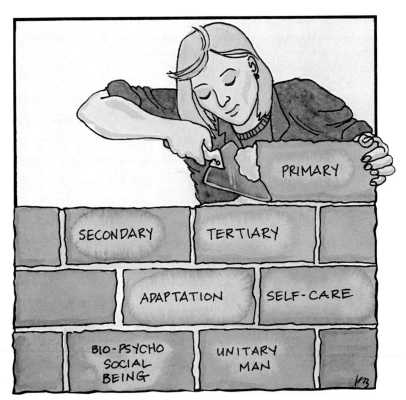

FIGURE 3–4 Nursing is in the process of building a body of scientific knowledge.

Theories that speak to the art and science of humanistic nursing were the earliest purely nursing theories developed. Some authors have looked back at the contributions of Florence Nightingale and have included her in that grouping. Among the others are Virginia Henderson and her *Definition of Nursing*, Faye Abdellah and the *Twenty-one Nursing Problems*, Lydia Hall and her *Core Care and Cure Model*, and Madeleine Leininger's *Transcultural Care Theory*.

Interpersonal relationship theories deal with interactions between and among people. Many of these theories were developed during the 1960s. Included in this grouping could be Hildegard Peplau's *Psychodynamic Nursing*, Joyce Travelbee's *Human-to-Human Relationship*, and Ernestine Wiedenbach's *The Helping Art of Clinical Nursing*.

Systems theories are so classified because they are concerned with the interactions between and among all the factors in a situation. A system is usually viewed as complex and in a state of constant change. It is defined as a whole with interrelated parts and may be a subsystem of a larger system as well as a suprasystem. For example, a person may be viewed as a system composed of cells, tissue, organs, and the like. The person is a subsystem of a family, which in turn is a subsystem of a community. In a systems approach, the person is usually considered as a "total" being or from a "whole" being viewpoint. Systems theories also provide for "input" into the system and "feedback" within the system. The systems approach became popular during the 1970s.

Stress adaptation models are based on concepts that view the person as adjusting or changing (adapting) to avoid situations (stressors) that would result in the disturbance of balance or equilibrium. The adaptation theory helps to explain how the balance is maintained and therefore points the direction for nursing actions. Included in this group one often finds Sister Callista Roy's adaptation model and Betty Neuman's work, but both may also be considered systems models.

One of the latest classifications of theories is by energy fields. These theories, although they may have been started earlier, have received increased recognition during the 1980s. Included in this group are the works of such persons as Myra Levine, Joyce Fitzpatrick, Margaret Newman, and Martha Rogers.

It is not our purpose to discuss and critique all the many approaches to nursing theory. The student who wants to pursue nursing theorists further is encouraged to consult the section on further reading at the end of the chapter. A brief discussion of the conceptual approach set forth by four nursing theorists who have developed theories used widely in nursing education programs follows.

Sister Callista Roy's Adaptation Model

This model is organized around concepts that describe how a person can adapt behavior to allow him or her to deal (cope) with stimuli from the environment that are stressors. Stressors disrupt the dynamic state of equilibrium and result in illness. Four adaptive modes, or ways in which a person adapts, are identified through: 1) physiologic needs; 2) self-concept; 3) role function; and 4) interdependence relations. Nursing's role is to assess a patient's adaptive behaviors and the stimuli that may be affecting the person and manipulate the stimuli in such a way as to allow the patient to cope or adapt.

Dorothea Orem's Self-Care Model

This model has a goal of "constancy" for the person and speaks to the concept of self-care. Self-care is the person's own action that has pattern and sequence and, when effectively performed, contributes to the way he or she develops and functions. Nursing's role is to help the person meet the self-care requisites, thus limiting self-care deficits.

Betty Neuman's Systems Model

Identified as a health care systems model, this approach to nursing is organized around stress reduction. It is primarily concerned with the effects of stress and the reactions to stress and the development and maintenance of health, and therefore also speaks to maintaining equilibrium. The person deals with stressors through "lines of defense" and is protected from stressors through "lines of resistance." Nursing's role is focused on reduction of stress factors and through prevention that is "primary, secondary, or tertiary."

Martha Roger's Unitary Man Theory

Although Martha Roger's theory of nursing may not be used to fashion conceptual frameworks in nursing education programs as frequently as some others, it represents a creative approach to nursing. Much of the language being incorporated into nursing education and practice is an outgrowth of Roger's work. Known as the science of unitary man, the essence of this model is the assumption that the person is a unified energy field that is continually interacting and exchanging matter and energy with the environment. These exchanges result in increasing complexity and innovativeness of the person. Health and illness are not viewed as separate states. Nursing's role is to re-pattern human beings and the environment to achieve maximum health potential. This model has been used by the North American Nursing Diagnosis Association (NANDA) in developing the nursing diagnosis taxonomy and the language used within that taxonomy. However, the group substituted the words "human response patterns" for the more unfamiliar "patterns of unitary man."

Key Concepts

⇨ Because education is key to the development of any profession, many studies focusing on nursing education have been conducted. The

Brown study, conducted in 1948, had a significant impact on the development of nursing education.

▷ Nursing education has also been influenced by the ANA Position on Nursing Education that advocated the baccalaureate degree as the minimum educational preparation for professional nursing. Many nursing educators, particularly those in diploma and associate degree programs, disagreed with this position.

▷ Many of the specialty organizations in nursing have supported the concept of the baccalaureate degree for professional practice. Criteria for credentialing in advanced practice are mandating the baccalaureate degree.

▷ Rising health care costs and the nursing shortage of the early 1990s have encouraged the development of models of differentiated practice in which graduates are employed in hospitals based on the competencies they learned in their nursing programs.

▷ Many other changes are anticipated in nursing education. These include greater computer literacy as well as education provided by computers and a shift to providing some clinical experience in a community setting.

▷ Critical to nursing is the decrease that has occurred over the past two decades in funds allocated to nursing education.

▷ The work of nursing theorists will continue to influence nursing education and nursing practice.

CRITICAL THINKING ACTIVITIES

1. Take a stand on the ANA Position on Nursing Education. Provide a rationale for the position you have taken. What do you see as the outcome of this decision? How would you see your position implemented in the future? What implications does it have for nursing practice?

2. Think about the unit where you are currently receiving clinical practice. What would be required to implement differentiated practice there? What would be the rationale for doing so? How might patients benefit?

3. If you were going to change the basic educational requirements for licensure, how would you go about implementing the change? How would you deal with the issue of "grandfathering." Explain the reasons for the approach you are suggesting.

4. What changes are currently happening in the nursing program in which you are enrolled? What was the basis for those changes? How do you think they will affect your performance as a new graduate? Be specific in the answers.

5. Select one nursing theorist. Describe what you find interesting and attractive about her nursing theory? Give the rationale for your decision.

References

ADNs, community college bar entry-level rules. Am J Nurs 85(8):921, 923, 1987

American Nurses Association's first position on nursing education. Am J Nurs 65(12):106–111, 1965

Brown EL. Nursing for the Future. New York: Russell Sage Foundation, 1948

Edge S. State positions on titling and licensure. *In* Looking Beyond the Entry Issue: Implications for Education and Service, NLN Publication No. 41-2173. New York: National League for Nursing, 1986

Hartung D. Organizational positions on titling and entry into practice: A chronology. *In* Looking Beyond the Entry Issue: Implications for Education and Service, NLN Publication No. 41-2173. New York: National League for Nursing, 1986

Harkness GA, Miller J, Hill N. Differentiated practice: A three-dimensional model. Nurs Management 23(12):26–30, 1992

Illinois RNs seek compromise on scope of practice. Am J Nurs 86(1):77, 84, 90, 1986

Kalisch BJ, Kalisch PA. Politics of Nursing. Philadelphia, JB Lippincott, 1982

National Council of State Boards of Nursing: A Study of Nursing Practice and Role Delineation and Job Analysis of Entry Level Performance of Registered Nurses. Chicago: National Council of State Boards of Nursing, 1986

Newman MA. Professionalism: Myth or reality. *In* Chaska N: The Nursing Profession: Turning Points. St. Louis: CV Mosby, 1990:49–52

NFLPN OKs "two nursing levels" 18 month curriculum for LPNs. Am J Nurs 84(10):1303, 1312, 1314, 1984

North Dakota rule changes require associate, baccalaureate education. Issues 7(2):1–3, 1986

Pennsylvania legislature bars change in entry rules. Am J Nurs 87:113, 126, 1987

Riehl JP, Roy SC. Conceptual Models for Nursing Practice. New York: Appleton-Century-Crofts, 1974

Stevens BJ. Nursing Theory: Analysis, Application, Evaluation, 2nd ed. Boston: Little, Brown, 1984

U.S. Public Health Service. Toward Quality in Nursing: Needs and Goals. Report of the Surgeon General's Consultant Group on Nursing. Washington, DC: U.S. Government Printing Office, 1963

Further Readings

A call for reform of our nursing education system. The AONE update. Nurs Management 24(1): 33, 1993

ADN "mavericks" found national group to fight title change. Am J Nurs 86(1):79, 82, 1986

A first for the nation: North Dakota and entry into nursing practice. Nurs Health Care 7(3): 135–141, 1986

Chaska NL. The Nursing Profession: Turning Points. St Louis: CV Mosby, 1990

Christ T. Entry into practice: A recurring issue in nursing history. Am J Nurs 80(3):485–488, 1980

Cross utilization of nursing staff. The AONE update. Nurs Management 24(7):38–39, 1993

Fishman DJ. Nursing informatics: The electronic information revolution in education and practice. *In* Strickland OL, Fishman DJ, eds: Nursing Issues in the 1990s. Albany, NY: Delmar Publishers, 1994:471–488

Fitzpatrick JJ, Whall AL. Conceptual Models of Nursing: Analysis and Application. Bowie, MD: Robert J Brady Co, 1983

George JB. Nursing Theories: The Base for Professional Nursing Practice, 2nd ed. Englewood Cliffs, NJ: Prentice-Hall, 1985

Marriner-Tomey A. Nursing Theorists and Their Work, 2nd ed. St. Louis: CV Mosby, 1989

Mathews JJ, Zadak K. Managerial decisions for computerized patient care planning. Nurs Management 24(7):54–56, 1993

McBeth A, Koerner J, Ethridge P. Advanced licensure/mandatory credentialing: A nurse executive point of view. Nurs Management 24(2):45–47, 1993

NLN seeks compromise on entry: ADNs hold out for RN licensure. Am J Nurs 87(1):113, 124–125, 1987

NLN members agree to shelve entry issues and call for steps to spur career mobility. Am J Nurs 89(8):1082–1083, 1989

Orem DE. Nursing: Concepts of Practice, 2nd ed. New York: McGraw-Hill, 1980

Primm PL. Entry into practice: Competency statements for BSNs and ADNs. Nurs Outlook 34(3):135–137, 1986

Roy SC, Roberts SL. Theory Construction in Nursing: An Adaptation Model. Englewood Cliffs, NJ: Prentice-Hall, 1981

Sharp N. Second license for the advanced practice nurse? Nurs Management 23(9):28–29, 1992

Simpson RL. The new careers in nursing informatics. Nurs Management 23(10):26–27, 1992

State boards declare "neutral stance" in entry-level debate. Am J Nurs 86(10):1180, 1986

Stull MK. Entry skills for BSNs. Nurs Outlook 34(3):138–139, 1986

Torres G. Theoretical Foundations of Nursing. East Norwalk, CT: Appleton-Century-Crofts, 1986

Town J. Changing to computerized documentation—plus! Nurs Management 24(7):44–48, 1993

Trofino J. Voice-activated nursing documentation: On the cutting edge. Nurs Management 24(7):40–42, 1993

II Legal and Ethical Accountability for Practice

As we examine legal, ethical, and bioethical issues in health care, we will first explore the issue of credentials for health care providers. Understanding some of the basic concerns related to credentialing and the rationale for the existence of credentials, will help to focus your attention on the responsibility of health care providers to the public.

The entire realm of law that guides the practice of any health occupation is a particular concern in a society where individuals often attempt to solve problems in a courtroom. A beginning understanding of rights and responsibilities when viewed from the focus of providing care is important to you.

Ethical and bioethical issues associated with health care constantly challenge us as professionals and as members of our society. Each new technological advance brings additional concerns to our attention. In this unit we try to provide you with a general background that will help you address legal, ethical, and bioethical concerns. In addition, we present some specific problems in the hope that considering them before you become directly involved will help you to address the issues more comfortably.

4

Credentials for Health Care Providers

Objectives

After completing this chapter, you should be able to

1. Define and discuss the concept of credentialing.
2. Differentiate between a diploma, certification, and licensure as credentials.
3. Explain the concepts of permissive and mandatory licensure for practice.
4. Outline the history of nursing licensure.
5. Identify the major content areas in laws regulating nursing practice.
6. Outline the role of the State Board of Nursing.
7. Discuss the process of revocation of a nursing license.
8. Differentiate between licensure by examination and licensure by endorsement.
9. Discuss the historical development of the licensing examination for nursing.
10. Discuss current trends in nursing licensure.
11. Describe the role of the Commission on Graduates of Foreign Nursing Schools.
12. Discuss the concept of certification in nursing.
13. Explain the problems associated with certification in nursing.

Ellis JR, Hartley CL: NURSING IN TODAY'S WORLD:
CHALLENGES, ISSUES, AND TRENDS, 5th ed.
© 1995 J.B. Lippincott Company

Credentials are written proof of qualifications. They communicate to others the nature of one's competence and provide evidence of one's preparation to perform in a specific occupation. The basic rationale for credentials in health care occupations is that the safety of the public is protected by providing a standard mechanism for judging competence. Further, those who are engaged in careers in health occupations want to be assured that the standards of practice in their discipline will remain high and that they will not be replaced by people with less educational preparation who would be willing to work for lower wages.

Types of Credentials in Health Care

Many types of credentials are used, for example, diplomas, degrees, licenses, and certificates. Each of these serves a different role. Not all are available for each different health occupation.

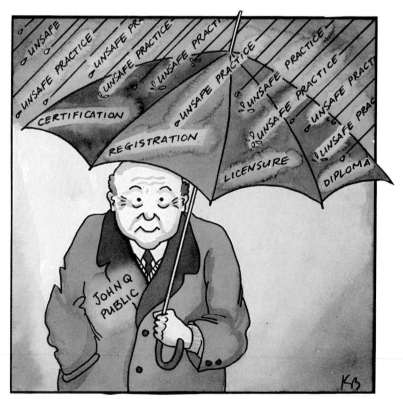

FIGURE 4–1 Various forms of credentialing ensure the public of qualified caregivers.

DIPLOMAS AND CERTIFICATES OF GRADUATION

A school or business conducting instruction awards a diploma or certificate to those who complete a designated program of study. An example is the diploma awarded on graduation from high school or college. A business that provides instruction in using computer programs might present a certificate to those who complete the course. When only a diploma or educational certificate is available, it is necessary to know about the educational institution and the specific educational program to evaluate the person's abilities.

CERTIFICATION

For some groups a standard credential is available in the form of certification provided by a nongovernmental authority, usually a professional organization. Workers with this type of credential are referred to as "certified" or sometimes as "registered." This type of credential should not be confused with a legal license. Certification usually is granted on completion of an educational program and the passing of a standardized examination, both of which are prescribed by a professional organization.

Some professional organizations provide certification for related occupational groups as well as their own. One such organization is the American Health Information Management Association (AHIMA), which examines and "*registers*" medical records administrators (Registered Records Administrators—RRA) and examines and "*certifies*" medical records technicians (MRT). In some professions a separate, independent organization has been formed with the sole purpose of providing credentialing. The board members of these credentialing organizations commonly include representatives from the profession, the educational setting, the public, and related professions. The National Accrediting Association for Clinical Laboratory Sciences (NAACLS) is such a group. Members of the various professional groups involved in laboratory science cooperated in setting up this association. The organization is incorporated as a private, voluntary entity and is not a governmental institution or department. The purpose of this organization is to make the laboratory science credentialing system more independent and as objective as possible. This organization awards the title medical laboratory technician (MLT) or medical technologist (MT) to those who have met the educational standard and passed the certification examination. These credentials are recognized by all groups in the field of laboratory science as professional credentials. Some states have made certification by this body the required criterion for practice in clinical laboratory sciences.

Some other bodies that currently accredit individual health occupations are investigating the possibility of setting up independent national entities with the sole purpose of credentialing. There are several reasons for this action. The first relates to the current consumer movement. In general, the public has not trusted the objectivity of people in professional groups that do not have consumer input. The creation of an independent credentialing body would ensure that those currently practicing a profession would not be the sole arbiters in determining who enters the field. A second rationale for this move is financial. By setting up a separate organization, which must be self-supporting through fees for its services, the professional groups are relieved of the financial burden that can result when an accrediting program grows rapidly and costs escalate. The third justification for an independent credentialing body is to provide a broader-based support for the credentialing process. A fourth reason relates to the complex federal laws governing non-profit organizations and their tax-exempt status.

LICENSURE

A *license* is a legal credential conferred by an individual state. A wide variety of health occupations are licensed in different states. Most states restrict licensing to those who have more direct contact with patients or clients. Physicians, dentists, pharmacists, and nurses are licensed in all states. The licensing of other health occupations varies. *Mandatory licensure* is a requirement that all individuals must obtain a license to practice. There is mandatory licensure for physicians and dentists in all states and mandatory licensure for nurses in all states but one. Mandatory licensure is instituted when there is believed to be a compelling public interest in licensure to protect the public.

Permissive licensure is a system whereby an individual may choose to become licensed to provide evidence of competence, but a license is not required to practice. Permissive and mandatory licensure are discussed in greater detail later in this chapter. Eligibility for licensure and the type of testing required are determined by the individual state or province. Most licensing laws specify completion of a state-approved educational program and require, in addition, the successful completion of a written examination prescribed by the state. Some professions, such as dentistry, require candidates to pass a practical examination as well as a written examination. Nursing is unique in having a standard licensure process in every state and territory in the United States. This was developed through the cooperative action of the state boards of nursing. A national examination may exist for other professions, but its application may vary. For example, there is a national licensing examination for pharmacy, but California prepares and administers its own examination and does not use the national pharmacy examination. There are national medical board examinations, but some states administer independent medical examinations. Even when the same examination is used for licensure, as in pharmacy, some states require that a person new to the state retake the licensing examination when applying for a license in that state.

Some states require completion of continuing education to renew a health care license. Pharmacists were one of the first groups required to pursue continuing education to remain licensed. Continuing education is required for relicensure of nurses and physicians in many states. The cost of the processes involved in monitoring continuing education has been a barrier to its adoption in other states.

The History of Credentialing in Nursing

Nursing leaders have historically maintained an ethical position that accountability to the public for quality nursing care is essential. The public, however, often has no method for evaluating the competence of an individual nurse. Therefore, the nursing profession has acted to try to ensure that nurses have credentials that can be recognized by anyone.

Credentials were not always available for nurses. Before the Nightingale schools became prevalent in England and nursing schools were established in the United States, little training was available to those who wanted to provide nursing care. Those who had received some training and those who had not worked side by side to deliver care. After schools of nursing became common, a rudimentary means of identifying the qualifications of caregivers was the certificate of completion that was issued by the nursing school. This was the first true credential for nursing practice.

However, because the quality of education that was offered in the nursing schools differed widely—programs varied in length from 6 weeks to 3 years—it became apparent that a completion certificate was not an adequate guarantee of competence. Nursing leaders were concerned about the situation. They believed that the patient had no way to judge whether a particular nurse's education was sound and might suffer from the quality of care administered by a poorly prepared nurse.

In 1896, the Nurses Associated Alumnae of the United States and Canada was created. This organization later evolved into the American Nurses Association (ANA). One of the major concerns of the association was the establishment of a credentialing system that was firmly based in laws passed by a legislative body. The route toward legal licensing for credentialing was long and difficult. Nurses, legislators, and the public had to be educated about the value of licensure for the profession and encouraged to support it. Table 4–1 presents a chronology of nursing licensure.

PERMISSIVE LICENSURE FOR NURSING

The ANA campaigned vigorously for the adoption of state licensure laws. These early laws provided for permissive licensure. The standards for permis-

TABLE 4–1 The History of Nursing Licensure

1867	Dr. Henry Wentworth Acland first suggested licensure for nurses in England
1892	American Society of Superintendents of Training Schools for Nurses organized and supported licensure in the United States.
1901	First nursing licensure in the world: New Zealand.
1903	First nursing licensure in the United States: North Carolina, New Jersey, New York, and Virginia (in that order).
1915	ANA drafted its first model nurse practice act.
1919	First nursing licensure in England.
1923	All 48 states had enacted nursing licensure laws.
1935	First mandatory licensure act in the United States: New York (effective 1947).
1946	Ten states had definitions of nursing in the licensing act.
1950	First year the same examination used in all jurisdictions of the United States and its territories: State Board Test Pool Examination.
1965	Twenty-one states had definitions of nursing in the licensing act.
1971	First state to recognize expanded practice in the nursing practice act: Idaho.
1976	First mandatory continuing education for relicensure: California.
1982	Change to nursing process format examination: National Council Licensure Examination for Registered Nurses (NCLEX-RN).
1986	First state to require baccalaureate degree for registered nurse and associate degree for licensed practical nurse: North Dakota (effective 1987).
1994	Computer adapted testing initiated nationwide.

sive licensure included graduating from a school that satisfied certain requirements and passing a comprehensive examination. Only those who had met
these standards could use the title "registered nurse." An employer or a member of the public could then differentiate between a registered nurse and an
individual who used the title "nurse" but had not met the standards required
to be registered. Under this system no one was required to have a license to
practice nursing.

With standards in place the community benefited because the established credential attested to a level of competence of the registered nurse. The
individual who was licensed as a registered nurse profited in regard to job
availability and salary when employers differentiated between those who were
licensed and those who were not licensed.

The first law providing for permissive licensure was passed in 1903 by
North Carolina. By 1923, all the existing 48 states had permissive licensure
laws. Alaska and Hawaii passed licensure laws while still territories and continued to recognize these laws when they became states. The set of laws regulating the practice of nursing is termed the *Nurse Practice Act.*

MANDATORY LICENSURE FOR NURSING

After permissive licensure laws came into being, nurses' activity regarding licensure became less intense because most nurses sought and received licenses to practice. However, there was still concern that some persons were practicing nursing without having demonstrated skill and knowledge. The majority of those functioning without licenses were nursing school graduates who had failed the licensing examinations. They were referred to as graduate nurses, as opposed to registered nurses. In addition, some individuals who had been educated as nurses in foreign countries and did not meet the licensure requirements in the state in which they were residing worked as nurses in health care settings.

To eliminate this situation and provide greater protection to the public, many nurses began to call for *mandatory* licensure. Mandatory nursing licen-

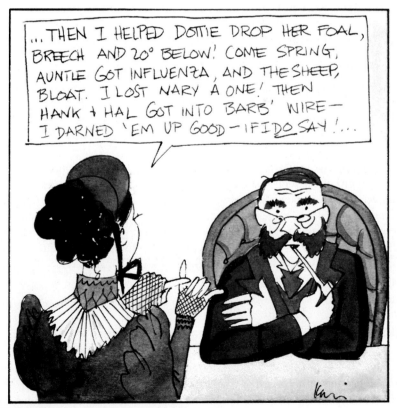

FIGURE 4–2 A standard credential makes hiring easier.

sure requires that all persons who wish to practice nursing meet established standards for education, pass standardized examinations, and secure a license to practice in the state, province, or territory in which they wish to work.

The first mandatory licensure law took effect in New York in 1947. Throughout the years additional states changed their laws relating to the practice of nursing and required licensure. Today, mandatory licensure is the standard in the United States and Canada as well as most other countries. Only the state of Texas allows for permissive licensure in some situations. Therefore, if you wish to work as a nurse in any state, territory, province, or other country you must obtain a license there before you begin working.

Current Nursing Licensure Laws

New legislation regarding nursing licensure is usually initiated through the nurses' association or through the State Board of Nursing at the instigation of the nursing community. The group initiating the action may spend months preparing and planning the content of the bill and gaining the support of legislators.

The proposed change in the law enters the legislative process through an elected member of the legislature who has been persuaded that the change is in the best interest of the public. The proposal must go through the entire legislative committee review, public hearing, and legislative voting procedure before it can become a law. The legislation when finally passed becomes part of the licensure law.

During the legislative process, individuals and organizations may affect the content of the proposed legislation by influencing the legislators. For example, in 1974 in New York a bill was introduced that would have changed the educational requirements for entry into practice to require a baccalaureate degree. During the legislative process a great deal of lobbying occurred and changes were made in the bill. Overall the support for the bill was diminished. The result was defeat of the bill and the proposed change in educational requirements was not enacted.

RULES AND REGULATIONS

Each state has its own set of rules and regulations to carry out the provisions of the law regulating nursing. These rules and regulations are established by the administrative body, usually the *State Board of Nursing*, that is given responsibility in the Nurse Practice Act. (See the section on the Role of the Board of Nursing.) Most states require that public hearings be held in regard to the proposed rules and regulations, but the board has the authority to make the final decision. The rules and regulations must be within the scope outlined by the legislation that was passed. Those that are accepted by the appropriate board have the force of law unless they are challenged in court and are found to be not in accord with the legislature's intent.

In some states the nursing practice act is detailed and specifies most of the critical provisions regarding licensure and practice. In other states the nursing practice act is broad, and the administrative body is given a great deal of power in making decisions through rules and regulations.

One example of the difference between what is contained in the enacted law and what is in rules and regulations in different states is in regard to the educational requirements for licensure. In some states the enacted law specifies that a diploma, an associate degree, or a baccalaureate degree is an acceptable preparation for registered nursing. In those states, for the educational requirements to change, the enacted law itself would have to be changed. In other states the educational requirement is not in the enacted law. In those states the educational requirement is established by the Board of Nursing through rules and regulations. This was the situation in North Dakota when the requirement for the registered nurse license was changed to the baccalaureate degree (see Chapter 3). Thus, both the actual Nurse Practice Act and the rules and regulations govern nursing in your state.

NURSING LICENSURE LAW CONTENT

Early in the 1900s, the ANA, as part of its leadership role in nursing licensure, formulated a model nurse practice act that could be used by state associations when planning legislation (Snyder and LaBar, 1984). This model was revised in 1981 by the ANA Congress for Nursing Practice and a more up-to-date approach to nursing licensure legislation was published (American Nurses Association, 1981). A year later the National Council of State Boards of Nursing (NCSBN) also developed a model nurse practice act (NCSBN, 1982). The NCSBN continues to update its model act as part of its role in supporting the state boards of nursing with the most recent revision being published in 1988 (NCSBN, 1988a). In addition the NCSBN has written a Model Nursing Administrative Rules (NCSBN, 1988b).

Most state nurse practice acts are periodically rewritten to more accurately reflect modern nursing practice. Often the state nurses association serves as the primary stimulus for legislators to consider nursing legislation. We recommended that you carefully read the Nurse Practice Act for the state in which you will be practicing. A copy of the act may be obtained from the State Board of Nursing (see Appendix A for addresses).

In some states one act covers both practical nursing and registered nursing, whereas other states have two separate, but similar, acts. Historically the role of the nursing assistant was not in law. As federal legislation mandating classes and certification for nursing assistants in long-term care takes effect, some states are modifying laws and rules and regulations to include the role of the nursing assistant. In other states regulations governing nursing assistants rest within a different department.

The following general topics are usually covered in state licensure laws.

Purpose

The purpose of regulating the practice of nursing is twofold: to protect the public and to make the individual practitioner accountable for actions. Note that the protection of the status of the licensed individual is not the reason for licensure. With this in mind you can better understand the inclusion of some other topics in the act.

Definitions

All the significant terms in the act are defined for purposes of carrying out the law. This is where the legal definition of nursing and the scope of practice are spelled out. The ANA model act suggests the following definition for the registered nurse:

> The practice of nursing means: the performance for compensation of professional services requiring substantial specialized knowledge of the biological, physical, behavioral, psychological, and sociological sciences and of nursing theory as the basis for assessment, diagnosis, planning, intervention, and evaluation in the promotion and maintenance of health; the casefinding and management of illness, injury or infirmity; the restoration of optimum function; or the achievement of a dignified death. Nursing practice includes but is not limited to administration, teaching, counseling, supervision, delegation, and evaluation of practice and execution of the medical regimen, including the administration of medications and treatments prescribed by any person authorized by state law to prescribe. Each registered nurse is directly accountable and responsible to the consumer for the quality of nursing care rendered (American Nurses Association, 1981).

In addition, the NCSBN has stated that "the focus of nursing practice is generally accepted to be individual human responses to actual or potential health problems" (Practice Questions, 1989).

Although no state uses the exact wording of any recommendation, among the concepts commonly included are the reference to performing services for compensation, the necessity for a specialized knowledge base, the use of the nursing process (although steps may be named differently), and components of nursing practice. Several states include some reference to treating human responses to actual or potential health problems. This definition first appeared in New York State's license law and was later incorporated in the ANA's "Nursing: A Social Policy Statement" (1980). Most states refer to the execution of the medical regimen, and many include a general statement about additional acts, which has been interpreted to recognize that nursing practice is evolving and that the nurse's area of responsibility can be expected to broaden.

Definitions of practical (vocational) nursing are more restrictive and usually designate that the individual must function under the supervision of a registered nurse or physician and in areas demanding less judgment and knowledge than is required of the registered nurse. The practical nurse standards usually focus on the assessment and intervention portions of the nursing process. Some states provide a list of specific functions appropriate to the practical nurse or list specific functions not permitted.

A variety of nursing assistants are employed in health care facilities. They may have other titles such as mental health technician, nurse aide, or medication technician. The preparation of and scope of practice for these individuals is a matter of serious concern to the public. With the current pressure to contain costs, these individuals may be assigned tasks and responsibilities beyond their educational preparation and competence. Adding legal requirements for education and defining their scope of practice in the law is one mechanism that has been used to control their practice.

Qualifications for Licensure Applicants

The qualifications for licensure may be described in detail in the law, or only general guidelines may be given, leaving the details up to the State Board of Nursing. The most common basic requirements are graduation from an approved educational program and proficiency in the English language. Some states make the educational requirements more specific, such as requiring high school graduation and either an associate or baccalaureate degree or a diploma in nursing for the registered nurse applicant.

All states require a passing score on a comprehensive examination but do not name the examination in the law. The current licensing examinations are discussed later in this chapter. Many states require that the applicant be of "good moral character" and some require "good physical and mental health."

Titling

This section of the law reserves the right to use specific titles for those who have met the requirements. In some states only the titles registered nurse and licensed practical nurse are specified. Other states also regulate the use of titles for advanced practice such as nurse practitioner or nurse midwife.

Grandfathering

Whenever a new law is written, a statement is usually included specifying that anyone currently holding the license may continue to hold that license, even if some requirements are changed. Without this provision the enactment of a new law would require that all individuals who are currently licensed reapply and show that they meet the new standards.

However, not all changes in the law are grandfathered. When new requirements are instituted that the legislature believes are important for the safety of the public, all currently licensed individuals may be required to meet that standard within a given period of time. For example, the legislature in Washington State passed a bill requiring all licensed health professionals to have evidence of 7 hours of education regarding acquired immunodeficiency syndrome that included certain specified topics. New applicants had to meet this requirement before a license would be granted. Current license holders were required to meet this requirement before a license would be renewed.

Renewal and Continuing Education Requirements

The length of time for which a license is valid is specified in the law, as well as any requirements for renewal. In some states license renewal requires only payment of a fee. Many jurisdictions require evidence of continuing education for renewal. Documenting continuing education may require submission of records or may be attested to by signing a form. In many states where the applicant is not required to submit records at the time of renewal, a procedure for random checking ensures compliance with the law. Continuing education requirements vary greatly, for example, from as many as 24 hours every year to as few as 15 hours every 2 years.

Financial Concerns

Although the act itself does not usually specify the fees to be charged, general restrictions on the method of calculating fees and on how the fees may be used are often included in the act. The act may specify how the expenses of the Board of Nursing are to be met and who has legal authority to make decisions regarding the use of funds.

Nursing Education Programs

Some state laws describe the requirements of a nursing education program in only the most general terms, leaving the details up to the Board of Nursing. In other states the law is specific. It may specify the number of years of education, the courses or content that must be included, and the approval process for a program. If the law is general, then the board sets more specific standards.

All nursing education programs in a state must fulfill the requirements of the state law.

Disciplinary Action

Disciplinary action refers to all penalties that may be enacted against an individual who has violated provisions of a licensing law. These actions may take the form of restrictions on practice, such as working only under supervision, suspension of a license for a specified period, or revocation of a license. Such disciplinary action can only be taken based on criteria stated in the law. In the past, most state acts contained general statements with regard to such matters as immoral and unprofessional conduct. Because of their vagueness, they proved to be unenforceable in court. In addition, most courts have only supported reasons for revocation of the license when the offense was in some way related to practice issues that affect the public. Therefore, most modern laws contain specific concerns such as:

> Fraud in obtaining a license
> Conviction of a felony
> Substance abuse
> Harming the public

Violations and Penalties

Specific power is provided to prosecute those who violate the provisions of the law. The board may be authorized to ask a court to halt a specific practice that it believes is contrary to the law until a full hearing can be held. This is called "injunctive relief." This term refers to the court order called an injunction that is presented to the individual or organization.

Exceptions

Certain provisions may allow those who are not licensed to act as nurses in specific situations. Performing as a student while in an educational program is usually the primary exception. In addition, those who are caring for family members or friends without pay are exempted. Those who are practicing nursing in a federal agency, such as a military hospital, are exempted from the local state law as long as they maintain a current license in another state.

Administrative Provisions

Each law requires administrative details that specify such aspects as when it will become effective and when the previous act will no longer be in force. Such provisions are usually of special interest when the law is first passed because nurses want to know when they will be affected by any changes.

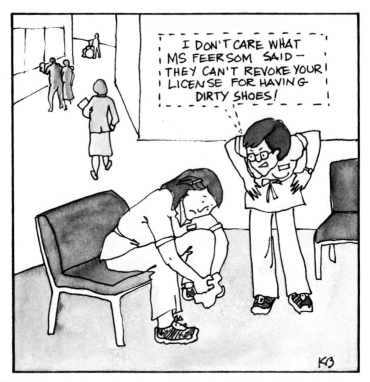

FIGURE 4–3 A nursing license may be revoked by the State Board of Nursing for reasons clearly spelled out in the law. These reasons may include fraud in obtaining a license, conviction of a felony, and conduct likely to harm the public.

EXPANDED NURSING ROLES

Some nurse practice acts provide for the practice of nurses in expanded roles, including nurse midwives, nurse anesthetists, and nurse practitioners. Often the law requires that the person be certified for advanced practice by the ANA or a nursing specialty organization (see section on certification later in the chapter). In some states no specific mention is made of expanded roles, but the Board of Nursing has approved specialty practice based on the provisions in the basic act. In still other states practice in special roles is not legally sanctioned. Contact the Board of Nursing in the state in which you are interested for information about specialty practice.

As part of *Nursing's Agenda for Health Care Reform* (ANA, 1991), nurses have been working actively to support advanced practice roles for nurses. The ANA does not believe that the inclusion of expanded practice in the licensure law is the best method of ensuring expanded practice. One concern is that some of the laws regulating specialty practice have provided for physician review of nursing's scope of practice. This takes autonomy away from nursing and allows medicine to control some aspects of nursing. Another concern is the rigidity, which may not allow for evolving nursing roles. The ANA holds the position that the licensure law should regulate minimum safe practice and that the profession should regulate advanced practice. This is the procedure in medicine, in which there is only basic licensure because a physician in specialty practice is regulated by specialty boards within the profession.

THE ROLE OF THE BOARD OF NURSING

The Board of Nursing is the group that is legally empowered to carry out the provisions of the law. The membership of the board, the procedure for appointment and removal, and the qualifications are important aspects of the Nurse Practice Act because the board has the power to write the rules and regulations that will be used in daily operations.

The members of the State Board of Nursing usually are appointed by the governor. The law specifies the occupational background of the candidates; nominations are often made by nurses, but the final membership is appointed. North Carolina is the only state in which the registered nurse members of the state board are elected by the registered nurses in the state.

Boards of nursing range in size from 7 to 17 members. Prerequisites regarding the educational background of nurses who serve as board members vary from state to state. Some states require that the board include nurses from differing occupational areas, such as education and nursing service. Most have at least one public member of the board. A few have at least one physician on the nursing board.

In the majority of states there is a combined board for registered nurses and licensed practical nurses. In the other states two separate boards exist. Each state board has a paid staff that usually is headed by a registered nurse who is employed as the executive director of the State Board of Nursing. The executive director is responsible for administering the work of the board and seeing that rules and regulations are followed. Some responsibilities related to professional licensure may be performed by a centralized state agency acting in relationship to all licensed occupations. These agencies range from those that have responsibility only for administrative matters, such as collecting fees, managing routine license renewals, and providing secretarial services, to those that have all decision-making authority, relegating the individual boards, such as the Board of Nursing, to advisory status.

Each state board must operate within the framework of its own state law regarding the practice of nursing, but all cooperate with one another through the NCSBN. They also cooperate with the ANA and the National League for Nursing (NLN) in some matters but maintain the separation that is required of a governmental body. For example, state boards acting together through the

NCSBN contract with the company that prepares the licensing examinations for registered nurses and practical nurses that are used throughout the United States.

Some of the activities for which the Board of Nursing is typically responsible include:

Establish standards for licensure
Examine and license applicants
Provide for interstate endorsement
Renew licenses, grant temporary licenses, and provide for inactive status for those already licensed who request it
Enforce disciplinary codes
Provide for revocation of license
Regulate specialty practice
Establish standards and curricula for nursing programs
Approve nursing education programs

Obtaining a Nursing License

There are two different procedures for obtaining a nursing license, one for applying for an initial license and the other for applying when one is already licensed in another jurisdiction. The initial licensure process is called "licensure by examination." Obtaining a license in a second jurisdiction is called "licensure by endorsement." In both instances, the applicant for licensure must meet all the provisions of the laws of the state in which he or she is seeking licensure such as educational preparation, language proficiency, and legal residency status. The difference is that in the original licensure process, the applicant must take and pass the standard licensing examination. In the licensure by endorsement process, the applicant is not required to take another examination. The licensure in another state is accepted as proof of minimum safe practice.

THE NURSING LICENSING EXAMINATION

The establishment of a licensing examination was an important part of early efforts to achieve a high standard for the registered nurse. When each state adopted a licensing law, it also established a mechanism for the examination of license applicants. A major achievement in the history of licensure was the formation of the Bureau of State Boards of Nurse Examiners, which eventually led to the use of an identical examination in all states in 1950. The original examination, called the State Board Test Pool Examination, was prepared by the testing department of the NLN under a contract with the state boards. Each state set its own standards for a passing score, although most states had a common accepted score for each test. Eventually all states accepted a common passing score for the State Board Test Pool Examination. The current examinations, called the NCLEX-RN for registered nursing and the NCLEX-PN for practical nursing, are used in all states and territories of the United States.

Content of the Examination

Historically, content of the examinations was divided into the subject categories of medical, surgical, obstetric, pediatric, and psychiatric nursing. Because nursing had changed in nature and these topics no longer reflected the totality of nursing practice, the NCSBN adopted a different plan for the examination, which was implemented in July 1982. For this new examination the National Council supported a research study that identified nursing behaviors critical to maintaining a safe and effective standard of care (Table 4–2). This research has been repeated periodically to ensure that the test plan remains relevant to current nursing practice.

In all of these studies newly licensed practicing registered nurses are studied to determine both the frequency and criticality of various behaviors. *Frequency* refers to how often the behaviors are required of the newly practicing registered nurse. *Criticality* refers to those actions that if performed incorrectly or omitted could cause serious harm to the client. These studies are called the "RN Job Analysis" and are reflected in the "Test Plan for the National Council Licensure Examination" (NCSBN, 1987).

The NCLEX-RN examination questions are organized into categories based on two sets of factors: client needs and steps of the nursing process. The client needs used are 1) safe, effective care environment (25%–31% of the questions); 2) physiologic integrity (42%–48% of the questions); 3) psychosocial integrity (9%–15% of the questions); and 4) health promotion–health maintenance (12%–18% of the questions) (NCSBN, 1987).

The nursing process is divided into the following five steps, each of which is tested in 15% to 25% of the questions: 1) assessing; 2) analyzing; 3) planning; 4) implementing; 5) evaluating. These two sets of behaviors form a matrix for questions (Table 4–3). The multiple choice questions in the examination are typically based on situations that require a nursing response. They are designed to test judgment and decision-making, not simply knowledge of facts (NCSBN, 1987).

Within these categories, then, behaviors that indicate safe practice are tested. For example one question might seek to determine the applicant's ability to assess a given situation to determine whether it was a safe care environment, while another question might determine whether the applicant would implement the correct action to maintain safety. In considering physiologic

TABLE 4–2 Critical Requirements for Practice

I. Exercises Professional Prerogatives Based on Clinical Judgment
A. Adapts care to individual patient needs.
B. Fulfills responsibility to patient and others despite difficulty
C. Challenges inappropriate orders and decisions by medical and other professional staff
D. Acts as patient advocate in obtaining appropriate medical, psychiatric, or other help
E. Recognizes own limitations and errors
F. Analyzes and adjusts own or staff reactions in order to maintain therapeutic relationship with patient

II. Promotes Patient's Ability to Cope with Immediate, Long-range, or Potential Health-Related Change
A. Provides health care instruction or information to patient, family, or significant others
B. Encourages patient or family to make decision about accepting care or adhering to treatment regimen.
C. Helps patient recognize and deal with psychological stress
D. Avoids creating or increasing anxiety or stress
E. Conveys and invites acceptance, respect, and trust
F. Facilitates relationship of family, staff, or significant others with patient
G. Stimulates, remotivates patient, or enables patient to achieve self-care independence

III. Helps Maintain Patient Comfort and Normal Body Functions
A. Keeps patient clean and comfortable
B. Helps patient maintain or regain normal body functions

IV. Takes Precautionary and Preventive Measures in Giving Patient Care
A. Prevents infection
B. Protects skin and mucous membranes from injurious materials
C. Uses positioning or exercise to prevent injury or the complications of immobility
D. Avoids using injurious techniques in administering and managing intrusive or other potentially traumatic treatments
E. Protects patient from falls or other contact injuries
F. Maintains surveillance of patient's activities
G. Reduces or removes environmental hazards

V. Checks, Compares, Verifies, Monitors, and Follows up Medication and Treatment Processes
A. Checks correctness, condition, and safety of medication being prepared
B. Ensures that correct medication is given to the right patient and that patient takes or receives it
C. Adheres to schedule in giving medication, treatment, or test
D. Administers medication by correct route, rate, or mode
E. Checks patient's readiness for medication, treatment, surgery, or other care
F. Checks to ensure that tests or measurements are done correctly
G. Monitors ongoing infusions and inhalations

(continued)

TABLE 4–2 Critical Requirements for Practice *(Continued)*

   H. Checks for and interprets effect of medication, treatment, or care, and takes corrective action if necessary.

VI. Interprets Symptom Complex and Intervenes Appropriately
   A. Checks patient's condition or status
   B. Remains objective, further investigates, or verifies patient's complaint or problem
   C. Uses alarms and signals on automatic equipment as adjunct to personal assessment
   D. Observes and correctly assesses signs of anxiety or behavioral stress
   E. Observes and correctly assesses physical signs, symptoms, or findings, and intervenes appropriately
   F. Correctly assesses severity or priority of patient's condition, and gives or obtains necessary care

VII. Responds to Emergency
   A. Anticipates need for crisis care
   B. Takes instant, correct action in emergency situations
   C. Maintains calm and efficient approach under pressure
   D. Assumes leadership role in crisis situation when necessary

VIII. Obtains, Records, and Exchanges Information on Behalf of the Patient
   A. Checks data sources for order and other information about patient
   B. Obtains information from patient and family
   C. Transcribes or records information on chart, Kardex, or other information system
   D. Exchanges information with nursing staff and other departments
   E. Exchanges information with medical staff

IX. Utilizes Patient Care Planning
   A. Develops and modifies patient care plan
   B. Implements patient care plan

X. Teaches and Supervises Other Staff
   A. Teaches correct principles, procedures, and techniques of patient care
   B. Supervises and checks the work of staff for whom she or he is responsible.

integrity, a question might focus on the appropriate assessment for a patient with an illness that threatens physiologic integrity and another would focus on evaluating the outcomes of actions taken to preserve physiologic integrity. In this way questions address two aspects of the matrix plan.

In 1993, the contract for preparing and administering the NCLEX examinations was awarded to Educational Testing Services of Princeton, New Jersey. In addition to administering the process of test preparation, the company scores the examinations and reports scores to the state boards. The testing service is authorized to sell statistical information related to the examination to the states and individual schools.

TABLE 4–3 Content Distribution of the NCLEX-RN Examination

	Client Needs			
Phases of the Nursing Process	Safe, Effective Care Environment 25%–31%	Physiologic Integrity 42%–48%	Psychosocial Integrity 9%–15%	Health Promotion– Health Maintenance 12%–18%
Assess 15%–25%				
Analyze 15%–25%				
Plan 15%–25%				
Implement 15%–25%				
Evaluate 15%–25%				

Preparing questions for the examination is a complex process. Individuals who teach in nursing programs across the country are brought together as item writers. Together these individuals write questions based on the test plan. Questions are then reviewed by content experts who are nurses in current practice who work with new graduates. A panel of individuals reviews the questions for bias. Each question is verified by using current nursing references. Additionally, test construction experts review all questions in regard to their structure. The final versions of all questions are then tested by inclusion as a nongraded part of the examinations being given to new graduates taking the licensure examination. The questions can then be evaluated for their appropriateness as part of a future scored examination.

Computerized Adaptive Testing (CAT)

All NLCEX examinations (both RN and PN) are now administered through computerized adaptive testing (CAT). The CAT consists of a bank of examination questions administered through a computerized system. CAT had its first field trials in 1990, testing across the country in 1993, and was adopted for all testing beginning in April 1994.

In this computerized test, the multiple choice questions are on a computer screen. The computer contains a large bank of questions and different

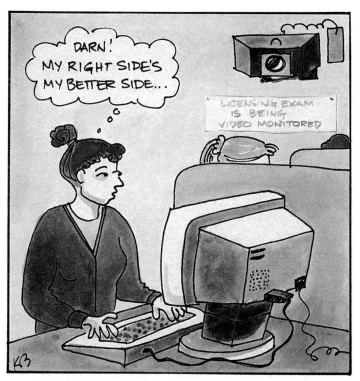

FIGURE 4–4 In computer adapted testing, security is closely monitored.

individuals may be presented with different questions. The development of questions and design of the computer program ensures that all tests are equivalent even when not identical. The computer program evaluates each response and then selects an appropriate question to present next, choosing a slightly harder question if the previous question was answered correctly or an easier one if the response was incorrect. The computer program ensures that all essential areas are tested and that the balance of hard/easy and differing aspects of the test matrix plan are all part of every examination. The maximum length of the examination is 5 hours, but it could be completed in as little time as an hour if the candidate performed especially well or very poorly. One break is required and others may be taken at the discretion of the applicant.

Each candidate for licensure makes an individual appointment at a testing site. At the testing site, the computers are located in a quiet room without distractions. Pencil and paper are provided for notes or calculations. (Calculators are not permitted.) Security is tightly monitored.

Each question along with its possible answers is presented on a separate screen. If there is a brief situation, it appears on the same screen as the question and answers. Only two keys are used throughout the examination. The space bar moves between the alternative answers and the "enter" key must be pressed twice to make a selection. A selection must be made to move to the next question. It is not possible to go back to a question previously answered. When the individual has completed enough questions for the computer program to determine either "pass" or "fail," the testing session is ended.

Scoring of the Examination

The computer computes the score as the applicant answers questions. Based on the computation made as the applicant progresses, additional questions are presented to clearly determine whether the applicant meets the standards for safe, effective practice. The score used for determining pass/fail is not a raw score (that is the number right) but one derived from a complex mathematical process. The test was not designed for the purpose of differentiating levels of excellence, only for demonstrating basic safe practice and this is what the pass or fail communicates.

Although the computer has determined the score, the individual is not notified of the result at that time. The scoring information is communicated to the Educational Testing Service, which then notifies the appropriate board. The individual is notified of "pass" or "fail" status by the appropriate board.

Preparing for the NCLEX

Each individual must determine how he or she can best prepare for the licensure examination. A review of the knowledge basic to nursing is important for most individuals. Those who become very anxious in testing situations may want to focus on anxiety-reducing exercises that may decrease anxiety at the time of the examination. Those who find the process of test taking difficult can gain greater self-confidence by practicing test-taking techniques. This can be done through printed tests in books or computerized test preparation programs.

To prepare applicants to take the examination, the NCSBN has authorized the preparation of a study book that explains the examination, how it was written, and the scoring system and provides sample questions to familiarize applicants with the way the test is written. Many companies also prepare review books, sample examination questions, and computerized practice examinations for preparing for the licensing examinations. Manuals that outline standard nursing practice relative to many different health care problems may be useful for reviewing nursing content. Live and videotaped review courses are available to those who want assistance with preparation.

THE LICENSURE EXAMINATION FOR PRACTICAL NURSING

The licensure examination for the practical nurse, the NCLEX-PN, has been designed in a similar manner. A new test plan based on the practical nurse job analysis done in 1986 and 1987 was adopted in 1989. New questions were then developed, and the new test plan was effective after 1990 (NCSBN, 1989). Client needs and the nursing process form the basis of this examination also. The practical nurse is expected to be in a dependent role in planning and evaluation and more independent in collecting data and implementing. The new test recognizes that numerous licensed practical nurses are employed in long-term care settings with clients older than 65 years of age. The percentages of questions in each category are shown in Table 4–4. The testing and scoring processes are similar to those used for the NCLEX-RN examination and a "pass" or "fail" is reported.

FUTURE TRENDS IN EXAMINATION

The NCSBN is investigating the potential for Clinical Simulation Testing (CST), a more complex form of computerized testing of nursing licensure applicants (Bersky and Yocom, 1994). In this type of test a client situation is

TABLE 4–4 Content Distribution of the NCLEX-PN Examination

	Client Needs			
Phases of the Nursing Process	Safe, Effective Care Environment 24%–30%	Physiologic Integrity 42%–48%	Psychosocial Integrity 7%–13%	Health Promotion– Health Maintenance 15%–21%
Collect Data 25%–35%				
Plan 15%–25%				
Implement 25%–35%				
Evaluate 15%–25%				

presented on the computer screen. The applicant is asked to determine the appropriate action and type the answer into the keyboard. The applicant receives points for correct actions and for the order or priority in which actions are chosen. Points are subtracted for inappropriate actions. Actions that might cause harm to the client are especially noted. Consideration is being given to putting the situations on a videodisc to provide visual cues as well as written information (Bersky and Brady, 1993). This type of testing is much more expensive to develop and administer than a multiple choice question examination. CST was first field tested in 1991. There are not specific plans as to when this type of testing will be initiated.

LICENSURE BY ENDORSEMENT

The process of obtaining a nursing license in another state after first being licensed in one state is called licensure by endorsement. There are no reciprocal agreements between states that provide for automatically moving licensure from one state to another. Each case is considered independently, based on the rules and regulations of the state. However, owing to the uniformity of licensing laws throughout most of the United States and its territories, nurses have enjoyed easy mobility between geographical areas.

Because the same licensure examination is used nationwide, no state requires that the examination be retaken. Basic educational requirements as well as additional requirements in the law must be met. Some states require that a nurse moving into the state meet the current criteria for new licensure. In other states a nurse must fulfill the requirements that were in effect at the time of the original licensure. A state may require a nurse to meet other criteria, such as those for continuing education, before granting licensure by endorsement. In all cases, appropriate paperwork must be completed, necessary fees paid, and a license obtained before beginning employment.

If a nurse wishes to maintain licensure in more than one state, this may be done once the license is secured by paying the renewal fees and meeting any other requirements for continued licensure such as continuing education.

A temporary license that allows the applicant for licensure by endorsement to be employed while credentials are being verified and processed is available in some states. Other states require that a permanent license be obtained before any employment is legal in those jurisdictions.

At the present time, North Dakota does not offer licensure by endorsement to all nurses licensed in other states. In North Dakota an associate degree is required for initial licensure as a licensed practical nurse and a baccalaureate degree is required for initial licensure as a registered nurse. All nurses registered in North Dakota were grandfathered into their licenses when this change in licensure regulations occurred. A registered nurse or licensed practical nurse from another state, who does not have the required degree and who seeks licensure by endorsement in North Dakota, must meet specific conditions and standards identified by the North Dakota Board, which may include enrollment in an educational program. North Dakota represents an exception to the general pattern of easy mobility for all registered nurses.

LICENSURE OF GRADUATES OF FOREIGN NURSING SCHOOLS

Nurses who have graduated from a nursing school in a foreign country and want to practice nursing in the United States must satisfy the Board of Nursing in their state that their education meets the requirements of the state and take the NCLEX-RN examination. To prevent the exploitation of foreign graduates who come to the United States to practice nursing and fail to pass the licensing examination, and to help ensure safety in health care for the U.S. public, the ANA and the NLN have sponsored an independent organization called the Commission on Graduates of Foreign Nursing Schools (CGFNS), which administers an examination to foreign-educated nurses. The examination covers proficiency in both nursing and English and helps the foreign-educated nurse to determine the possibility of passing the actual licensing examination. Nurses may take the CGFNS examination while still in their own country, although it is also given in selected cities in the United States and Canada.

To obtain a nonimmigrant preference visa from the U.S. Immigration and Naturalization Service or a work permit from the U.S. Labor Department, the foreign-educated nurse must first pass the CGFNS examination. The majority of states also require the CGFNS examination as a preliminary step for foreign-educated nurses before taking the NCLEX examination for licensure.

In addition to its role in preparing and administering the CGFNS examination, the CGFNS organization also investigates and validates credentials held by graduates of foreign nursing schools for boards of nursing and other appropriate organizations. Nursing education throughout the world is varied and offers differing titles and types of education. Those who are not familiar with a foreign nursing education and licensure system and who lack foreign language proficiency may have difficulty interpreting transcripts, diplomas, and other documents and determining whether the credentials presented are the equivalent of the licensed practical nurse or of the registered nurse in this country. CGFNS maintains current data on nursing from around the world as well as having a staff who are involved full time with this process. This enables this organization to provide an accurate evaluation of credentials of graduates of foreign nursing schools (Schaefer, 1990).

FEES FOR LICENSURE

All states charge a fee for processing an application for licensure. At the time of initial licensure there are also fees for taking the licensing examination and a fee to the company that prepares and scores the examination. The total cost for initial examination and license is usually more than $100. In addition, there is a fee each time a license is renewed. For specific information on licensure fees, temporary permits, and continuing education requirements, write to the Board of Nursing of the state in which you are interested.

Revocation of a License

A license to practice any occupation becomes a property right of the individual after the state has awarded it. As long as the individual renews by paying the appropriate fees and meets any requirements, such as continuing education, a license cannot be revoked without cause. The possible reasons for revoking a license are spelled out in the law. (The common reasons are listed earlier, in the discussion of disciplinary action.)

The procedure for revoking a license includes a fact finding process amd a hearing, which functions in many ways like a court proceeding. The state board or a specially designated hearing board is responsible for conducting the hearing and making a decision. The board may provide a license with conditions, suspend a license until certain conditions are met, or revoke a license completely. For example, an individual being faced with charges based on chemical dependency might be directed to enter a treatment program, to not be employed in any nursing position with direct responsibility to clients or access to drugs, and to be monitored for compliance. If these conditions are met, the individual may then be reinstated to full rights and privileges of licensure when treatment is completed. The board's decision may be appealed to a court of law in most states. The individual being threatened with revocation of a license should have an attorney for legal counsel throughout the proceeding. If a board of nursing finds that the individual's actions constitute a felony, the board is obligated to report that to the criminal authorities for prosecution.

SUNSET LAWS

Most laws remain in effect until the legislature votes to rescind or replace them. Because this has resulted in archaic laws remaining in effect for years and years, some states have passed what are known as "sunset laws." Sunset laws provide that any regulatory act, such as the Nurse Practice Act, will automatically be rescinded if not reauthorized. In states with sunset laws, nurses cannot wait for an opportune time when they would like to support changes in the Nurse Practice Act. Instead they must identify when sunsetting will occur and work in advance to sustain the current law and/or make changes. The advantage of sunset laws is that they guarantee that the legislature will review and evaluate agencies and programs.

International Nursing Licensure

Throughout the world nursing education and nursing licensure differ greatly. In Australia nursing education has been moved into university settings and future applicants for licensure in that country will be required to have university education. In Italy nursing education is now consolidated under broad programs administered by university nursing departments. The nations of Eastern Europe are facing many drastic changes in their health care systems as they move into different relationships with the West. Nursing education was restricted during Soviet domination and many nurses had limited educational opportunities with basic nursing education occurring at the high school level in some instances. These nurses are now seeking ways to broaden nursing education in their countries.

Based on these wide differences, nursing credentials are not easily transferred internationally. The International Congress of Nurses (ICN) has supported the development of effective licensure legislation worldwide. In 1988, the ICN launched a project called "Nursing Regulation: Moving Ahead," which was funded by the W. K. Kellogg Foundation. This ongoing project has involved nurses and officials from 77 countries in seminars and studies. The publications produced by the project have been used as countries examine the regulations involving nursing (Affara and Styles, 1990).

Individuals who are interested in international nursing need to consider their own language proficiency as well their educational backgrounds. Not all countries welcome nurses educated elsewhere. They may have a surplus of nurses and wish to avoid displacing local nurses. Others are concerned that nurses educated in affluent societies such as the United States and Canada may understand little about health care needs and practice in a developing country. Organizations actively working in the international health field will usually provide information on opportunities and licensure requirements in various countries. The ICN in Geneva can provide addresses of appropriate governmental authorities to contact regarding licensure in specific countries.

Certification in Nursing

Certification in nursing is primarily a professional, not a legal, credential. The definition of certification adopted by the Interdivisional Council on Certification of the ANA (1978) states: "Certification is the documented validation of specific qualifications demonstrated by the individual registered nurse in the provision of professional nursing care in a defined area of practice." Certification is available from a variety of professional nursing and health care organizations.

ANA CERTIFICATION

Currently, ANA certification is a method of recognizing nurses who have special expertise. Applicants must demonstrate current practice beyond that required for licensure as a registered nurse. The applicant must take a national examination and submit evidence of completing any other requirements, such as educational preparation, for the specific clinical area. Certificates are valid for a period of 5 years, after which the nurse must meet specific criteria to renew the certification for another 5 years. Table 4–5 lists the various certification credentials available from the ANA. A baccalaureate degree in nursing is required for initial certification in many areas and a master's degree in nursing often is required for initial clinical specialist or nurse practitioner certification.

OTHER CERTIFICATION PROGRAMS

Certification as a registered nurse anesthetist is provided by the American Association of Nurse Anesthetists (AANA). Since 1952 the AANA, with the approval of the American Hospital Association, has accredited programs for preparing nurse anesthetists and has administered an examination for certification of graduates of these programs. According to the AANA, certified registered nurse anesthetists administer more than half of all anesthetics. Nurse anesthetists were the first nurses to be certified beyond the basic level.

The National Association of Pediatric Nurse Associates/Practitioners (NAPNAP) offers certification for the pediatric nurse practitioner. This has resulted in two certificates being awarded in the same area by two organizations. NAPNAP and the ANA have had joint conferences regarding certification, and it was hoped that one jointly sponsored certification might result. Fundamental differences still exist, however, between the two organizations on how authority for determining standards should be established.

The Association for Women's Health, Obstetric, and Neonatal Nursing (AWHONN) formerly called Nurse's Association of the American College of

TABLE 4–5 ANA Certification Areas Available

Community Health Nurse (RN, C)
General Nursing Practice (RN, C)
Gerontological Nurse (RN, C)
Medical–Surgical Nurse (RN, C)
Nursing Administration (RN, CNA)
Nursing Administration, Advanced (RN, C)
Perinatal Nurse (RN, C)
Pediatric Nurse (RN, C)
Psychiatric and Mental Health Nurse (RN, C)
School Nurse (RN, C)

Nurse Practitioner Certification
  Adult Nurse Practitioner (RN, C)
  Family Nurse Practitioner (RN, C)
  Gerontological Nurse Practitioner (RN, C)
  Pediatric Nurse Practitioner (RN, C)
  School Nurse Practitioner (RN, C)

Clinical Specialist Certification
  Clinical Specialist in Adult Psychiatric Mental Health Nursing (RN, CS)
  Clinical Specialist in Child and Adolescent Psychiatric and Mental Health
    Nursing (RN, CS)
  Clinical Specialist in Community Health Nursing (RN, CS)
  Clinical Specialist in Gerontological Nursing (RN, CS)
  Clinical Specialist in Medical–Surgical Nursing (RN, CS)

Obstetricians and Gynecologists (NAACOG) provides certification for nurses working in women's health care, obstetrics, or neonatal nursing. The American College of Nurse Midwives provides a certification program for nurses specializing in nurse midwifery. Nurses graduating from approved midwifery programs apply for certification through this organization. Approved programs may be at a basic level or at a master's degree level. The license to practice as a midwife depends, however, on the state licensure laws. Some states do not allow the practice of nurse midwives; in other states the law recognizes the certification as an appropriate credential for practice; and in still other states no decision has been made.

Many other specialty organizations in nursing have certification programs (Table 4–6). Most of these are administered by a separately titled and funded certification organization that is closely related to the specialty organization. This administrative structure is set up to protect the sponsoring organization from economic liability, to preserve tax-exempt status, and to provide a more objective approach to the credentialing process. Information on any of these specialty certification programs can be obtained by writing directly to the organization (see Appendix B).

Some organizations of health care workers offer credentialing to individuals in specific occupations that may include nurses. For example, the Society

TABLE 4–6 Certification Available Through Specialty Organizations*

Addictions Nursing (CARN)	CARN Certification, National League for Nursing
Critical Care Nursing (CCRN)	American Association of Critical Care Nurses Certification Corporation
Diabetes Educator (CDE)	National Certification Board for Diabetes Educators
Emergency Nursing (CEN) Flight Nursing (CFRN)	Board of Certification for Emergency Nursing
Enterostomal Therapy (CETN)	Enterostomal Therapy Nursing Certification Board
Gastroenterology (CGC)	Certifying Board of Gastroenterology Nurses and Associates
Hemodialysis Nurse (CHN) Peritoneal Dialysis Nurse (CPDN) Infection Control (CIC)	Board of Nephrology Examiners Nursing and Technology Certification Board of Infection Control
Intravenous Nursing (CRNI)	Intravenous Nurses Certification Corporation
Lactation Consultant (IBCLC)	International Board of Lactation Consultants Examiners
Maternal/Child Specialities Ambulatory Women's Health Care Nurses (RNC) High-risk Obstetric Nurse (RNC) Inpatient Obstetric Nurse (RNC) Low-Risk Neonatal Nurse (RNC) Maternal Newborn Nurse (RNC) Neonatal Intensive Care Nurse (RNC) OB/GYN Nurse Practitioner (RNC) Reproductive Endocrinology/ Infertility Nurse (RNC)	National Certification Corporation for the Obstetric, Gynecologic, and Neonatal Nursing Specialities
Neuroscience Nurse (CNRN)	American Board of Neuroscience Nursing Professional Examination Service
Nurse Administrator— Long-Term Care (RN, C)	Center for Credentialing Services NADONA/LTC Professional Exam Review System
Nurse Anesthetist (CRNA)	Council on Certification of Nurse Anesthetists
Nurse Midwife (CNM)	Association of Certified Nurse Midwives Certification Council
Nutrition Support Nurse (CNSN)	National Board of Nutrition Support Certification

(continued)

TABLE 4–6 Certification Available Through Specialty Organizations*
(*Continued*)

Occupational Health Nursing (COHN)	American Board for Occupational Health Nurses
Oncology Nursing (OCN)	Oncology Nursing Certification Corporation
Ophthalmic Nursing (CRNO)	National Certifying Board for Ophthalmic Registered Nurses
Orthopedic Nursing (ONC)	Orthopaedic Nurse Certification Board
Pain Management (CNOR)	American Academy of Pain Management
Pediatric Specialties General Pediatric Nurse (CPN) Pediatric Nurse Practitioner (CPNP)	National Certification Board of Pediatric Nurse Practitioners & Nurses
Perioperative Nurse (CNOR)	National Certification Board of Perioperative Nursing
Plastic and Reconstructive Surgical Nurse (CPSN)	Plastic Surgical Nursing Certification Board
Post-Anesthesia Nurse (CPAN)	American Board of Post-Anesthesia Nursing Certification Professional Examination Service
Rehabilitation Nurse (CRRN)	Rehabilitation Nursing Certification Board
School Nurse (CSN)	National Board for Certification of School Nurses
Urology Nurse (CURN)	American Board of Urologic Allied Health Professionals

*See Appendix B for addresses of organizations.

of Gastroenterostomal Assistants offers certification to individuals employed in gastroenterology laboratories. This certification is available to both registered nurses and licensed practical nurses. The Association for Practitioners in Infection Control certifies individuals who are professionals in infection control and include nurses in this group.

CERTIFICATION AS A BASIS FOR LICENSURE

Some states are using certification as a means of identifying competence in an expanded or specialized role for the registered nurse and thus are giving legal recognition to the nurse possessing this certification. The requirements and methods for obtaining certification remain under the control of the organization granting the certification. The nurse receives a license from the state to practice in the expanded role. This is true of certified nurse anesthetists who are all certified through the AANA but who receive legal status to practice in anesthesia by the appropriate authority in their state. This may be the Board of Nursing, although in some states nurse anesthetists practice under the Board of Medicine.

Titles being used in these expanded roles vary from state to state. Some current titles are advanced registered nurse (ARN), specialized registered nurse (SRN), nurse practitioner (NP), independent nurse practitioner (INP), advanced nurse practitioner (ANP), advanced registered nurse practitioner (ARNP), and certified registered nurse (CRN). In some states the specialized nurse uses the title of the specific certification, such as family nurse practitioner (FNP) and pediatric nurse practitioner (PNP).

PROBLEMS RELATED TO CERTIFICATION

Not all of the problems associated with certification have been resolved. Programs that prepare nurses in various specialties lack uniformity. The situation is reminiscent of the early years of nursing education. Some advanced programs accept any registered nurse and are completed in 6 to 9 months. Other programs that prepare nurses for the same specialty may be at the master's degree level. Thus, the title awarded by the program is not a reliable indication of the degree of competence achieved by the nurse specialist. It is hoped that certification programs will improve the situation by defining the common standard of performance that must be demonstrated to attain the certificate.

Another concern is the disparity that occurs from state to state in credentialing nurses in specialty areas. This can hamper mobility and interfere with meeting the health care needs in areas of the United States where these nursing specialists are not recognized. Some believe that the certification program will be of help because it sets national standards that states may adopt. When different states adopt certification as an appropriate way of credentialing, movement between those states is facilitated.

A third problem has been related to the equivalency of certificates in different specialties. In the past not all specialty certifications have required the same educational, testing, or practice requirements. To remedy this the American Nurses' Credentialing Center has established the master's degree as the requirement for initial certification of clinical specialists or nurse practitioners and a baccalaureate degree for initial certification in other specialty practice areas. Those who already are certified will retain certification as long as they continue to meet the practice and continuing education requirements.

THE FUTURE OF CERTIFICATION IN NURSING

Both the public and nurses have been confused because credentialing in nursing involves so many aspects related to education, licensure, and certification. Because the ideal credential clearly communicates qualifications and competence, it is important for nursing to have a credentialing system that can be understood by others.

In 1988, the ANA established a credentialing center titled the American Nurses' Credentialing Center, bringing together all of its credentialing activities. They invited all other organizations providing credentialing to join. Some organizations joined but most retained their individual programs.

Then in 1991, eight national nursing certification programs joined to establish the American Board of Nursing Specialties. These organizations were the American Nurses' Credentialing Center of the ANA, the American Board for Occupational Health Nursing, American Board of Neuroscience Nursing, Association of Rehabilitation Nurses, Council on Certification of Nurse Anesthetists, National Board of Nutritional Support Certification, Nephrology Nursing Certification Board, and the Orthopaedic Nurses Certification Board. According to their report, these eight organizations represent more than 65% of the total number of registered nurses certified in specialty practice (Specialty Certification, 1991). The goal of this board is to ensure quality in specialty nursing and to increase the public's ability to identify individuals who bring a consistent standard of education and experience to their practice. This is a major breakthrough in the entire certification process for nursing.

The Future of Credentialing in Health Care

Numerous new health care occupations related to new procedures and processes in medical care are developing. There continues to be pressure to license these additional health care providers by those who believe the state should take positive action to protect the public. Those who oppose credentialing of additional individual groups of health care workers believe that modern-day employers are able to assess workers and differentiate between them on the basis of competence. Some of those who oppose credentialing of individual health occupations believe that licensing the institution that hires the employees would be an adequate safeguard for the public.

Another approach to credentialing in health care being advocated is certifying specific competencies rather than an entire field of practice. Those advocating this approach believe that it would facilitate the development of individuals with a broad range of competencies suited to a particular setting. For example, in a rural area one individual might be certified as competent to perform certain basic x-ray examinations (such as for simple fractures), basic laboratory studies (such as complete blood count and urinalysis) and some basic patient care procedures (such as bathing, toileting, feeding, and positioning). Because more complex procedures are sent to a larger center and there is no need for a full-time person in any of these positions, basic care would be made available in a convenient and low-cost manner. Certification of specific competencies by the employing agency is sometimes referred to as *site-based examination* and *site-based certification*. One concern about this method of certifying competencies is the focus on technical skills without adequate recognition of the knowledge base needed for decision-making and judgment. Another concern is the complexity of keeping track of the many specific competencies and the difficulty with job mobility when competencies are not standardized. Credentialing in the various other health occupations will remain an important concern.

Key Concepts

- ▷ Credentials are written proof of qualifications and may include diplomas conferred by educational programs, certification or registration by professional groups, and legal licenses conferred by governmental agencies.
- ▷ Permissive licensure allows for those meeting certain standards to be licensed, whereas mandatory licensure requires that all individuals who wish to practice in the field must be licensed to practice.
- ▷ Nursing leaders began efforts to obtain legal licensure in 1896. The first permissive licensure law was passed in 1903 by North Carolina and the the first mandatory licensure law was passed in New York in 1947.
- ▷ Legal rules governing nursing practice are found in the licensure law passed by a legislative body. Further provisions governing nursing are found in the rules and regulations established by the administrative agency in whom the legislation vests authority.
- ▷ The nursing practice act usually contains a definition of nursing, qualifications for licensure applicants, use of titles, renewal and continuing education requirements, grandfathering, financial concerns, nursing education programs, disciplinary action, violations and penalties, administrative provisions, and expanded nursing roles.
- ▷ The Board of Nursing is the administrative agency with the authority to carry out the provisions of the Nurse Practice Act.
- ▷ A license to practice nursing must be obtained from the state or province in which you wish to work. An initial license is termed licensure by examination and subsequent licenses may be obtained in other jurisdictions through licensure by endorsement.
- ▷ The NCLEX-RN examination is administered through a computerized plan that includes five steps of the nursing process and four areas of client needs.

▷ Graduates of foreign nursing schools may be required to take the CGFNS examination, which reviews both nursing content and English language ability.

▷ A license may be revoked by the State Board of Nursing, a designated disciplinary board, or a court of law based on specific reasons stated in the Nurse Practice Act.

▷ Certification provides evidence of specialized clinical knowledge and ability beyond the basic level. Certification as a nurse practitioner may be used as a basis for legal approval to practice in an expanded role.

CRITICAL THINKING ACTIVITIES

1. A student about to graduate from a registered nursing program in New York, wishes to practice nursing in New Jersey. What steps should she take to ensure that she may legally practice nursing in New Jersey?
2. A registered nurse who has been working in Indianapolis, Indiana for 10 years decides to relocate to Orlando, Florida. What steps should the nurse take to ensure that she is able to work as a registered nurse in FLorida?
3. A registered nurse is interested in working in the critical care unit of a hospital in your community. What would he have to do to be considered for such a position?

References

Affara F, Styles M. Nursing regulation moves ahead. Int Nurs Rev 37(4):307–311, 1990

American Nurses Association. Nursing: A Social Policy Statement. Kansas City, MO: American Nurses Association, 1980

American Nurses Association. Nursing's Agenda for Healthcare Reform. Washington, DC: American Nurses Publishing Co., 1991

American Nurses Association. The Study of Credentialing in Nursing: A New Approach, vol 1. The Report of the Committee. Kansas City, MO: American Nurses Association, 1978

American Nurses Association Congress for Nursing Practice. The Nursing Practice Act: Suggested State Legislation. Kansas City, MO: American Nurses Association, 1981

Bersky A, Brady D. A new generation of competence assessment in nursing: Computerized clinical simulation testing (CST). Issues 14(1): 1–8, 1993

Bersky AK, Yocom CJ. Computerized clinical simulation testing: Its use for competence assessment in nursing. Nurs Health Care 15(3):120–127, 1994

National Council of State Boards of Nursing. Test Plan for the National Council Licensure Examination for Practical Nurses. Chicago: National Council of State Boards of Nursing, 1989

National Council of State Boards of Nursing. Model Nurse Practice Act. Chicago: National Council of State Boards of Nursing, 1988a

National Council of State Boards of Nursing. Model Nursing Administrative Rules. Chicago: National Council of State Boards of Nursing, 1988b

National Council of State Boards of Nursing. Test Plan for the National Council Licensure Examination for Registered Nurses. Chicago: National Council of State Boards of Nursing, 1987

National Council of State Boards of Nursing. Model Nurse Practice Act. Chicago: National Council of State Boards of Nursing, 1982

Practice questions: A framework for thinking. Issues 10(3):3–5, 1989

Schaefer B. International credentials review: Crucial and complex. Nurs Health Care 11(8):431–432, 1990

Snyder ME, LaBar C. Issues in Professional Practice, Vol. 1, Nursing: Legal Authority for Practice. Washington, DC: American Nurses Publishing Co., 1984

Specialty certification groups form organization. Am Nurse 23(4):20, 1991

Further Readings

Birkholz G. Implications of the National Practitioner Data Bank for nurse practitioners. Nurse Pract 16(8):40, 42–43, 46, 1991

Edwards S, Edmondson P, Giesey C, Payne G, Raper J. NCLEX-RN review courses: Are they working? Nurs Management 22(11):54, 1991

Fiesta J. Why nurses lose their licenses, Part I. Nurs Management 24(10):12, 14, 1993

Fiesta J. Why nurses lose their licenses, Part II. Nurs Management 24(11):14–15, 1993

Fiesta J. Why nurses lose their licenses, Part III. Nurs Management 24(12):16, 1993

Henry PF. Your due process rights in a disciplinary action. Nurse Pract Forum 2(4):210–211, 1991

Konradi D, Stockert P. Preparing for the NCLEX-RN. Imprint 40(1): 6–9, 1993

Providing for the needs of handicapped candidates. Issues 10(5):8–9, 1989

Spanier A. The development process of NCLEX-PN and NCLEX-RN pools. Issues 9(3):3–6, 1988

Tharp C. Computerized clinical simulation testing: The future is happening today. Issues 11(1):1, 10–11, 1990

Wall DM, Miller DE, Widerquist JG. Predictors of success on the newest NCLEX-RN. West J Nurs Res 15(5):628–643, 1993

5 | Legal Responsibilities for Practice

Objectives

After completing this chapter, you should be able to

1. Differentiate between the terms ethics and law.
2. Identify two general sources of law and describe their differences.
3. Explain the role of institutional policies and protocols in legal decision-making.
4. Differentiate between civil law and criminal law.
5. Describe some situations in which nurses may be involved in criminal law.
6. Define negligence, torts, and malpractice.
7. Define liability, identifying situations in which liability is shared by employers or supervisors.
8. State points to be considered in the purchase of professional liability insurance.
9. List the most commonly recurring legal issues in nursing.
10. Explain how informed consent, advance directives, and the Patient Self-Determination Act support the patient's rights.
11. Discuss the nurse's responsibility in the specific issues that can constitute malpractice.
12. Identify factors that contribute to a suit being instituted against a health care professional.
13. Discuss a variety of actions by the nurse that might prevent the initiation of a lawsuit.
14. Explain the various aspects of testifying for a legal proceeding.

Karine Guard, RN, MN, JD, served as a consultant regarding the legal material presented in this chapter.

Ellis JR, Hartley CL: NURSING IN TODAY'S WORLD:
CHALLENGES, ISSUES, AND TRENDS, 5th ed.
© 1995 J.B. Lippincott Company

Discussion about the individual nurse's responsibility and accountability for personal actions is appearing more frequently in nursing literature. Certainly as a nurse you will need to be aware of your responsibilities. You will also want to understand clearly to whom you are accountable for your actions. Your professional responsibilities rest on a dual framework of legal and ethical constraints.

Ethics vs. Law

Ethics are the principles of conduct governing one's relationships with others—basic beliefs about right and wrong. For example, ethics are at the basis of a decision regarding whether you will lie to your charge nurse about why you decided to stay home from work when you were not ill. There are no laws determining your action in such a situation. You make a personal decision in regard to the right action. However, because the community as a whole might agree that to pretend illness to escape work was inappropriate behavior, the employer would be supported in a decision to dismiss you from your job if you should do this on a continuing basis. Ethical decisions, therefore, have consequences both for oneself and for others. In this simple case there are multiple consequences: the employer did not have anyone to do the necessary work, patients were deprived of care, and you lost your job.

Law includes those rules of conduct or action recognized as binding or enforced by a controlling authority such as the local, state, or national government. Ethics and the law may go hand in hand, with one supporting the other. Situations in which this occurs are not difficult to understand. For example, if you choose to steal money from your employer, that would be considered unethical behavior. It would also be a violation of the law. Many laws were written to provide a basis for the community to enforce those ethical principles of conduct that were believed to be essential to the well-being of the community as a whole.

In some instances ethics may address entirely different questions than does the law. The first example of not reporting to work as expected is an instance that would not be addressed by laws, although most people would have a similar view of right and wrong in that instance.

In still other situations some people will find that the law and their own ethics are divergent. These are the most difficult circumstances in which to make decisions. An example of the law setting different standards than those set by ethics occurs in the case of a member of the armed forces killing an enemy soldier during a war. No country considers this to be an illegal act, but some people believe that such action is unethical and have therefore become conscientious objectors during times of war.

The purpose of this chapter is to show how the law affects nursing practice. Ethics are discussed more completely in Chapters 6 and 7. Examples and situations are given throughout this chapter to help you understand the specific concepts discussed. Many more factors were considered than can be presented in a brief paragraph. It is the interaction of these multiple factors that makes it impossible to make absolute predictions regarding legal outcomes in specific situations that occur in the real world of practice. The specific factual data in each case may also contribute to different decisions although they may appear similar on the surface. Different judges and juries may also interpret facts and law in various ways, resulting in dissimilar outcomes for cases that appear to be alike. To help you see how actual cases occur, summaries of actual legal cases are presented for your consideration throughout the chapter.

If you have a question about a specific personal situation, you would be well advised to consult an attorney who is experienced in medicolegal matters. The facility where you are employed may have a legal counsel who is available to you. Another source of legal aid is your nurses association attorney. If you desire private counsel, suitable names may be recommended by your local bar association.

Sources of Law

There are two general sources of law: statutory law and common law.

STATUTORY LAW

Statutory law is composed of enacted law and regulatory law. Enacted law includes laws enacted by legislative bodies such as a county or city council, a state or provincial legislature, the U.S. Congress or Parliament and carry the greatest weight in court. Nurse practice acts are in this category and are passed by state legislatures.

Regulatory law includes the rules and regulations established by governmental agencies such as licensing boards and other rule-setting bodies. Rules and regulations formulated by the State Board of Nursing are in this category. These agencies are authorized through enacted laws to establish rules and regulations. These rules and regulations have the same force as enacted law unless found by a court to be outside the scope of or contrary to the intent of the enacted law.

COMMON LAW

Common law derives from common usage, custom, and judicial decisions or court rulings. Previous judicial decisions or court cases are used to establish precedents for interpretations of both statutory and common law. These decisions are binding within the jurisdiction of that particular court but are used in a more general way for guidelines in other jurisdictions. Common law is fluid and cannot be defined with precision. In general, statutory law carries more weight in the court than does common law.

The circumstance of abandoning a patient demonstrates how common law applies to nursing. There are no statutory laws dictating that nurses cannot leave a seriously ill patient unless they ensure that someone else will provide care, but common practice and custom, which could be supported through testimony of nurses and other health care workers, require this of a nurse. Failure to meet this standard might be deemed a violation of common law.

RULINGS

A *ruling* made by a state attorney general is an attempt to provide guidelines based on an interpretation of the statutory and common law relative to a specific situation and is not a final legal decision. Different attorneys general might vary in their opinions. The validity of an opinion only stands until a court rules on the situation. The final decision in any legal issue rests with a court.

THE ROLE OF INSTITUTIONAL POLICIES AND PROTOCOLS

Institutional policies provide guidance as to the proper actions to be taken in specific situations and identify the individuals responsible for taking action. Established hospital policies may be considered by the court as indications of common usage (common law) and therefore may become important as a basis for legal decisions. They may protect the institution itself and the employees of the institution from legal difficulties if they are based on current practice and sound legal advice.

Most often policies are developed by members of the hospital staff who have expertise in the practice area under consideration. An attorney may also be consulted to ensure that policies conform to legal requirements. Final approval of policies often rests with the board of trustees, directors, or commissioners who have ultimate responsibility for the financial and legal management of the organization.

Institutional policies are changed in response to new situations and new expectations occurring in society. Usually there is an established institutional route for the change or expansion of hospital policy. Nurses may be in a position to recognize the need for such a change as they use policy and compare it with the latest professional information.

A *protocol* or *procedure* provides specific guidelines on performing a task. The purpose of protocols and procedures is to ensure that there is consistent, sound practice in an institution. Just as policies must be updated, so too should protocols or procedures.

Classification of Laws

Law can be divided into civil and criminal components. Both statutory law and common law may be subdivided in this way.

CRIMINAL LAW

The term *criminal law* applies to law that affects the public welfare as a whole. A violation of criminal law is called a *crime* and is prosecuted by the government. On conviction, a crime may be punished by imprisonment, parole con-

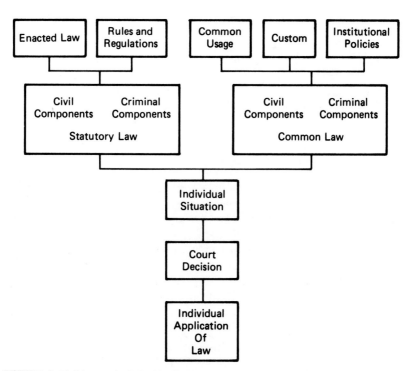

FIGURE 5–1 Civil law and criminal law both may affect a nursing situation.

ditions, a loss of privilege (such as a license), a fine, or any combination of these. The punishment is intended to deter others from committing the crime as well as to punish the violator.

CIVIL LAW

Civil law applies to laws that regulate conduct between private individuals or businesses. A *tort* is a violation of a civil law in which another person is wronged. Private individuals or groups may bring a legal action to court for breach of civil law. Judgment of the court results in a plan to correct the wrong and may include a monetary payment to the wronged party. Nurses may find themselves involved with both civil and criminal laws, either separately or within the same situation.

Criminal Law and Nursing

Because a violation of any law governing the practice of any licensed profession may be a crime, you must be aware of the extent of the Nurse Practice Act. In instances in which the Nurse Practice Act requires that actions be taken only under the direction of a physician (such as administering a drug), that explicit authorization must exist.

Standing orders that refer to specific situations as well as the usual orders written for an individual patient may be adequate authorization. However, custom or usual practice will not substitute for the specific authorization required by law. A violation of a professional practice act may be prosecuted as a crime even if no actual harm occurred to the patient.

Violation of a State Practice Act

Rowland, a registered nurse, served as the primary care provider for a woman in childbirth. She was found to be practicing midwifery without the proper certification, and the court ordered a trial on a misdemeanor complaint for the illegal practice of medicine. Practicing nurse midwives in California had to have a certificate in midwifery to provide primary care in cases of normal childbirth. The court noted that California's statute specifically prohibited individuals without the appropriate credential from treating, diagnosing, operating on, or prescribing for a woman undergoing normal pregnancy or childbirth.

Rowland v. Municipal Court of Santa Cruz County, 556 P.2d 1081, 1089 (1977) California

Situation: Violation of a Practice Act

A nurse in a physician's office is contacted by a patient. The patient describes an urgent problem that the physician commonly treats. The physician is unavailable, and there are no standing orders. The nurse proceeds to give the medication she believes the physician would have prescribed.

The Nurse Practice Act does not give the nurse the authority to diagnose disease and prescribe the medication to treat it regardless of whether this is an urgent situation. The Medical Practice Act contains this authorization. This, then, is a violation of the law and is a crime, even though the patient was not harmed.

Violation of laws related to the care and distribution of controlled substances is also a crime.

Situation: Violation of Narcotic Laws

In making the routine check of the narcotic record before going off duty, the night nurse notes that the record does not match the actual count of morphine in the supply. She is tired and does not wish to spend the time searching the record and correcting the mistake. Instead she makes a false entry for a patient who did not receive a narcotic so that the record appears correct.

Because the laws regulating the controlled substances are rigid, this would be a violation of the law.

It is costly to the state to undertake criminal prosecution; therefore, even when discovered, some violations of criminal law are not prosecuted in court. Knowing this, some nurses make the error of believing that "minor" violations are acceptable. Even when not prosecuted in court, criminal action could result in the loss of a job and in loss of a license to practice nursing.

Nurses have also been charged with such serious crimes as murder and assault that were committed while in the role of caregiver. These serious crimes are investigated, prosecuted, and tried by the criminal courts. A license to practice nursing may be temporarily withdrawn while such charges are investigated and tried. If the individual is found innocent, the license may then be restored. If the individual is convicted of the crime, the nursing license may be revoked along with other sentencing and penalties being assigned.

Civil Law and Nursing

Civil law relates to legal disputes between private parties. Malpractice actions brought in health care situations involve civil law.

TORTS

Torts are civil wrongs committed by one person against another (Bernzweig, 1990). The wrong may be physical harm, psychological harm, or harm to reputation, livelihood, or some other less tangible value. The action that causes a civil wrong may be either intentional or unintentional. An intentional tort is one in which the outcome was planned although the person involved may not have believed that the intended outcome was harmful to the other person.

Situation: Intentional Tort

An elderly, oriented, and competent patient decides to leave the hospital in the evening without medical consent, although additional treatment has been planned.

The evening nurse decides that this patient needs the planned treatment and should not be allowed to leave. She removes the patient's clothes from the room, disconnects the telephone so that the patient cannot call for a taxi, and tells the patient that he will not be allowed to leave.

The patient expresses anger and states that he will leave as soon as he finds a way. The next morning he makes a call to his son and leaves the hospital.

The nurse purposefully acted to keep the patient in the hospital against his will. This was her planned intent. Even though she thought it was in the patient's best interests, the patient felt wronged by losing his liberty and freedom of action. A court would generally agree that loss of liberty is a wrong. If legal action is taken, the nurse may be found to have committed an intentional tort (that is, a planned wrong to another person occurred).

An unintentional tort is a wrong occurring to another person or property, although it was not intended to happen. The most common cause of an unintentional tort is negligence.

NEGLIGENCE

Negligence is the failure to act as a reasonably prudent person would have acted in a specific situation (Guido, 1992). If harm is caused by negligence, it is termed an *unintentional tort* and damages might be recovered. *Negligence* is a broad term that has many applications throughout society. All negligence has the following four essential characteristics (Fiesta, 1994):

1. Harm must have occurred to an individual.
2. One person must be in a situation where he or she had a duty toward the person harmed.
3. The person must be found to have failed to fulfill his or her duty. This is called "breach of duty." This might include either doing what should not have been done (commission of an inappropriate action) or failing to do what should have been done (omission of a necessary or appropriate action).
4. The harm must be shown to have been caused by the breach of duty.

Each of these points must be addressed in any legal action. The presence of harm is often clear. For example, if a person has a fractured hip, no one would dispute that this was harm. When the harm is so clear that anyone would agree on it, the term *res ipsa loquitur* is used. This is Latin for "the thing speaks for itself." In this case the harm does not need to be "proved" to the court because all would agree that a fractured hip is a harm. However, all harm is not so straightforward. For example, when a person claims emotional suffering, the court must determine whether harm actually occurred.

Situation: Negligence

A homeowner fails to repair a broken step at the entrance to his home. He fails to warn a guest of the broken step and the guest trips on the broken step in the dark and is injured.

Negligence could be charged. The injury is the harm; the homeowner has a duty toward a guest to safeguard that guest from foreseeable harm; a reasonably prudent person would have repaired the step or at least warned the guest; and the injury can be shown to be a direct result of the homeowner's failure to act prudently.

Res Ipsa Loquitur

The patient underwent an appendectomy and awakened with sharp pain between his neck and his right shoulder. He received diathermy treatments, but the pain increased and then began to radiate down his right arm. Eventually he was unable to lift or rotate muscles on the right. After the patient brought suit, two physicians testified that the injury was caused by a trauma or strain applied to his right shoulder and neck during surgery. At the time of the trial no operating room personnel offered any reason for the injury. It could not be proven that the patient was under one person's exclusive control when the injury occurred.

The court found that in a case in which an unconscious patient receives injury during the course of treatment, all of those involved in the treatment may be found negligent under the doctrine of *res ipsa loquitur* (the thing speaks for itself). In other words, the injury occurred and the hospital personnel were responsible for the patient during the time when it occurred; therefore, hospital personnel were responsible for the injury.

Ybarra v. Spangard 154 P.2d 687 (1945) California

MALPRACTICE

Malpractice is a term used for a specific type of negligence. It refers to the negligence of a specially trained or educated person in the performance of his or her job. Therefore, *malpractice* is the term used to describe negligence by nurses in the performance of their duties.

The definition of malpractice is almost the same as the definition of negligence with one modification. The professional person must have had a *professional duty* toward the person injured. For example, the nurse is acting as a nurse for the person (this may be either a paid or volunteer activity). Additionally the harm that occurred to the injured person or to the property must be based on failure to act as a reasonably prudent *professional* would have acted in the situation. This is a higher standard than required of the general public (Bernzweig, 1990).

Just as all parts of the situation are clear in some general negligence situations and not in others, the professional duty is similarly clear in some instances and not in others. The nurse who is assigned to care for a patient in a hospital clearly owes a duty to that patient. In some situations duties overlap and more than one nurse might have a duty toward the same patient. Whether a supervisor, another nurse on the unit, or a nurse visitor has a professional duty might be in dispute. Again the court would decide whether a duty was present.

A breach of duty is a failure to act according to the standards of the profession for that situation (Fiesta, 1994). To determine that a breach of duty was present, the court would have to determine what represents the standard of professional practice for that situation.

The final question then becomes one of identifying the cause of the harm that occurred. Malpractice is only present if the breach of duty was the cause of the harm. In the case of a fractured hip, if the nurse failed to raise the side rail and turned the patient to the side of the bed and off onto the floor, the failure to safeguard the patient (breach of duty) could be shown to be a direct cause of the fall and fractured hip (the harm). The cause of harm is not always so clear and may be part of the dispute in a legal action.

Situation: Omission of Correct Action

An elderly, disoriented person is admitted to an acute care facility. The nurse fails to establish a plan for monitoring and maintaining safety for this person. The patient falls out of bed, sustaining a fractured hip.

This could be found to be malpractice. The nurse was working in a professional capacity and had a duty to this patient. The patient can be shown to

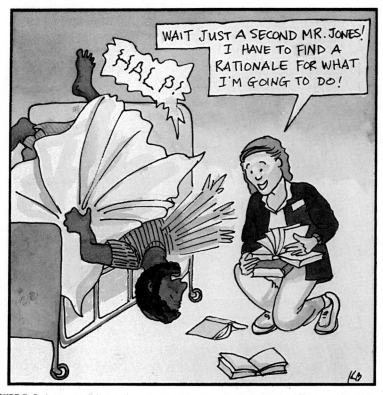

FIGURE 5–2 A reasonably prudent nurse uses common sense as well as nursing theory.

have an injury. It may be demonstrated through testimony by nurses and by reference to standard nursing texts that a reasonably prudent registered nurse would have been expected to take action to protect this patient from falls. It was this failure to act that caused the fall and fracture. This failure to act could then constitute malpractice.

Situation: Commission of Inappropriate Action

A postoperative patient has an order to ambulate. The nurse assigned to this patient finds that the patient's condition has changed drastically since the order was written. The patient has a fever and a rapid pulse and is complaining of severe acute abdominal pain. The nurse proceeds to have the patient ambulate. The patient faints, sustaining a head injury in the fall. This necessitates additional hospitalization, x-ray films, and diagnostic procedures.

Direct Causation of Harm in Malpractice

A patient developed a postoperative infection of the eye following cataract surgery. Scarring of the cornea developed, and after years of unsuccessful treatment for the infection the eye was removed. The patient and a witness both stated that a nurse had picked up an eye patch that had fallen on the floor and applied it directly to the patient's eye. The infection that developed after this event was due to the cultured organisms of *Enterobacter* (a common bowel pathogen) and *Staphylococcus albus* (a common skin pathogen). Despite the testimony about the nurse's action, the patient lost his suit because he was unable to prove that the organisms came from the floor (a lack of causality between the act and the harm that resulted).

DeFalco v. Long Island College Hospital, 393 N.Y.S. 2d 859 (1977) New York

Again, this could be found to be malpractice. The nurse was working as a professional with a duty to this patient. The patient can be shown to have sustained injury. It may be demonstrated that a reasonably prudent nurse would have recognized that the change in the patient's condition called for altering the plan of care and not ambulating at this time. This was the breach of duty. Ambulating the patient in that condition was the cause of the fall and the head injury. Therefore, malpractice could be found owing to inappropriate action on the part of the nurse.

Liability

A person found guilty of any tort (whether intentional or unintentional) is considered legally *liable*, or legally responsible, for the outcome. The person legally liable usually is required to pay for damages to the other person. This may include actual costs of care, legal services, loss of earnings (present and future), and compensation for emotional and physical stress suffered. A *liability*, then, is an obligation or debt.

PERSONAL LIABILITY

As an educated professional, you are always legally responsible or liable for your actions (Bernzweig, 1990). Thus, if a physician or supervisor instructs you to do something that is contrary to your best professional judgment and says, "I'll take responsibility," that person is acting unwisely. The physician or supervisor giving the directions may also be liable if harm results, but that would not remove your personal liability.

Situation: Personal Liability

The registered nurse giving medications on a large medical unit notes that an order for digoxin (a heart medication) is considerably larger than the usual dose. She looks up the medication in a reference book and finds her view of the dose size confirmed. The ordered dose is several times the usual dose. The nurse then calls the supervisor and explains the situation.

The supervisor double checks the order with the registered nurse and then states: "Dr. Jones is an outstanding physician. I am sure he has a good reason for ordering this dose. Go ahead and give the medication as ordered." The nurse then gives the medication, and the patient suffers a toxic reaction.

The registered nurse would likely be held liable for giving the incorrect amount of medication. She had the knowledge and judgment to recognize the dose as erroneous and failed to check with the physician. A statement by the supervisor does not remove the nurse's personal responsibility for her own actions. Because even a competent physician might make an error, the nurse had a responsibility to clarify that order. The supervisor and the physician could be held liable in addition to the nurse but not instead of her.

Although each person is legally responsible for his or her own acts, the example above illustrates that there are also situations in which a person or organization may be held liable for actions taken by others.

EMPLOYER LIABILITY

The most common situation in which a person or organization is held responsible for the actions of another is the employer–employee relationship. In many instances the employer can be held responsible for the torts committed by an employee. This is called the doctrine of respondeat superior (let the master respond). The law holds the employer responsible for having hired qualified persons, for establishing an appropriate environment for correct functioning, and for providing supervision or direction as needed to avoid errors or harm. Therefore, if the nurse, as an employee of the hospital, is guilty of malpractice, the hospital may also be be named in the suit. The employer's liability may exist even if the employer appears to have taken precautions to prevent error.

It is important to understand that this doctrine does not remove any responsibility from the individual nurse, but it extends responsibility to the employer in addition to the nurse. If, for example, a hospital has a procedure that does not conform to good nursing practice as you know it and you follow that procedure, you will still be liable for any resulting harm. You are expected to use your education and training to make sound judgments regarding your work.

Situation: Employer Responsibility for a Staff Nurse

A nurse working in a long-term care facility is giving medications at night. In an attempt to not disturb the patient, she gives an injection in a darkened room, gives it in the wrong location, and hits a nerve.

Both the nurse in this situation and the long-term facility might be found liable for the harm that resulted. The nurse had a personal, professional responsibility in giving medications. The facility also had a responsibility for making sure that employees carry out procedures safely and correctly.

CHARITABLE IMMUNITY

In some states nonprofit hospitals have "charitable immunity." This means that the nonprofit hospital cannot be held legally liable for harm done to a patient by its employees. The employees of that nonprofit hospital are still legally liable for their own actions. The trend in legislation is toward the repeal of laws providing for charitable immunity. Those active in the consumer movement have argued that no institution should be relieved of responsibility in such a blanket fashion. If you are employed by a nonprofit institution, it is important that you know whether the law in your state provides for charitable immunity for the institution.

SUPERVISORY LIABILITY

When a nurse is in the role of charge nurse, head nurse, supervisor, or any other category in which the job involves supervision or direction of other persons, there is a potential for liability for the actions of others. The supervising nurse is responsible for exercising good judgment in a supervisory role. This includes making appropriate decisions about assignments and delegation of tasks. If an error occurs and the supervising nurse is shown to have exercised sound judgment in all decisions made in that capacity, the supervising nurse may not be held liable for the error of a subordinate. If poor judgment was used in assigning an inadequately prepared person to an important task, the supervisory nurse might be liable for resulting harm. The extent of the subordinate's responsibility would rest on his or her level of education and training. Persons without education or training might not be liable for some errors. The more education subordinates have, the more likely they will be liable also.

Situation: Supervisory Responsibility for an Educated Staff Member

Two sudden admissions to the coronary care unit create a situation in which additional help is needed to care for the patients in the unit.

The staff supervisor calls the person whose name appears first on the list of temporary placement registered nurses. This nurse agrees to come in immediately. The nurse is not asked whether she has education or experience in coronary care, nor does she volunteer this information. She has no background or experience in coronary care.

While working in the coronary care unit, the temporary nurse is assigned the complete care of two patients. Because of her lack of ability to read the monitors, a potentially life-threatening problem is not identified until the patient "arrests." Resuscitation efforts are successful, but the patient suffers some brain damage.

Both the staffing supervisor who placed the inadequately prepared nurse in the unit and the temporary nurse herself could be found liable—the supervisor for incorrectly assigning the nurse and the nurse for not recognizing her own limitations. The educational preparation of the temporary nurse gave her the background to understand that expertise was needed in this situation and that she herself did not possess that expertise. If that situation were changed so that the temporary nurse was reviewed for expertise in coronary care and found to have that expertise, then the supervisor might not be liable for the error of the temporary nurse. The supervisory function of ascertaining level of preparation and ability to meet the standards of the job would have been carried out.

> ### Situation: Supervisory Responsibility for Staff Member With Limited Education
>
> The evening nursing supervisor is responsible for adjusting personnel assignments when employees are absent. She decides to send an extra aide to the emergency department to assist. This aide has never been assigned to the emergency department before and has no education or training other than the orientation to direct care given by the hospital. The supervisor instructs the aide to take care of the desk and answer the phone while others are busy.
>
> While the aide is alone at the desk, a family enters the emergency department with an infant in acute distress. The aide instructs the family to sit down and wait until a nurse comes out of one of the rooms.
>
> It is a long time before the nurse appears and care for the infant is instituted. The infant has a complicated recovery that later could be shown to be due to the delay in initial treatment.

The supervisor might be found negligent in this case for assigning the aide to emergency department duties without proper direction or supervision. The aide might not be found negligent because she had no basis for recognizing the seriousness of the situation nor for recognizing her own lack of ability to meet the responsibilities involved in being at the desk in an emergency department.

Liability Insurance

Liability insurance transfers the costs of being sued and of any settlement from the individual to a large group. The expectation is that most individuals would not be sued and that therefore the pool of premiums will adequately cover the costs of those who are sued, the administrative costs of managing the policies, and the profit for the insurance company. The individual benefits by transferring risk from himself or herself to the insurance company for the cost of the insurance policy.

Currently a liability insurance crisis exists in the United States. The cost of liability insurance has escalated at an extraordinary rate. Some of the factors that have caused this to happen are the large judgments that have been made, the number of suits that have been brought, the large fees that attorneys receive, and the high profits of insurance companies. Nurses in advanced practice have been especially affected by the increase in premiums because their incomes have traditionally been moderate and they cannot raise fees enough to cover insurance costs that may equal those of physicians.

The American Nurses Association (ANA) has initiated a data bank related to legal claims against nurses. The organization is asking all registered nurses to provide information to it regarding legal action in which they have been named as a defendant. The ANA's purpose is to have adequate records to support its contention that the low level of suits against nurses should translate into low-cost liability insurance.

Some states have initiated legislation that allows for awards to cover actual losses and costs of care, while limiting awards for pain and suffering and other nontangible factors. Sometimes this has been accompanied by restrictions on insurance company rates. Some laws are also being amended to restrict the monetary liability of any party to the percentage of responsibility. For example, if damages were set at $10,000 and each of two defendants were determined to be responsible for 50% of the problem, one party could not be made to pay more than $5000, even if the other party had no assets and could not pay. Liability laws continue to be a major concern for nurses because nurses are being named in an increasing number of suits.

INSTITUTIONAL AND INDIVIDUAL INSURANCE

When a suit is brought, liability insurance pays for attorney's fees and the costs of your defense as well as for a settlement or judgment up to the limits of the policy. Many hospitals or other institutional employers carry liability insurance that covers both the institution and its employees. Some hospitals may limit the coverage that their policies provide for individual employees in an effort to hold down costs.

Even if an employer carries liability insurance, it is often advisable for the individual professional to carry an independent policy. An independent policy may cover the person in voluntary activities as well as on the job. It also will follow the person who moves from one employer to another. If a legal action is instituted against the professional, the individual liability insurance policy may provide independent legal counsel.

Some nurses state that they do not carry insurance because it might encourage people to bring suit against them. They are under the mistaken assumption that persons will not sue if it means financial hardship for the person being sued. This is an error because most individuals who sue do not know whether the nurse carries individual insurance. In addition, insurance is not the only source of payment for a judgment. Judgments may be levied against most tangible assets, such as a house, a car, or savings, as well as against future earnings. Married nurses who reside in community property states should realize that one half of the assets of the family may be vulnerable to a judgment reached. Community property states at this time include Arizona, California, Idaho, Louisiana, Nevada, New Mexico, Texas, and Washington. These factors combine to support the need for the individual professional to carry liability insurance that will provide legal counsel and protection in the case of any judgment.

ANALYZING INSURANCE COVERAGE

Individual liability insurance for registered nurses is available from a variety of insurance companies directly through their agents and through professional organizations that offer coverage as a service to members. When investigating individual liability insurance, ask the agent or company the following questions:

1. In what situations would I, as an individual, be covered?
2. In what situations would I not be covered?
3. How is my coverage affected by my actions? For example, if I failed to follow hospital policy, would I still be covered?
4. What are the monetary limits of the policy?
5. Does the policy provide me with an attorney?
6. Is the policy renewable at my option? What factors affect renewability?
7. Does the insurance cover incidents that occurred while the policy was in force, regardless of when the claim is brought (*claims occurred insurance coverage*), or does it cover incidents only if I am currently insured (*claims brought insurance coverage*)?
8. What is the cost compared with other policies?

Liability insurance coverage that is carried by the hospital should be carefully investigated by the nurse employee. "Full coverage" is not a very informative statement. Questions 1 through 4 above apply to institutional policies as well as to individual policies. In addition, you should ask the following questions in regard to an institutional policy:

1. Does the policy provide me with an individual attorney, or will the same attorney be working for the hospital?
2. At what point would the hospital no longer be responsible and would I become personally responsible?
3. How would my job be affected if a lawsuit is filed or payment is awarded based on the action against me? (Check institutional policy as well as the insurance company policy.)

4. Does the insurance company have the right to seek restitution from me if it pays a claim based on my actions?

It is important that you have accurate answers to these questions so that you can make an informed decision regarding your need for an individual policy.

INSURANCE COST AND COVERAGE

The ANA has a group policy providing $500,000 per claim and $1 million total in 1 year as basic coverage for the registered nurse. Optional higher limits are available. The cost for basic coverage in 1994 was approximately $89 per year. Inflation can be expected to increase this cost. Since the 1970s, the cost of the basic coverage provided by the ANA policy rose from approximately $12 per year to its current amount.

Liability insurance coverage for specialty practice as a nurse practitioner, nurse anesthetist, or nurse midwife is a much greater problem. Some insurance companies have refused to cover these groups. Others have dramatically increased costs. Nursing organizations are working to resolve this problem. Group policies are available for some of these individuals through professional organizations. Other individuals are covered by institutional policies and do not try to maintain individual policies.

Legal Issues in Nursing

Some individual issues recur continually in nursing practice. It is wise for the nurse to consider and try to understand these particular issues as they relate to individual practice.

DUTY TO REPORT OR SEEK MEDICAL CARE FOR A PATIENT

A nurse who is caring for a patient has a legal duty to ensure that the patient receives safe and competent care. This duty requires that the nurse maintain an appropriate standard of care and also that the nurse take action to obtain an appropriate standard of care from other professionals when that is necessary. For example, if a nurse identifies that a patient needs the attention of a physician and fails to make every effort to obtain that attention, the nurse has breached a duty to the patient.

Situation: Failure to Seek Medical Care for Patient

The registered nurse is caring for a postoperative patient during the night. The patient's blood pressure begins to drop and the pulse begins to rise. The nurse's assessment indicates that the patient may be bleeding internally. The nurse institutes a plan for close nursing monitoring and calls the surgeon to describe the situation. The surgeon gives a telephone order to increase the intravenous fluid rate and states that he will see the patient in the morning. The patient's condition continues to deteriorate, but the nurse does nothing further to ensure that a physician examines the patient.

If the outcome is unfavorable, the nurse can be found to have breached a duty to the patient. The patient relies on the nurse to provide appropriate care and to identify when a physician is needed. The nurse could have made other telephone calls to the surgeon and failing the success of that could have followed the facility's procedure for asking another physician (such as the emergency department physician) to see the patient.

The nurse has a duty to continue all efforts to try to obtain appropriate medical care for the patient. If the nurse had followed all procedures, sought another physician, and continued efforts when initial attempts were unsuccessful, the nurse would not have breached a duty. The nurse cannot guarantee a physician's care but can guarantee that the patient will not be left without an advocate.

CONFIDENTIALITY AND RIGHT TO PRIVACY

Confidentiality and the right to privacy with respect to one's personal life are basic concerns in our society. This right has been inferred from interpretation of the federal constitution, but is explicitly stated in some state laws. With increased computerization of records, which can result in easier retrieval and cross-referencing of records from a variety of sources, the general public is becoming more concerned about potential invasions of privacy.

All information regarding a patient belongs to that patient. A nurse who gives out information without authorization from the patient or from the legally responsible guardian can be held liable. If you have any question about who the legally responsible guardian is, be sure to consult with your administrative authority. There may be a court-appointed legal guardian, or the situation may be governed by specific state laws regarding who becomes the responsible guardian when the person is unable to give personal consent. The hospital administration should be able to ascertain the correct guardian.

Only those professional persons involved in the patient's care who have a need to know about the patient can be allowed routine access to the record. A physician who is not involved in the patient's care or who does not have an administrative responsibility relative to that care is not allowed routine access. Persons not involved in care can only be allowed access to the record by specific written authorization or by court order.

You should be cautious about what information you share verbally and with whom. In some instances, especially those involving treatment for alcoholism, drug abuse, and acquired immunodeficiency syndrome, even revealing the diagnosis or reasons for hospitalization would be considered a legal violation of confidentiality.

A directory information policy has been adopted by many acute care hospitals. This policy gives specific guidelines about what must be revealed according to freedom of information laws but will not violate confidentiality. Usually you are allowed to reveal the patient's name and gender and a general statement of condition (satisfactory, serious, and so on). If your hospital has no written policy, this is a wise standard to follow.

Medical records professionals state that it is not uncommon for attorneys, family members, media representatives, or law enforcement officials to request access to patient records or specific patient information without having express consent of the patient or a legal court order to view the record or be given information. Those unfamiliar with laws regarding privacy sometimes reveal information inappropriately. If you are ever approached for patient information by someone who purports to have authority, your best course of action is to refer that individual to appropriate administrative personnel who can determine the validity of the request.

Situation: Breach of Confidentiality

A well known political figure is hospitalized for a hysterectomy. The registered nurse in charge on the evening after the surgery answers the telephone. The call is from a man who identifies himself as a reporter from the community newspaper. He states that he has heard of the hospitalization and wonders how the patient is doing. The nurse responds that the patient is doing as well as could be expected for someone who has just had a hysterectomy for possible cancer. The column written in the paper suggests that because the political figure has cancer, she is an inappropriate candidate for office in the next election, and this becomes a major campaign issue.

The nurse could be held liable in a suit charging breach of privacy and confidentiality for revealing this information to the press.

DEFAMATION OF CHARACTER

Any time that shared information is detrimental to the person's reputation, the person sharing the information may be liable for defamation of character. Written defamation is called libel. Oral defamation is called slander. Defamation of character involves communication that is malicious and false. Sometimes such comments are made in the heat of anger. Occasionally statements written in the chart are libelous. Severely critical opinions may be stated as fact. An example of such a statement might be "The patient is lying," or "The patient is rude and domineering." Patients may charge that these comments in the chart adversely affected their care by prejudicing other staff against them. The prudent nurse will chart only objective information regarding patients and give opinion in professional terms, well documented with fact. In conversations the prudent nurse avoids discussing patients.

Situation: Slander

Two registered nurses are leaving the floor for their coffee break. They are discussing the patients in their care as they wait for the elevator. They enter the elevator with a number of other people and continue their conversation. The first nurse says: "That Mrs. Johnson in room 201. I don't know whether I can take another day of her! She's impossible!" The other nurse replies: "I know just what you mean. I had her last week and she was just on the bell all the time. If you ask me, there's nothing wrong with her that a good swift kick wouldn't cure!" First nurse: "Do you really think she's faking?" Second nurse: "I'm sure of it. Have you ever watched her when her husband comes to visit?"

A relative of the patient is one of the people in the elevator and overhears the conversation. The relative reports the conversation to the patient.

If the patient brings suit, the nurses involved might be found guilty of slander. The nurses were discussing the patient in a place where others could hear the conversation. The comments clearly identified the patient, reflected opinions that were not supported with fact, and potentially could jeopardize the patient's reputation and standing in the community.

Defamation of character may also be charged by a health care provider who believes that statements made by another professional are false, malicious, and have caused harm. There are accepted mechanisms for confidentially reporting inappropriate care or errors. These should be used rather than making critical statements to uninvolved third parties. In many states licensed professionals are required to report poor practice or illegal acts on the part of other professionals. Criticism reported without malice and in good faith through appropriate channels is protected from legal action for defamation of character.

Defamation of Character

A nurse in an emergency department made derogatory remarks about certain hospital physicians during a committee meeting. She was asked to resign because of her statements. She filed suit stating that this was an infringement of her rights of free speech. The court upheld the hospital in asking for her resignation because it was not her comments but the place in which she voiced them that was inappropriate.

Bach v. Mount Clemens General Hospital, Inc., 449 F. Suppl 686 (1978)

The federal government is now maintaining the National Data Bank on licensed health care providers. All judgments paid or convictions for malpractice and situations in which privileges to practice are curtailed or withdrawn must be reported to this data bank. All institutions must consult this data bank for information before giving any health care provider privileges. The purpose of the National Data Bank is to protect the public from incompetent professionals who continue to practice by moving from one place to another.

PRIVILEGED INFORMATION

Privileged communication refers to information shared with certain professionals that does not need to be revealed even in a court of law. All states consider certain types of communication between client and attorney, between patient and doctor, or between an individual and a member of the clergy as privileged. Not all states recognize the nurse–patient relationship as one in which privileged communication exists. Even in those states that recognize nurse–patient communication as potentially being privileged, *all* communication between patients and nurses is not considered privileged. It is important that you understand that privilege is a limited concept. Only a court can determine if privilege exists in any specific case. If the court does not determine information to be privileged, then you are legally obligated to testify about the communication.

INFORMED CONSENT

Everyone has the right to make decisions about oneself. Part of the right to make one's own decisions is the right to either consent to or refuse medical treatment.

Legal Requirement

The law requires that the person give voluntary and informed consent. *Voluntary* means that no coercion existed; *informed* means that the person clearly understood the choices being offered. Included in the discussion must be the alternatives for treatment, the risks of any treatment proposed, the relative value of any treatment proposed, and the risks of not having treatment. This consent may be either verbal or written. Written consent usually is preferred in health care to ensure that a record of consent exists, although a signature alone does not prove that the consent was informed. A blanket consent for "any procedures deemed necessary" is not usually considered adequate consent for specific procedures. The form should state the specific proposed medical procedure or test.

The patient's medical condition is usually not accepted by the courts as a valid reason for not giving complete and accurate information. Currently there are no clear guidelines as to what constitutes complete information. Courts have generally supported the idea that usual risks need to be disclosed but that rare or unexpected risks do not have to be discussed.

The law places the responsibility for obtaining consent for medical treatment on the physician. It is the physician's responsibility to provide appropriate information, and he or she is liable if the patient charges that the appropriate information was not given.

Responsibility for Informed Consent

An elderly woman came to the hospital for cataract surgery. She signed the usual hospital consent form. After the surgery the woman became blind. She brought suit against the physician and the hospital contending that she had not been informed that this was a possible complication of the surgery. The court held that the hospital was not liable because the responsibility for informed consent rested with the physician.

Cooper v. Curry, 589 P.2d 201 (New Mexico, 1978)

The nurse may present a form for the patient to sign, and the nurse may sign the form as a witness to the signature. This does not transfer the legal liability for informed consent for medical care to the nurse. If the patient does not seem well informed, it would be prudent for the nurse to notify the physician so that further information can be given. Although the nurse would not be legally liable for the lack of informed consent, the nurse has ethical obligations relative to assisting the patient to exercise his or her rights and to assisting the physician in providing appropriate care.

Advance Directives

Advance directives are legal documents attesting to the wishes of an individual in regard to health care in situations where he or she is no longer capable of giving personal informed consent. They are completed in "advance" of the situation in which they might be needed and "direct" the actions of others. Advance directives may specify a person assigned to provide consent when the individual is incapacitated. A *durable power of attorney for health care* is a document that legally assigns responsibility for making health care decisions to a person chosen for that role. This document may also contain specific advance directives such as whether tube feedings, intravenous fluids and nutrition, ventilator support, and other such treatments should be instituted if the individual is found to be terminally ill or in a persistent vegetative state.

Situation: An Advance Directive in Action

An elderly person was admitted with terminal cancer. He indicated that he had discussed his wishes with his family and had decided that he did not want to be resuscitated if "anything" happened. With the help of his attorney, the patient had prepared an advance directive stating his wishes. The nurse informed the patient that he had the right to make these decisions, but that it was important to discuss them with his physician as well. The advance directive was placed on the patient record. She notified the physician who met with the patient and family members. The physician then noted this family meeting in the patient's record and on the physician's orders wrote "Do Not Resuscitate in accord with advance directive."

In 1990, the Patient Self-Determination Act (PSDA) was passed by the U.S. Congress. It took effect in 1992 and required that on admission to any health care service (hospital, long-term care center, or home care agency) clients be given an opportunity to determine what lifesaving or life-prolonging actions they wanted to be carried out. The agency must provide adequate information for the individual to make an informed decision regarding these important matters. As a result of this legislation, agencies reviewed and revised policies and protocols regarding consent. In many agencies a nurse has the responsibility to provide the education and obtain a signature on a document indicating preferences.

Information regarding the results of the PSDA is being analyzed by several government agencies to determine whether there has been a change in practice. Some have suggested that the manner in which self-determination and the possible alternatives are explained greatly influences the patient choices made. One suggestion for change has been that these matters first be discussed in the health care provider's office before admission. When this is possible, it would allow for more time to consider alternatives and consult significant others. The final decision could then be made away from the pressure of the health care environment.

Consent for Nursing Measures

Nurses must obtain consent for nursing measures undertaken. This does not mean that exhaustive explanations need to be given in each situation because courts have held that patients can be expected to have some understanding of usual care. Consent for nursing measures may be verbal or implied. The nurse may ask, "Are you ready to ambulate now?" The patient answers, "Certainly," providing verbal consent. Alternatively the nurse may state, "I have the injection the doctor ordered for you. Will you please turn over?" If the patient turns over, this is implied consent.

The nurse should remember that the patient is free to refuse any aspect of care offered. However, just as in the case of the physician, the nurse is responsible for making sure that the patient is informed before making a decision. Good nursing care requires that you use all means at your disposal to help the patient comprehend the value of the proposed care. For example, the postoperative patient needs to understand that getting into a chair is part of the plan of care, not a convenience for the nurse or simply a change to prevent boredom. Thus, a patient's refusal of care is accepted after the patient has been given complete information so that an informed decision was made.

Right to Refuse Treatment

A 23-year-old woman who was a Jehovah's Witness refused to have a blood transfusion because of her religious beliefs. The hospital asked the court to require that she have the transfusion because it was necessary to save her life. The court upheld her right to refuse the transfusion because an adult of sound mind has a right to refuse treatment.

St. Mary's Hospital v. Ransey, 465 So2d 666 (Fla. App. 1985)

The confused or disoriented patient presents a different problem in terms of consent. If the person truly is not capable of making decisions, then the nurse should attempt to present necessary nursing actions in a way that elicits cooperation and avoids confrontation over decisions. When this is not possible, consent may be obtained from the legal guardian.

Withdrawing Consent

Consent may be withdrawn after it is given. People have the right to change their minds. Therefore, if after one intravenous infusion the patient decides not to have a second one started, that is his or her right. As a nurse you have an obligation to notify the physician if the patient refuses a medical procedure or treatment.

Consent and Minors

For a minor, consent usually is given by a parent or legal guardian. You should also obtain the minor's consent when he or she is able to give it. Courts are emphasizing increasingly that minors be allowed a voice in their own lives when it concerns matters that they are capable of understanding. This is especially true for the adolescent, but you need to consider it with any child who is 7 years of age or older. When the minor refuses care and the legal guardian has authorized that care, you should not proceed until legal clarification is given. Your nursing supervisor should be consulted.

Minors who live apart from their parents and are financially independent or who are married are termed *emancipated minors*. In most (but not all) states an emancipated minor can give consent to his or her own treatment. Some states have additional specific laws allowing minors to give personal consent without also obtaining parental consent for treatment of sexually transmitted disease or for obtaining birth control information and supplies. You would need to be sure of the law in your own state if you practice in an area where this would be a concern. Most institutions have developed policies to guide employees in making correct decisions in this and other areas dealing with consent.

Consent and the Mentally Incompetent

For a person who is legally determined to be mentally incompetent, consent is obtained from the legal guardian. A legal guardian is constrained from making some types of decisions. For example, if the health care action could be identified as injurious to the individual involved, a court may need to be consulted regarding consent. An example of this would be sterilization. This could be interpreted as injurious because it permanently removes the potential of becoming a parent.

Health care providers often encounter those for whom no legal determination of competence has been made but who do not seem able to make an informed decision. This might include the very confused elderly person, the inebriated person, or the unconscious person. The law in each state specifies who is allowed to give consent in such situations. There are also guidelines to follow in making the decision that the person cannot give his or her own consent. Your facility policy should contain directions to guide you in obtaining a legal consent. If it does not, you should consult an administrative person for a decision. Determining who is able to give legal consent in such a situation is not a nursing responsibility.

EMERGENCY CARE

Care in emergencies has many legal repercussions. If a true emergency exists, consent for care is considered to be implied. The law holds that if a reasonable person were aware that the situation was life threatening, he or she would give consent for care.

An exception to this is made if the person has explicitly rejected such care in advance, such as a Jehovah's Witness who is carrying a card stating his personal religion and that he does not wish to receive blood or blood products. This is one reason emergency department nurses should check a patient's wallet for identification and information related to care. If this is done with another person and a careful inventory of contents is made and signed by both, there should be little concern for liability for taking such an action.

Institutional Emergency Care

The judgment that an emergency exists is important because certain actions may be legal in emergencies and not legal in nonemergency situations. The issue of consent is affected by the determination that an emergency exists. Standards of practice for emergencies also differ from those for nonemergency situations.

Most facilities that provide emergency care have policies designed to ensure that there is adequate support for claiming that an emergency exists. Thus, the policy will often state that in the emergency department at least two physicians must examine the patient and concur that the emergency requires immediate action without waiting for consent. This ensures maximum legal protection for the physician and the institution.

In hospital emergencies the nurse sometimes may be in the position of identifying an emergency and that the needed action is one that only a physician usually performs. If "life or limb" is truly in danger, the courts have held that the nurse can do those immediate things necessary even if they usually are considered a medical function, provided the nurse has the essential expertise to perform the action safely and correctly. The hospital would be expected to have a policy, which the nurse would follow, to verify and document the situation fully. This usually involves consultation with a supervisory nurse and verification of the emergency situation as well as attempts to obtain medical assistance.

Situation: Nursing Action in a Hospital Emergency

In an orthopedic unit it is common to care for patients with new casts. A young man with a newly applied long-leg cast is admitted via the emergency department at 6 PM. The nurse assigned to this patient's care carefully makes all the appropriate observations throughout the evening and documents his findings. He notes that the leg is beginning to swell and that the edges of the cast are beginning to cut into the skin. At that time the nurse notifies the supervisor that a problem is developing and that he thinks the physician should be notified. The supervisor agrees and the nurse begins to try to contact the physician. Continuous observations are made, noting increasing swelling, color changes in the exposed toes, and loss of sensation. The physician cannot be reached and no other physician is immediately available. After consultation with the supervisor, the nurse decides that an emergency exists and that the cast needs to be cut open to relieve the pressure. Cutting a cast open is considered a medical procedure in this hospital. The nurse has been taught to use a cast cutter and is familiar with the procedure. The nurse, with the supervisor's approval, cuts open the cast and secures it in place with an elastic bandage. All observations made, consultations carried out, attempts to notify the physician, and the final action taken are carefully documented in the chart. Hospital policy was followed throughout the situation to ensure that all necessary steps had been taken.

Although going beyond usual nursing practice, this would not be considered a violation of either the nursing or the medical practice acts because an emergency existed and the results of inaction would have been serious. Additionally, the nurse had the expertise and was prepared to carry out the necessary action safely. This emergency care is usually limited to specific technical procedures that the nurse has learned. It does not include diagnosing disease or prescribing medication unless there are specific standing orders relative to the situation.

Noninstitutional Emergency Care

Emergencies encountered outside the health care environment present other problems. Anyone rendering aid in an emergency is expected to behave as a reasonably prudent person would in such a situation. The nurse rendering aid in an emergency must behave as a reasonably prudent nurse in that situation. Thus, the standard is higher than for the nonprofessional person, although the nurse is not expected to perform as if he or she were in an institutional setting. The physical situation and the psychological situation are both considered when determining what is reasonably prudent nursing action.

All states and Canadian provinces have "Good Samaritan" statutes that encourage health care professionals to give aid in emergency situations. The first of these statutes was enacted in California in 1959 (Bernzweig, 1990). These statutes vary in content and comprehensiveness but relieve a professional of some liability when reasonable care is used. These laws often make people feel more secure when rendering aid.

Each nurse must make an individual decision about rendering emergency aid in a specific situation. This involves ethical as well as legal considerations. If the profession of nursing is a public trust and nurses are truly involved in the business of caring, then failure to come to the aid of an individual who is in serious danger is an ethical violation of that trust. To this date there has been no instance of a nurse being sued for coming to the aid of someone in an emergency situation (Bernzweig, 1990; Fiesta, 1994). Professional liability insurance does provide coverage when the nurse assists in this way and that fact may make you feel more comfortable about rendering emergency aid.

In many states emergency personnel must render all possible aid including all resuscitative measures when they are called to an emergency situation. This has resulted in situations in which a family member of a terminally ill person has called 911 because of a concern, rescuers arrived, and the person was resuscitated although he or she had clearly stated that resuscitation was not desired. As more individuals receive terminal care in their homes, this has become an increasing concern. Legislation allowing for patient self-determination in regard to emergency responders has now been passed in some states. The law usually stipulates the precise circumstances in which an individual may provide an advance directive in regard to emergency procedures and how that must be documented for emergency personnel to be able to honor these wishes.

FRAUD

Fraud is a deliberate deception for the purpose of personal gain and is usually prosecuted as a crime. Situations of fraud in nursing are not common. One example would be trying to obtain a better position by giving incorrect information to a prospective employer. By deliberately stating that you had completed a nurse practitioner program to obtain a position for which you would otherwise be ineligible, you are defrauding the employer. This may be prosecuted as a crime because you also put members of the community in danger of receiving substandard care. You may also commit fraud by trying to cover up a nursing error to avoid legal action. Courts tend to be more harsh in decisions regarding fraud than in cases involving simple malpractice because fraud represents a deliberate attempt to mislead others for your own gain and could result in harm to those assigned to your care.

Situation: Fraud

A registered nurse is giving medications to the patients to whom she is assigned. When presenting a patient with his pills he states that he was sure the doctor had discontinued the red pill because he had a reaction to it the evening before. The nurse states that she is sure these are the correct medications. The patient takes the pills and the nurse charts the medications. The patient subsequently has a reaction. The nurse becomes frightened, goes back, and alters the medication record to make it appear that the medication was not given.

This situation could be considered fraud. The deception was the changing of the record and the personal gain was freedom from responsibility for the error.

ASSAULT AND BATTERY

Assault is saying or doing something to make a person genuinely fear that he or she will be touched without consent. Battery is unconsented or unlawful touching of a person. Neither of these terms implies that harm was done. Harm may or may not have occurred.

For an assault to occur, the person must be afraid of what would happen, even if the threatening person would not or could not carry out the threat. "If you don't take this medication, I will have to put you in restraints" is an example of an assault. For battery to occur, the touching must occur without consent. Implied consent is acceptable. Therefore, if the patient extends an arm for an injection, he cannot later charge battery, saying that he was not asked. But if the patient agreed because of a threat (assault), the touching would still be considered battery because the consent was not freely given.

If you have an order to give a patient an iron injection and the patient says, "No. I had one of those before and they hurt!" and you persist and give the injection, a charge may be filed against you for battery. This is true even though the iron greatly benefited the patient and was a valid physician's order. The patient always has the right to refuse treatment.

Assault and Battery

A patient was involuntarily committed to a mental hospital. She was a practicing Christian Scientist. When she refused to take medications, she was held down and given an injection by a nurse. She brought suit and recovered damages for assault and battery because the court found she was not dangerous to herself or others and had not been found incompetent and therefore she could not be compelled to take medication.

Winters v. Miller, 446 F2d 65 (1971)

FALSE IMPRISONMENT

Making a person stay in a place against his wishes is false imprisonment. The person can be forced to stay by using either physical means or verbal means. It is easy to understand why restraining a patient or confining a patient to a locked room could constitute false imprisonment if proper procedures were not first carried out.

Keeping a patient confined by nonphysical means is perhaps less clear. If you removed a patient's clothes for the express purpose of preventing his leav-

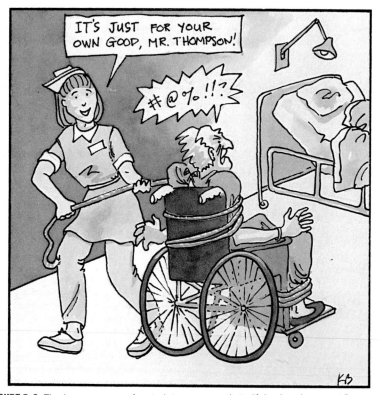

FIGURE 5–3 The improper use of restraints may constitute "false imprisonment."

ing, you could be liable for false imprisonment. Threats to keep a person confined, such as "If you don't stay in your bed, I'll sedate you," can also constitute false imprisonment. Any time a patient needs to be confined for his or her own safety or well-being, it is best to help the person understand and agree to that course of action. If the patient is not responsible, the guardian or legal representative may give permission. (This returns to the issue of who may give consent.) The third alternative is to objectively document the need in the patient's record and obtain a physician's order as soon as possible. Be sure to follow the policies of the facility.

In the conventional care setting you cannot restrain or confine responsible adults against their wishes. All persons have the right to make decisions for themselves, regardless of the consequences. The patient with a severe heart condition who defies orders and walks to the bathroom has that right. You protect yourself by recording your efforts to teach the patient the need for restrictions and by reporting the behavior to your supervisor and the physician.

In the same context, the patient cannot be forced to remain in a hospital. If a patient wants to leave against medical advice, that is the patient's right. Again, you document your efforts in the record and follow applicable policies to protect the facility, the physician, and yourself from liability. The example of an intentional tort given earlier in this chapter involved false imprisonment.

A hospital may not detain a patient for nonpayment of a bill. The hospital is free to take legal action against the person who does not pay, but refusing discharge would also constitute false imprisonment.

False imprisonment suits are a special concern in the care of the psychiatric patient. Some particular laws relate to this situation. In the psychiatric setting you may have patients who have voluntarily sought admission. The same restrictions on restraint or confinement that apply to the patients in the general care setting apply to these patients. Other patients in the psychiatric setting may have been committed involuntarily through the applicable laws of the state. Specific measures may be used to confine the involuntarily committed patient. These are usually defined by law in terms of situations covered, type of restraint allowed, and length of time restraining may be used. If you work in a psychiatric setting, you should review the specific policies that have been developed about restraint to protect clients and assist staff in functioning within the legal limits.

Factors That Contribute to Malpractice Claims

When poor results or harm do occur in the course of nursing practice, they usually are not followed by a suit. An understanding of some of the factors that enter into whether a suit is instituted may help you.

SOCIAL FACTORS

Much is being written about changes in the public's attitudes toward health care personnel. Health care is big business, and patients complain increasingly of not being known individually. This results in a patient being more willing to bring suit against someone who is part of the large, impersonal system.

Health costs are high, and some people see hospitals and physicians as having the ability to pay a large settlement, whether directly or through insurance. If the patient's own income is lessened or disrupted by the illness, he or she might bring suit as a solution to economic difficulties. Increased public awareness of the size of monetary judgments that have been awarded may also be an economic incentive to instituting a suit.

SUIT-PRONE PATIENTS

Some people are more likely to bring suit for real or imagined errors. If these people are recognized as being suit-prone patients, it is possible for you to protect yourself through increased vigilance in regard to care and by special emphasis on thorough record-keeping. Although we would warn you to guard against stereotyping, these general descriptions may help you to avoid problems. Suit-prone patients usually are identified by overt behavior in which they are persistent fault finders and critics of personnel and of all aspects of care. They may be uncooperative in following the plan of care and sensitive to any perceived slight.

Persons who exhibit hostile attitudes may extend their hostile feelings to the nurses and other health care persons with whom they have contact. The nurse who becomes defensive in the face of hostility only widens the breach in the nurse–patient relationship. It is necessary to pay careful attention to those principles for care learned in psychosocial nursing that dealt with how to help the hostile patient. Assisting patients to solve their own problems and supporting the patients are the best protection for the nurse.

Another type of patient who appears more suit-prone is the very dependent person who uses projection to deal with anxiety and fear. These individuals tend to ascribe fault or blame for all events to others and are unable to accept personal responsibility for their own welfare. Again, meeting these patients' needs with a carefully considered plan of care is the answer.

A common error when confronting a suit-prone patient is for staff to become defensive and withdraw. This is done partly because the situation is unpleasant and partly because staff members feel personally threatened by the patient's behavior. This increases the likelihood of a suit if a poor result occurs.

Another possible nursing response to the suit-prone patient is to become more directive and authoritarian. This tends to increase the patient's feeling of separation and distance from the staff and again increases the likelihood of suit.

If the staff is helped to view the patient as a troubled person who manifests his or her problems in this manner, sometimes they find it easier to be objective. The patient is in need of all the nursing skill that the prepared nurse can bring to the emotional problems. The suit-prone patient does not always end up suing. Much depends on the response of health care personnel.

SUIT-PRONE NURSES

Nurses may also be suit-prone. A nurse who is insensitive to the patient's complaints, who does not identify and meet the patient's emotional needs, or who fails to identify the limits of his or her own practice may contribute to suits instituted not only against the nurse but also against the employer and the physician. The nurse's self-awareness is critical in preventing suits.

Preventing Malpractice Claims

The most significant thing you can do to prevent malpractice claims is to maintain a high standard of care. To do this you may work at improving your own nursing practice and also the general climate for nursing practice where you work. You can do this in a variety of ways.

SELF-AWARENESS

Identify your own strengths and weaknesses in practice. When you have identified a weakness, seek a means of growth. This may include education, directed experience, or an opportunity for discussion with colleagues.

Be ready to acknowledge areas of weakness to supervisors, and do not accept responsibilities for which you are not prepared. The nurse who has not worked in pediatrics for 10 years and accepts an assignment to a pediatric unit without orientation and education is setting the stage for an error to occur. Lack of current familiarity with the area is not a defense against liability. As a professional you should not accept the position if you cannot meet the criterion of being a reasonably prudent nurse in that setting. In instances of true emergency (eg, disaster, flood), courts may be more lenient, but "we need you here today" is not an emergency.

ADAPTING PROPOSED ASSIGNMENTS

Nurses may find themselves assigned to units where they have little or no experience with the types of patient problems they will encounter. It is reason-

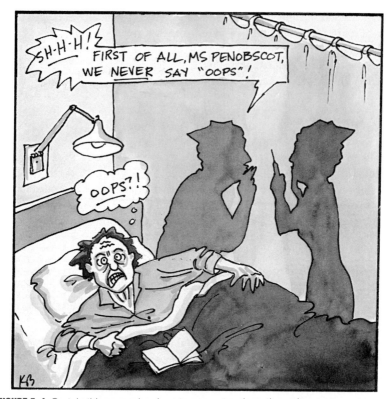

FIGURE 5–4 Certain things can be done to prevent malpractice suits.

able to be assigned to assist an overworked nurse in a special area if you can assume duties that are within your own competence and allow the specialized nurse to assume the specialized duties. It is not reasonable or safe for you to be expected to assume the specialized duties. Thus, if you are not prepared for coronary care, you might go to that unit, monitor the intravenous lines, take vital signs, and make observations to report to the experienced coronary care nurse. The experienced nurse would then be able to check the monitors, administer the specialized medications, and make decisions. Note that this does fragment the patient's care and would not be appropriate as a permanent solution but could alleviate a temporary problem in a safe manner.

FOLLOWING POLICIES AND PROCEDURES

It is your responsibility to be aware of policies and procedures of the employing institution. If they are sound, they can be an adequate defense against a claim, providing they were carefully followed.

For example, the medication procedure may involve checking all medications against a central medication Kardex. If you have done this and there was an error in the Kardex, you might not be liable for the resulting medication error. You had followed all appropriate procedures and acted responsibly. The liability would rest with the person who made the error in transcribing the medication from the physician's orders to the Kardex. If, however, you had not followed procedure in checking, you might also be liable because you did not do your part in preventing error. As discussed previously, policies are often designed to provide legal direction.

CHANGING POLICIES AND PROCEDURES

As nursing evolves, changes are needed in procedures. Part of your responsibility as a professional is to work toward keeping all procedures up to date. These are part of nursing expertise. Are there written policies to deal with emergency situations? Statements such as "Oh, we've always done it this way" are not adequate substitutes for clearly written, officially accepted policies. Often facilities that are reluctant to make changes based on the suggestions of individual nurses are much more receptive to new ideas when the legal implications of outmoded practice are noted.

DOCUMENTATION

Nurses' records are unique in the health care setting. They cover the entire period of hospitalization, 24 hours a day, in a sequential pattern. Your record can be the crucial factor in avoiding litigation. Documentation in the record of observations made, decisions reached, actions taken, and the evaluation of the patient's response are considered much more solid evidence than verbal testimony, which depends on one's memory.

For legal purposes, observations and actions that are not recorded may be assumed not to have occurred. Properly kept records may also protect you from becoming liable for the error of another by demonstrating that you did all in your power to prevent harm, including consulting with others. Because each case is determined by the facts as well as by the applicable law, clear documentation of all relevant data is important.

One concern expressed regarding problem-oriented records and charting "by exception" is that these formats may provide less detailed information and may be less helpful in defense against litigation. This does not have to be the case. You can use any system of charting and record-keeping to provide appropriate and adequate documentation of care. If you identify something that needs to be recorded and cannot find a provision within your system to make that recording, you can be sure that others have experienced the same difficulty. You might begin inquiries toward establishing a clear mechanism for the record-keeping that concerns you. When nurses serve on committees to review and plan charting procedures, it is wise for them to seek consultation with the attorney for the facility. This would help ensure that the plan for record-keeping is legally sound as well as professionally useful.

The Nurse as Witness

In the course of your practice as a registered nurse a time may arise when you will be asked to serve as a witness in a legal proceeding. There are two kinds of cases that would involve the nurse as a witness to the facts in a specific case.

The first type is a personal injury action in which a person has been injured, for example, in an automobile accident and you or your organization has been involved in the care of that person. Your testimony in that case might be on behalf of the person to help describe the injuries and the care received for those injuries. For example, you may be asked to testify regarding the care given in a burn center to a victim of an electrical accident who received considerable nursing care during the recovery period.

The second type of lawsuit that involves the nurse as witness to specific facts is one in which a patient brings a lawsuit against persons or organizations who have provided health care that the patient believes was below the standard of the community. Medical malpractice is therefore alleged. The nurse may be included in those who are charged with malpractice. For example, you may have to give evidence regarding medical record notes or care given to the patient in the days before the alleged malpractice occurred. In both of these situations the concern is with the specific factual details of that particular case.

The nurse may also be involved in a lawsuit as an expert witness. An expert witness, under Rule 702 of the Federal Rules of Evidence, accepted in the federal courts and many state courts, is defined as "a witness qualified as an expert by knowledge, skill, experience, training, or education" who may testify in the form of an opinion or otherwise. The purpose of testimony as an expert witness is to provide information and opinion that can be used by the court in making a decision. When you appear as an expert nursing witness, your testimony provides an opinion that will assist the judge or jury to understand complex areas of nursing care. This includes a professional opinion that relates to your area of expertise on the appropriate care for a given situation. For example, if you are an operating room nurse, you may be given medical records from another hospital and asked to render an opinion, on the basis of your expertise, whether the standard of nursing care given at the first hospital was within the standards of the community. Your role as an expert may not be accepted without question in a legal action. You may have to clearly state the qualifications, both education and experience, that enable you to make a judgment.

When you become involved in any legal action, you should be sure that you understand both your rights and your obligations in regard to legal action.

DISCOVERY

In a civil lawsuit, one between parties for the recovery of money damages, a lengthy discovery process leads up to the trial itself. Often cases are settled before trial by the testimony developed in the discovery process. Discovery involves gathering information through document examination, interrogatories (written questions answered under oath), and depositions.

A deposition is a formal proceeding in which each attorney has an opportunity to question the witness, and a sworn verbatim record is made by a court reporter (Guido, 1992). Depositions are often held in attorneys' offices or in the health care facility for the convenience of the health care providers. Sometimes depositions are taken to preserve the testimony of a witness for trial under certain circumstances and are used in place of live testimony at trial. Most depositions in which you would participate, however, would be depositions for discovery purposes.

TESTIMONY AS A WITNESS IN DEPOSITION OR AT TRIAL

When you are being asked to consult as an expert witness, your role is based on your knowledge of nursing practice. When you are asked to testify as a witness to *fact*, you will be testifying to the exact situation and circumstances of the event or events in question. You should always consult an attorney before talking to anyone about a matter in which you have been asked to testify, especially a malpractice action.

The attorney who asks you to testify as an expert witness should be able to provide you with information you need about your testimony. Feel free to inquire of that attorney what your role is in the case and in which areas your testimony is expected. The attorney is likely to discuss at length what questions will be asked of you and ask you what your answer would be to those questions.

When nurses are asked to testify as to the facts of a situation, they sometimes believe that because they have done nothing wrong they do not need legal counsel. The law is complex, and you could jeopardize the position of an institution for which you work, or even jeopardize yourself and your professional future, with unwise statements. The person who is bringing suit may alter or amend the original complaint to involve new defendants including you. If you have liability insurance, you should advise your insurance company and an attorney will be assigned to talk with you. If you are covered by an employer's policy, you should consult with the appropriate administrative representative immediately to obtain legal counsel. This attorney should assist you in understanding the questions in the case, your role, and how you can protect yourself in the situation.

As a witness, you will be required to swear or affirm to tell the entire truth. Failure to do this is perjury. You are expected to answer the questions asked of you to the best of your ability; however, you do not have to provide an answer that would incriminate yourself, nor do you have to answer a question for which you do not remember or know the answer. It is perfectly permissible to state "I do not remember" or "I do not know" if you do not.

It is helpful if you use words and terms that can be understood by those who are not familiar with medical terminology or explain medical terminology where its use is essential. If hypothetical situations or cases are presented for your response, be sure to note the differences between the hypothetical case and the one currently under consideration before you respond.

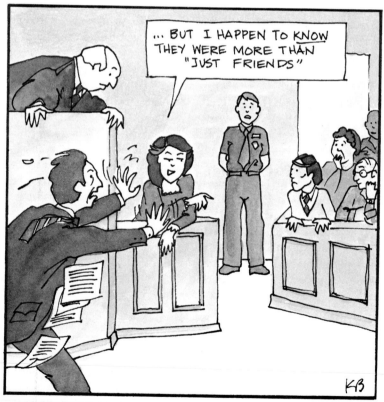

FIGURE 5–5 When testifying in court you should answer only the questions asked. Do not introduce other information.

Be brief and direct when answering questions. Do not volunteer additional information that has not been asked for by the attorney. You may open up entire areas of inquiry that would not be considered without your comments. It is the attorney's job to ask the question so as to bring out the facts to which he or she wants you to testify. The opposing attorney will have an opportunity on cross-examination to ask you additional questions that the attorney believes are necessary for the facts of the case. However, be cautious about simply answering "yes" or "no." In some instances an explanation is essential if the simple answer is not to sound as if you did not perform appropriately (Aiken, 1994).

Key Concepts

▷ Ethics are principles of conduct governing one's relationships with others. Law includes those rules of conduct or action recognized as binding or enforced by government.

▷ Statutory law is enacted by legislative bodies, whereas regulatory law includes those rules and regulations established by administrative bodies within the government.

▷ Civil law encompasses those laws regulating private conduct between individuals. Criminal law regulates actions having to do with the safety of the community as a whole. Violations of criminal law are considered crimes, whereas violations of civil law are considered torts.

▷ Malpractice actions brought against health care workers involve civil law. Nurses may be involved in cases related to torts, negligence, or malpractice.

▷ In any situation in which a person is found guilty, the individual is legally liable. Liability may be focused at the individual, the supervisor, or the employer.

▷ Liability insurance may be purchased that transfers the cost of being sued and the cost of any settlement from the individual to a large group.

▷ A number of legal issues recur in nursing. Among these are the duty to report or seek medical care for a patient, protection of the patient's confidentiality and the right to privacy, defamation of character, privileged information, the various issues related to informed consent, and issues related to different types of emergency care.

▷ Nurses can also be involved in cases related to fraud, assault and battery, and false imprisonment.

▷ A number of factors contribute to malpractice claims. These include social factors, suit-prone patients, and suit-prone nurses.

▷ A nurse can do many things to prevent malpractice claims. Being aware of your own practice, accepting only those assignments for which you are prepared, following policies and procedures, and doing proper documentation are among the most important.

▷ Nurses may be called as witnesses in trials because of their expertise in a particular area or because of personal involvement in the case being tried. It is important that you understand both your rights and your obligations in regard to legal action.

CRITICAL THINKING ACTIVITIES

1. At what point in accepting a new position in a community hospital would you think it appropriate to ask to review the hospital policy manual? How would you go about this process? How would you proceed if the person you asked acted as though you were out of line in your request?

2. After observing a colleague for several months you believe her practice is such that she might be in jeopardy of being sued one day. What is your responsibility in this case? Should you discuss this with your colleague? If yes, how?

3. After you have obtained your first job, will you purchase personal malpractice insurance? Why or why not?

4. You have been called as a witness to testify in a malpractice case against a local orthopedic surgeon. You are anxious about testifying. How can you best prepare for this? From whom can you seek assistance and guidance?

5. A good neighbor friend experiences some unfortunate episodes of extremely poor care in a local hospital where you are employed. She discusses these with you and asks your advice regarding initiating a suit. What are your obligations in this situation, both as a friend and as a professional? If you need help reaching a decision, to whom can you turn?

References

Aiken TD. Legal, Ethical, and Political Issues in Nursing. Philadelphia: FA Davis, 1994

Bernzweig EP. The Nurse's Liability for Malpractice, 5th ed. St. Louis: C.V. Mosby, 1990

Fiesta J. The Law and Liability, 2nd ed. New York: John Wiley & Sons, 1994

Guido GW. Legal Issues in Nursing: A Source Book for Practice. Norwalk, CT: Appleton-Lange, 1992

Further Readings

Calderon E. 1989 Immigration Nursing Relief Act. J Nurs Adm 23(1):5–6, 1993

Carson W. Nursing and professional boundaries: Legal barriers to practice. Am Nurse 25(2):24, 1993

Edmunds MW. Council's pursuit of national standardization for advanced practice nursing meets with resistance. Nurse Pract 17(10): 81–83, 1992

Horty JF. Healthcare law. Mod Health Care (regular column)

Lawsuits: An ounce of prevention. Nursing 20(5):146, 1990

The legal side. Am J Nurs (regular feature)

Regan Reports on Hospital Law. Providence: Medica Press (quarterly publication)

Regan Reports on Medical Law. Providence: Medica Press (quarterly publication)

Regan Reports on Nursing Law. Providence: Medica Press (quarterly publication)

Regan WA. Legally speaking. RN (regular column)

Regan WA. OR nursing law. AORN J (regular column)

Rx: Avoid "speculation" & "admissions" in charting. Regan Reports on Nursing Law 30(10):2, 1990

Sangermano C. The Patient Self-Determination Act. Semin Perioperative Nurs 1(4):232–239, 1992

Schirm V, Gray M, Peoples M. Nursing personnel's perceptions of physical restraint use in long term care. Clin Nurs Res 2(1):98–110, 1993

Tammelleo AD. Court upholds nurse's refusal to float. Case in point: Winkleman v. Beloit Memorial Hospital (483 N.W. 2d 211—WI[1992]). Regan Reports on Nursing Law 33(2):2, 1992

Varga K. How to protect yourself against malpractice. Imprint 36(5):33–34, 36–37, 1989

Weiler K. Patient self-determination: Is anyone really listening? J Gerontol Nurs 19(10):42, 1993

Wold JL. The living will: Legal and ethical perspectives. J Neurosci Nurs 24(1):50–53, 1992

6

Ethical Concerns in Nursing Practice

Objectives

After completing this chapter, you should be able to

1. Explain how personal religious and philosophical viewpoints, the Code for Nurses, and the Patient's Rights document are used as bases for ethical decision-making.

2. Analyze the relationships between basic ethical concepts in ethical decision-making.

3. Describe four ethical theories that may be used when considering ethical problems.

4. Explain how sociocultural factors affect ethical decision-making for nurses.

5. Discuss the various occupational factors that influence decision-making.

6. Outline a framework for ethical decision-making.

7. Discuss how ethics relates to commitment to the patient/client, commitment to personal excellence, and commitment to nursing as a profession.

8. Review the ethical and legal obligations related to the chemically impaired nursing colleague.

Ellis JR, Hartley CL: NURSING IN TODAY'S WORLD:
CHALLENGES, ISSUES, AND TRENDS, 5th ed.
© 1995 J.B. Lippincott Company

Concerns about right and wrong and good and evil are ethical issues that relate to fundamental beliefs in our society. These concerns have always been with us, and each generation has examined its own issues and the setting in which they occur and has made its own decisions. In our generation, the advent of advanced technology has created problems that previous generations could not have imagined. In the same way, future generations may confront ethical concerns that we have not yet envisioned. Because of a number of societal factors that have placed these problems squarely before us, ethical issues are being intensively discussed and debated.

Many of the issues discussed in this chapter and the next are controversial and emotionally charged. Controversy often creates conflict. Conflicts may exist in values, in opinions, in solutions, and in judgments. As you read about these issues and discuss them in your classroom or with a classmate, we urge you to respect others by carefully listening to them and honestly attempting to understand their position with its accompanying values and beliefs. Only by considering all aspects of an issue can we seek and find understanding for ourselves. Understanding the issues involved allows us to deal more positively with the personal stress we may experience in our own lives as we attempt to find answers to ethical questions.

Throughout these chapters we emphasize personal decision-making as the basic task when confronted with an ethical question. Ethical decision-making cannot be avoided in nursing. Issues constantly confront us. Some nurses are tempted to back away and say, "That is not my concern," but the old saying "Not to decide is to decide" was never more true. Doing nothing is indeed making a decision. Decision-making is often uncomfortable because we are left with a choice between alternatives, of which none is good or desirable. Dealing with the pain as well as the joy of life is part of being human. As we personally confront difficult decisions we can learn to become more supportive and caring toward the clients, families, and coworkers with whom we work.

A Basis for Decision-Making

All persons must determine their own basis for making ethical decisions. Some people rely on formal philosophical or religious beliefs that define matters in relation to what is believed to be the truth or good and evil. Others make a decision by attempting to weigh what will result in the greatest good for the greatest number. Still others reach a decision on the basis of personal life experience or on the basis of the experience of someone dear to them. By these and other mechanisms people come to different conclusions when confronted with ethical problems.

A dilemma may be created when you find that different values, each of which is important to you, would lead to opposing actions. Conflict may be created when you and another individual are led to differing ethical conclusions regarding the same set of facts. Many times it is possible and appropriate for you to accept another person's ethical decision as appropriate for that person; however, at other times your own position will cause you to say, "I must oppose this action." This may bring you into direct conflict with others. When this occurs, we urge you to be constructive not destructive in the methods you choose to work toward your personal goals.

PERSONAL RELIGIOUS AND PHILOSOPHICAL VIEWPOINTS

Your personal viewpoint certainly will be a major factor influencing your ethical decision-making. Achieving self-understanding in values is a lifelong learning task, and undoubtedly your position on various issues will change as you move through life. Values represent the concepts, ideals, behaviors, social principles, and major themes that give meaning to our personal life and make us unique. Values are the product of our life experiences and are influenced by family, friends, culture, environment, education, and many other conditions. Because of this our values may change.

Values clarification is a process that includes assessing, exploring, and determining personal values. It also includes identifying the priority a particular value holds in our process of personal decision-making. Often we do not fully explore our own values until we are confronted with a specific situation in which a decision is necessary. Recognizing your own value system before being confronted with a personal problem is a goal of the classes, seminars, and books on the topic of values clarification. Although you should not feel pressured to alter your personal value system, it is important for you to seriously explore your own feelings and beliefs about various issues.

Religious beliefs form the basis for ethical decision-making for some people. However, a person who is a member of a particular religious group may not ascribe to all of the beliefs of that group. Individuals make their own decisions with regard to each situation, and that attitude may not parallel the doctrine of their religious group. For example, some Muslims maintain that women should be completely separated from men and wear veils when in the presence of men. They would find any health care setting that did not respect this belief to be in conflict with basic values. Other Muslims do not adhere to this strict interpretation of Islamic law, and women wear modest clothing but do not wear veils. They would be more comfortable in most Western health care settings because they would not feel a conflict with their personal values.

Nursing offers a wide variety of job opportunities to the new graduate. In choosing a job, certainly you cannot expect to avoid all conflict or problem situations, but you probably would want to avoid working in an area in which

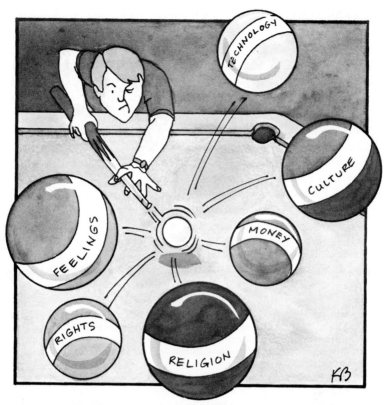

FIGURE 6–1 Decisions made in relation to one aspect of an ethical situation will affect all other aspects of the problem.

there was constant conflict. Before you accept a position, you may want to consider whether it holds the potential to create conflict with your basic beliefs. For example, if you are ethically opposed to abortion, it would be wise to avoid employment on an obstetric unit where therapeutic abortions are routinely performed. In this situation, making your views known and refusing certain assignments after you had begun employment might result in termination because the employer may justifiably assert that you agreed to fulfill all the responsibilities of the position when you accepted employment.

Similarly, your personal value system might lead you to work in a particular area in which you have identified a strong ethical commitment. For example, the hospices for the dying in England were begun by religious groups who saw value in the life of the person who was dying. Their religious beliefs were and have continued to be part of their approach to care. If you strongly value your own ethnic or cultural approach to health care, you might choose to work in a health care setting where that approach is part of the philosophy.

CODES FOR NURSES

Through their professional organizations, nurses have developed some common guidelines to use in making ethical decisions. They are contained in the American Nurses Association's (ANA) Code for Nurses, and the International Council of Nurses Code for Nurses. Each attempts to outline the nurse's responsibilities to the client and to the profession of nursing.

The ANA code is somewhat unique among professional codes because it addresses fairly specific issues and does not confine itself to matters of etiquette or broad general statements. Warren T. Reich, editor in chief of the *Encyclopedia of Bioethics*, was quoted as stating, "This is probably the most interesting and responsive code I have ever read" (New Encyclopedia, 1977, p 8). Tentative codes were presented by nurses in the 1920s, the 1930s, and the 1940s. Finally, in 1950, a code of ethics was adopted. It has been revised several times since then, most recently in 1976. Early versions stated that the

---

A. N. A. CODE FOR NURSES

1. The nurse provides services with respect for human dignity and the uniqueness of the client unrestricted by considerations of social or economic status, personal attributes, or the nature of health problems.
2. The nurse safeguards the client's right to privacy by judiciously protecting information of a confidential nature.
3. The nurse acts to safeguard the client and the public when health care and safety are affected by the incompetent, unethical, or illegal practice of any person.
4. The nurse assumes responsibility and accountability for individual nursing judgments and actions.
5. The nurse maintains competence in nursing.
6. The nurse exercises informed judgment and uses individual competence and qualifications as criteria in seeking consultation, accepting responsibilities, and delegating nursing activities to others.
7. The nurse participates in activities that contribute to the ongoing development of the profession's body of knowledge.
8. The nurse participates in the profession's efforts to implement and improve standards of nursing.
9. The nurse participates in the profession's efforts to establish and maintain conditions of employment conducive to high quality nursing care.
10. The nurse participates in the profession's effort to protect the public from misinformation and misrepresentation and to maintain the integrity of nursing.
11. The nurse collaborates with members of the health professions and other citizens in promoting community and national efforts to meet the health needs of the public.

(Reprinted by permission of the American Nurses' Association)

FIGURE 6–2 ANA Code for Nurses.

nurse had an obligation to carry out physician's orders; later versions, however, stress the nurse's obligation to the client. This includes protecting the client from incompetent, unethical, or illegal practice.

The International Council of Nurses' Code was most recently revised in 1973. The introductory section of this code speaks of the general responsibilities of the nursing profession. Five sections follow, dealing with the more specific concerns of people, practice, society, coworkers, and the profession. In addition, the International Council of Nurses has written a Pledge for Nurses, which is a statement of affirmation and acceptance of the personal and ethical responsibilities of being a member of the nursing profession. Both of these documents can serve as guidelines for ethical conduct.

THE PATIENT'S RIGHTS

The patient's rights are another consideration in decision-making. Ideally we have always recognized this in some ways. As early as 1959, the National League for Nursing formulated a statement regarding patient's rights. However, for many years health care professionals assumed the attitude that they knew what was best for patients and made many decisions without consulting with or considering the rights of the patient/client. For example, the patient with a specific disease was not offered information about possible treatment alternatives, even when valid alternatives did exist. The patient's physician made the decision regarding which treatment method was preferable, and that was the only one presented to the patient. Today we consider this an example of paternalism.

As the health consumer movement became more active, greater attention was paid to the rights of the patient. Today patients may expect to be informed of all alternatives for treatment and often want to participate in making the decision about type of treatment, including both the possible benefits and the risks of the treatment methods presented. The law has also supported the right to informed decision-making.

In 1973, the American Hospital Association published A Patient's Bill of Rights, which outlines the rights of the hospital patient and serves as a basis for making decisions about hospitalized patients. Some have criticized this document, saying that it is rather innocuous because it simply reminds patients of their rights (such as privacy, confidentiality, and informed consent) but says nothing of hospitals that fail to act in accordance with these rights. The AHA revised this document in 1992. In the Introduction, hospitals are encouraged to modify and adapt the AHA document to their individual situations and communities. The revised document speaks more forcefully regarding the hospital's responsibility for providing medically indicated care and services. In addition, it emphasizes the collaborative nature of health maintenance which requires patient responsibility as well as provider responsibility.

Introduction

Effective health care requires collaboration between patients and physicians and other health care professionals. Open and honest communication, respect for personal and professional values, and sensitivity to differences are integral to optimal patient care. As the setting for the provision of health services, hospitals must provide a foundation for understanding and respecting the rights and responsibilities of patients, their families, physicians, and other caregivers. Hospitals must ensure a health care ethic that respects the role of patients in decision making about treatment choices and other aspects of their care. Hospitals must be sensitive to cultural, racial, linguistic, religious, age, gender, and other differences as well as the needs of persons with disabilities.

The American Hospital Association presents A *Patient's Bill of Rights* with the expectation that it will contribute to more effective patient care and be supported by the hospital on behalf of the institution, its medical staff, employees, and patients. The American Hospital Association encourages health care institutions to tailor this bill of rights to their patient community by translating and/or simplifying the language of this bill of rights as may be necessary to ensure that patients and their families understand their rights and responsibilities.

Bill of Rights*

1. The patient has the right to considerate and respectful care.
2. The patient has the right to and is encouraged to obtain from physicians and other direct caregivers relevant, current, and understandable information concerning diagnosis, treatment, and prognosis.

   Except in emergencies when the patient lacks decision-making capacity and the need for treatment is urgent, the patient is entitled to the opportunity to discuss and request information related to the specific procedures and/or treatments, the risks involved, the possible length of recuperation, and the medically reasonable alternatives and their accompanying risks and benefits.

   Patients have the right to know the identity of physicians, nurses, and others involved in their care, as well as when those involved are students, residents, or other trainees. The patient also has the right to know the immediate and long-term financial implications of treatment choices, insofar as they are known.
3. The patient has the right to make decisions about the plan of care prior to and during the course of treatment and to refuse a recommended treatment or plan of care to the extent permitted by law and hospital policy and to be informed of the medical consequences of this action. In case of such refusal, the patient is entitled to other appropriate care and services that the hospital provides or transfer to another hospital. The hospital should notify patients of any policy that might affect patient choice within the institution.

These rights can be exercised on the patient's behalf by a designated surrogate or proxy decision maker if the patient lacks decision-making capacity, is legally incompetent, or is a minor.

(continues)

FIGURE 6–3 The Patient's Bill of Rights.

4. The patient has the right to have an advance directive (such as a living will, health care proxy, or durable power of attorney for health care) concerning treatment or designating a surrogate decision maker with the expectation that the hospital will honor the intent of that directive to the extent permitted by law and hospital policy.

   Health care institutions must advise patients of their rights under state law and hospital policy to make informed medical choices, ask if the patient has an advance directive, and include that information in patient records. The patient has the right to timely information about hospital policy that may limit its ability to implement fully a legally valid advance directive.

5. The patient has the right to every consideration of privacy. Case discussion, consultation, examination, and treatment should be conducted so as to protect each patient's privacy.

6. The patient has the right to expect that all communications and records pertaining to his/her care will be treated as confidential by the hospital, except in cases such as suspected abuse and public health hazards when reporting is permitted or required by law. The patient has the right to expect that the hospital will emphasize the confidentiality of this information when it releases it to any other parties entitled to review information in these records.

7. The patient has the right to review the records pertaining to his/her medical care and to have the information explained or interpreted as necessary, except when restricted by law.

8. The patient has the right to expect that, within its capacity and policies, a hospital will make reasonable response to the request of a patient for appropriate and medically indicated care and services. The hospital must provide evaluation, service, and/or referral as indicated by the urgency of the case. When medically appropriate and legally permissible, or when a patient has so requested, a patient may be transferred to another facility. The institution to which the patient is to be transferred must first have accepted the patient for transfer. The patient must also have the benefit of complete information and explanation concerning the need for, risks, benefits, and alternatives to such a transfer.

9. The patient has the right to ask and be informed of the existence of business relationships among the hospital, educational institutions, other health care providers, or payers that may influence the patient's treatment and care.

10. The patient has the right to consent to or decline to participate in proposed research studies or human experimentation affecting care and treatment or requiring direct patient involvement, and to have those studies fully explained prior to consent. A patient who declines to participate in research or experimentation is entitled to the most effective care that the hospital can otherwise provide.

11. The patient has the right to expect reasonable continuity of care when appropriate and to be informed by physicians and other caregivers of available and realistic patient care options when hospital care is no longer appropriate.

FIGURE 6–3 *(Continued)*

12. The patient has the right to be informed of hospital policies and practices that relate to patient care, treatment, and responsibilities. The patient has the right to be informed of available resources for resolving disputes, grievances, and conflicts, such as ethics committees, patient representatives, or other mechanisms available in the institution. The patient has the right to be informed of the hospital's charges for services and available payment methods.

The collaborative nature of health care requires that patients, or their families/surrogates, participate in their care. The effectiveness of care and patient satisfaction with the course of treatment depend, in part, on the patient fulfilling certain responsibilities. Patients are responsible for providing information about past illnesses, hospitalizations, medication, and other matters related to health status. To participate effectively in decision making, patients must be encouraged to take responsibility for requesting additional information and instructions. Patients are also responsible for ensuring that the health care institution has a copy of their written advance directive if they have one. Patients are responsible for informing their physicians and other caregivers if they anticipate problems in following prescribed treatment.

Patients should also be aware of the hospital's obligation to be reasonably efficient and equitable in providing care to other patients and the community. The hospital's rules and regulations are designed to help the hospital meet this obligation. Patients and their families are responsible for making reasonable accommodations to the needs of the hospital, other patients, medical staff, and hospital employees. Patients are responsible for providing necessary information for insurance claims and for working with the hospital to make payment arrangements, when necessary.

A person's health depends on much more than health care services. Patients are responsible for recognizing the impact of their life-style on their personal health.

Conclusion

Hospitals have many functions to perform, including the enhancement of health status, health promotion, and the prevention and treatment of injury and disease; the immediate and ongoing care and rehabilitation of patients; the education of health professionals, patients, and the community; and research. All these activities must be conducted with an overriding concern for the values and dignity of patients.

A patient's Bill of Rights was first adopted by the American Hospital Association in 1973. This revision was approved by the AHA Board of Trustees on October 21, 1992.

©1992 by the American Hospital Association, 840 North Lake Shore Drive, Chicago, Illinois 60611. Printed in the U.S.A. All rights reserved. Catalog no. 157759.

FIGURE 6–3. *(Continued)*

Other groups have also formulated statements regarding rights of the health consumer, nurses' associations among them. In some states, rights of the health consumer are being formalized into legal statements.

Basic Ethical Concepts

Basic concepts that are involved in most ethical situations include beneficence, nonmaleficence, autonomy, justice, fidelity, and veracity. Identifying how they apply to a particular situation and balancing their competing claims often present a challenge.

BENEFICENCE AND NONMALEFICENCE

Beneficence refers to the obligation to do good, not harm, to other people. Further it is to act in the best interests of another person (Cohen, Cohen, and Thomasma, 1988). It is difficult to decide who will determine what is good for a person. In most instances we expect that people will make their own deci-

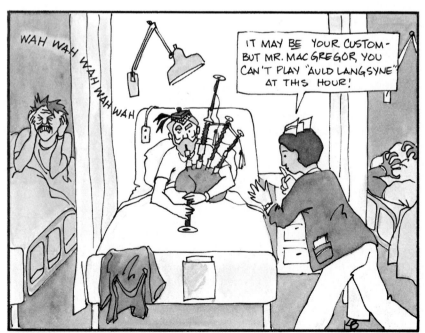

FIGURE 6–4 The nurse in providing care respects the beliefs, values, and customs of the individual.

sions. But who decides for the infant, the mentally incompetent, and others who are unable to make decisions? Another problem centers around what is good. Is all life good, or are there situations when not living is better than life? Is it better to sustain life in the face of all disability, or is it better to allow a person to die and have suffering ended? There are no simple answers, and the answers may not be the same for everyone.

A term related to beneficence is *nonmaleficence*, which means to do no harm. As far back as Hippocrates, physicians were entreated to do no harm. Florence Nightingale stated that the patient should be no worse for having been nursed. In health care we recognize that sometimes we do harm to individuals although that is not intended. Nosocomial infections, adverse drug reactions, and side effects of such treatments as irradiation and chemotherapy for cancer are certainly harmful to the individuals who experience them. The ethical mandate is that we refrain from intentionally inflicting harm. Sometimes it is difficult to accept situations in which a side effect of a particular treatment results in harm to the patient. In some cases, given the alternatives, a patient will opt not to have the treatment (eg, irradiation).

AUTONOMY

Autonomy refers to the right to make one's own decisions and, conversely, to respect the choices that others make for themselves (Cohen, Cohen, and Thomasma, 1988). However, there are limitations on the right to choose. What should those limitations be? How is autonomy affected by interpersonal relationships and strong familial ties? Are there instances when people with more background and understanding should make decisions for others? In what instances should the legal system interfere with personal decision-making? How does autonomy relate to professionals as well as to patients and their families? For some individuals autonomy may be a less central value than are values related to the family. Is this acceptable? Who decides how much autonomy is "enough?"

JUSTICE

Justice refers to the obligation to be fair to all people. We must ask "How is fairness defined?" Does fairness mean that people should be treated the same? Is it just for one person to receive more resources than another? If so, what makes it "just" and how does that relate to the distribution of scarce medical resources? Does age make a difference in what we consider just? Should it? Does justice imply that the government should provide what individuals cannot provide for themselves? What are the rights of one person when those rights affect the rights of another? Can we measure fairness in any objective sense? These issues will be discussed in greater detail in Chapter 7.

FIDELITY

Fidelity refers to the obligation to be faithful to the agreements and responsibilities that one has undertaken. What are the responsibilities of health care personnel to individuals, employers, the government, society, and self? When these responsibilities conflict, which should take priority? In reality, which does take priority? Do circumstances alter which should have priority? What if the health care provider and the client disagree as to the obligations and responsibilities? Who makes the decision as to what constitutes fidelity?

VERACITY

Veracity refers to telling the truth. From childhood we are all admonished to tell the truth and to avoid lying. When we are children this seems straightforward. As we become adults, we see more and more instances where the choices are less clear. For example, do you tell the truth when you know it will cause harm to an individual? If you do, you have then abandoned the principle of nonmaleficence. Do you tell a lie when it would make someone less anxious and afraid? You might see this as beneficence (doing good), but then you have abandoned the principle of veracity.

Sissela Bok, an ethical philosopher, has written an extensive treatise entitled *Lying: Moral Choice in Public and Private Life* (Bok, 1978). In this book she explores the ethical principles that relate to lying and then relates these to specific areas of concern, one of which is lies to the sick and dying. Her conclusions are that lying, by its very nature, is detrimental to the liar as well as to the person to whom the lie is told. She recognizes that justification for lying does exist in some situations. These situations are when the truth will cause greater harm than the lie.

She concludes that rarely is lying to the sick and dying justified. The loss of trust in caregivers, the anxiety created by not knowing the truth, the loss of opportunity to deal with personal and family concerns, and other adverse consequences of not being told the truth far outweigh the perceived benefits of lying. She points out that the damage associated with sad news or risks is usually less than physicians or other caregivers perceive it will be. She states that lying should be seen as an unusual step and one that requires reasons to be set forth and debated and alternatives to be carefully weighed.

As we present a variety of ethical concerns, try to relate these concepts to the problem and identify which ethical concept is presenting the greatest difficulties. Identify whether the conflict is one in which two general values conflict. Try to determine from your own viewpoint which value should have greater weight in that particular situation.

Ethical Theories

It is not our intent to delve with any depth into the writings of early philosophers. However, some ethical theories are mentioned frequently enough in the literature that surrounds bioethical issues that some background seems appropriate.

An ethical theory is a moral principle or a set of moral principles that can be used in assessing what is morally right or morally wrong in a given situation. Over the years we have called on the theories of philosophers to guide us in considering the various factors affecting our decision-making.

UTILITARIANISM

Utilitarian ethics is found most prominently in the works of Jeremy Bentham (1748–1832) and John Stuart Mill (1806–1873). Utilitarian philosophy is also referred to as a "teleological theory," for the Greek word *teleos*, which means "end." The basic concept is that an act is right if it is useful in bringing about a good outcome or end. Furthermore, when issues compete they are weighed to determine which will bring the greatest good for the greatest number. The act is preferable that produces more total good.

This ethical theory would encourage us to act in ways that would produce the greatest balance of good over evil and is sometimes said to be "the greatest happiness principle." The philosophers who used this term did not consider happiness to be a superficial concept but rather one that reflected true well-being. Using this theory would lead one to weigh consequences of actions. The action with the most positive consequences and the least negative consequences would be the preferred action. People use this approach when they support budget decisions to provide vaccines to thousands of children instead of an organ replacement to one.

DEONTOLOGY

Another prominent ethical theory is based on a concept of moral duty or obligation. This is termed *deontology* (from the Greek word for duty). Immanuel Kant (1724–1804), who is associated with this position, strongly opposed utilitarianism. He argued that the moral rightness or wrongness of human action should be considered independently of the consequences of the action. According to Kant it is not the consequences that makes an action right or wrong but the principle or motivation on which the action is based that determines right or wrong.

As a society, we use this theory when we determine the motivation for killing before charging an individual with the crime. For example, a homeowner may shoot an intruder who is personally attacking him. In another situation, a robber may shoot a store clerk in the course of a robbery. Although the consequence of both acts is the same (a person is dead), the motive is the deciding factor in whether the state charges a person with murder. The homeowner who shot the intruder would be found to be motivated by self-defense and therefore not guilty of murder. The robber would be found to have been motivated by criminal intent and therefore be charged with murder.

According to Kant, individuals should be guided by concepts of duty to others in determining what actions to take. He believed that some duties are binding. To be considered binding a duty must be universal (ie, applicable to every individual), unconditional (ie, acted on without reservation), and imperative (ie, demanding of action). These three aspects of duty can be applied to an individual situation. For example, when determining the moral action when being the first to arrive at the scene of an automobile accident, you would determine universality by asking "Should every individual be asked to help those injured in an automobile accident?" You would determine the unconditional situation by asking "Should this action apply in every such accident?" Whether action was imperative would be determined by asking "Does this situation require action by those present?" If you answered yes to all of these questions, you would have a binding moral duty to act.

Another fundamental principle of Kant's work is what he called the "categorical imperative." A person, according to Kant's imperative, should always be considered as an end, never as a means to achieve another end. Therefore, according to Kant, we are not justified in using people as research subjects without their knowledge even if the result would be great scientific advance. That would be using them as means and failing to respect their fundamental humanness.

Major concepts of Kant's work are its universal application and its respect for the person. Those using this theory would seek to determine their duty toward others in a given situation regardless of who that individual might be.

NATURAL LAW

The "natural law theory" is found in the writings of St. Thomas Aquinas (1223–1274). The fundamental concept of his theory is that actions are morally right when they are in accord with our nature and end as human beings and are morally wrong when they are not in accord with our nature and end as human beings. Basically this states that good should be promoted, evil should be avoided, and ethics should be grounded in our concern for human good. The word "good" was not defined in a way that might be clear to all of us, but Catholic theologians conceive of natural law as inscribed by God, endowing all things with potentials that serve to define their natural end. Thus, natural rules can be discovered that should be used to guide action.

SOCIAL EQUITY AND JUSTICE

Rawls proposed a concept of social equity as an approach to justice. He believed that if people of reason were placed in a situation of ethical choice without knowing which position they had in society (a situation he called the original position), they would choose the alternative that supported the most disadvantaged person. Using this approach, the concern of society should be directed toward the most disadvantaged because they are the ones least able to speak for themselves.

Social Factors That Influence Ethical Decision-Making

Ethical decisions are not made in a vacuum. Many factors exert pressure and demand response as we search for appropriate answers to the dilemmas that face us. All facets of today's world are experiencing change, and nursing is no exception. The "truths" of yesterday are being challenged by the realities and new problems confronting us today.

In studying ethical issues it is important for you to understand the many forces that are operating. These forces are not independent or mutually exclusive but act and react on one another in a constantly changing milieu, causing evolutionary changes in all segments of society.

SOCIAL AND CULTURAL ATTITUDES

Changes in the attitudes of society as a whole profoundly influence each of its segments. For example, the shifting roles of women and of attitudes toward marriage and the family and the changing status of minorities have all required nurses to reexamine their personal feelings and alter their way of providing nursing care.

Ethical concerns are the by-products of a number of factors at work in our society today. The rights of the individual have been increasingly emphasized in all aspects of living and, more recently, in dying. In the health care field this is most pointedly illustrated by the use of the terminology "health care" as opposed to "medical care." Health care suggests much greater involvement of others and places the client in the center of the activity, whereas medical care places the physician in the key role. The meaning of "consumer unit" is shifting from an individual to a total family or even a whole community. The focus of care also has changed from one that was primarily disease oriented to one that is strongly preventive.

The size of the group being affected by ethical decisions has a bearing on the decision-making process. The smaller the group, organization, or society that is involved in the decision-making, the easier the process of arriving at an acceptable alternative. Many of our ethical considerations now involve our society as a whole or, in some cases, the world; therefore, solutions are difficult. For example, an individual couple may choose rhythm and abstinence as their family planning method. If it is not successful for them, they must cope with the reality of having a child. If we mandate this as the only acceptable family planning method for a nation, then there will be thousands of unplanned children and the society will have obligations for support. Thus, the issue becomes much more complex applied to wider society.

The value a society places on the individual or the family directly influences the standard of care. In Western society we believe in each person's right to exercise choice based on individual beliefs and conscience. We also place high value on preserving individual life. Therefore, we often use tremendous resources to try to achieve additional years, months, or even days of life for a person who chooses that care. Another society that places greater emphasis on the community good than on the individual may not choose to use resources in that way. The standard of care might reflect comfort without use of expensive treatment modalities.

A culture's religious values and belief in an afterlife directly affect ethical issues. The Hindu belief in rebirth after death and the immutability of fate affects decisions about using health care resources. Those who believe that the outcome is predetermined by fate will not choose to commit major resources and efforts toward altering that outcome.

The population, or, more accurately, the overpopulation, of a country relative to its resources may also have a direct bearing on the value placed on life. The material resources to provide many health services may not be available. Decisions may be made to eliminate certain costly health care procedures even though they are known to be effective and desired by individuals.

SCIENCE AND TECHNOLOGY

Scientific advancement and technology have left us wrestling with concerns that would have been considered science fiction 50 years ago. Before the development of kidney dialysis, we accepted the fact that people with nonfunctioning kidneys would soon die. After machines that would filter body wastes became available, a genuine dilemma arose over who of the many candidates would have dialysis and who would not and would consequently die. More people needed treatment than equipment, time, and personnel available to treat them. As the technology became available, the ethical questions refocused on decisions to end treatment rather than on issues related to initiating treatment.

Other technology has had similar effects. The advent of machines that could artificially breathe for someone challenged the medical and legal professions to examine their definitions of life and brought into focus problems of whether and when to turn off a ventilator. Heart and lung machines that could adequately perfuse the body while the heart was stopped for surgical procedures enabled operations to be performed that were unheard of 50 years before. Fetal monitors, which can be attached to women while they are in labor, provide a continuous readout of the status of the fetus. Such monitoring has resulted in an increase in the number of infants delivered by cesarean section. The implantation of an artificial heart in a human being received worldwide attention. This technology is extremely costly, and the survival of patients after implantation has been limited, leading to many ethical discussions regarding the appropriateness of using artificial hearts or funding further research. Individuals with acquired immunodeficiency syndrome have a limited life expectancy even with the best of health care. Should they be encouraged to participate in sometimes risky research to advance scientific knowledge and the possibility of future benefit to others? Thus, scientific and technological advances continue to present ethical questions for which often no answers are readily apparent.

LEGISLATION

Social change and legislation are constantly interacting. Legislation may follow changes in society's attitudes, converting new ideas into law. For example, the social change of increased acceptance of infants born of single mothers resulted finally in legislation that changed the wording of birth certificates and dropped the word "illegitimate."

When social change is desired, legislation may be actively sought to require people to behave in new ways. This was true for much of the civil rights legislation. A change in society was desired, and supporters of civil rights sought legislation as one step in the change. Recent legislative action that speaks to the needs and opportunities available to the disabled has brought about changes in policies, procedures, and even architecture. It has opened many peoples' eyes to the ethics of how the disabled are treated.

JUDICIAL DECISIONS

The judicial system also provides a major avenue for debating and trying to solve ethical problems. We find that more and more issues are taken to court and judicial decisions are used as the basis for determining the appropriate action. As you continue to study this topic, note that we have often cited a landmark decision in regard to an ethical issue. The process does not stop there, however. Some people may disagree with a judicial decision and continue to oppose it. Judicial decisions may also be overturned by higher courts. Meanwhile, the questions regarding the individual person's role in carrying out a judicial decision remain. For example, although the law in the past forbade abortions, some physicians believed so strongly in the right of the individual to have the procedure done and were so upset by the results of nonprofessional abortions that they were willing to perform them despite the law prohibiting them. These physicians were, of course, liable to prosecution if they were caught, and some were prosecuted for performing illegal abortions. Now that abortion is legal, in many instances decisions must be made by individuals about participating in care and by society about funding.

FUNDING

The financing of health care represents a major area of conflict that has ethical dimensions. The government has become more and more involved in providing funds for health care. Some people are asking how much time, money, and energy we should allocate to health care and how that money should be divided. How obligated are we as a society to make some form of health care available to all? What is it that health care can and cannot provide? Which is more important, prevention or cure? Health care includes controversial procedures, such as abortions and sterilization. Some taxpayers do not ethically sanction these procedures and do not want their tax dollars used to fund them. Thus, decisions about funding challenge basic values.

Occupational Factors That Influence Decision-Making

By virtue of the positions they hold in the health care system, nurses have special pressures influencing them as they try to make decisions. An awareness of these factors may help you as you struggle with personal problems in decision-making.

STATUS AS AN EMPLOYEE

Most nurses are not in independent practice but are employed by hospitals, nursing homes, community agencies, or outpatient facilities. Pressures divide the nurse's loyalty among patient, employer, and self. You will notice that codes do not speak of responsibilities to the employer, yet certainly you have certain loyalties and obligations to the employer who pays your salary and makes decisions in regard to your work. It is not unusual for an ethical decision to involve conflict between the best interests of the employer and the patient.

When discussing ethical decisions in the abstract, most people say that, of course, the patient's best interest should be the only priority. In real situations, however, the issues often are not so clearly defined. If a nurse's decision affects the employer adversely, the result may be job loss, poor references, and a severely curtailed economic and career future. As an example, one physician was known to routinely require his patients to sign blank surgical permits on admission to the hospital. One of the staff nurses became upset with this procedure after learning that the patients often did not understand what was being planned. Eventually she discussed the matter with the physician, pointing out that she did not believe that it was ethical to require the patients to sign the blank documents, especially because they were not informed of alternative methods of treatment. The physician became angry and complained to the hospital administration, threatening to take his surgeries elsewhere. This would have created a considerable economic loss for the hospital and, depending on the action of the administrator, the nurse might have been labeled a troublemaker and even discharged to placate the physician.

COLLECTIVE BARGAINING CONTRACTS

Collective bargaining contracts can protect nurses in making ethical decisions. By formalizing reasons and procedures for termination of employment and outlining grievance measures so that individual nurses have a mechanism for protecting themselves, the contract may provide greater freedom. (See Chapter 9 for more discussion of collective bargaining and grievance measures.)

Some people believe that contracts hamper individual freedom. The supervisor who believes that an employee does not deliver optimal care may feel unable to do anything about the situation because the correction and termination processes under a contract are so complex. Often many specific steps related to notifying the employee of unsatisfactory work and providing assistance for employee improvement are required before a person can be discharged.

COLLEGIAL RELATIONSHIPS

Relationships among nurses who work together as effective colleagues and support one another, share in decision-making, and present a unified approach to others can provide an excellent climate for ethical decision-making. All too often such relationships are lacking in health care institutions. Nurses feel alone and are not experienced in seeking out and providing support to one another. Greater effort on the part of all nurses in this area might be rewarding and is certainly long overdue.

AUTHORITARIAN AND PATERNALISTIC BACKGROUNDS

The historically authoritarian and paternalistic attitudes of physicians and hospitals often have relegated nurses, most of whom are women, to dependent and subservient roles. These role differentiations have in the past inhibited nurses from taking independent stands on issues, and they continue to affect relationships in the health care field. In some settings ethical decisions are made in a context that does not include nursing participation and yet nurses are expected to implement whatever decisions are made.

Nurses increasingly are speaking out against an approach that leaves them out of the decision-making process. Nurses of today might expect a physician to discuss a problematic situation related to possibly futile treatment with the critically ill patient, with the family, and with the nursing staff. The patient would be encouraged to express personal needs, the family's views would be included, and the nurses' input would be part of the decision-making process regarding the medical plan of care.

If a nurse makes an ethical decision on the basis of the patient's best interest but contrary to the physician's or hospital's interest, public support may be forthcoming. The public increasingly sees health care as big business and tends to support those who champion consumer interests that conflict with the institution's interests. This support may be short lived and therefore should not be relied on for protection against the adverse consequences of an ethical decision.

ETHICS COMMITTEES IN HEALTH CARE

Many hospitals have had ethics committees for years. Such committees were traditionally composed of physicians and were for the purpose of monitoring the behavior of physicians. They acted when a physician's inappropriate behavior, such as arriving at the hospital intoxicated, was reported to them. Today the scope of ethics committees has enlarged considerably. Membership has grown, and, representatives of the hospital administration, the community, and a variety of health care disciplines are being included. An ethicist may serve as a consultant or as a member of the committee. If nurses participate, they then have a formal mechanism to share in ethical decision-making.

The widespread consumer movement has become a significant factor in health care. Consumers are demanding a greater voice in all aspects of their own health care delivery. Part of this involvement is at the decision-making level and through ethics committees.

Bringing a wide variety of expertise and experience, the members of an ethics committee may help individuals who must make an ethical decision to identify whether they have all the relevant information, help them to determine other options they have not considered, and provide assistance in comparing the situation with basic ethical principles and theories. Often the committee acts in an advisory capacity to medical staff members and families struggling with difficult decision-making. Ethics committees may also help institutions establish policies in regard to ethical concerns that tend to recur in that setting.

CONSUMER INVOLVEMENT IN HEALTH CARE

With consumers involved in decision-making, nurses again may face a situation in which they are expected to take action or no action based on the conclusions of others. Modern nurses may find this as problematic as action based on a physician's decision. For example, an obstetric patient who has hemorrhaged severely may refuse blood transfusions because of religious beliefs. The nurse, recognizing the benefit of the transfusion, may have difficulty maintaining effective communication and rapport with the patient and family because of her own convictions that a transfusion is the best treatment.

A Framework for Ethical Decision-Making

When faced with ethical decisions, most of us hope to find the "right" answer. Unfortunately, often no right answer exists for everyone or every situation. The answer must often be that human beings do the best they can in the situation in which they find themselves and continue to struggle with feelings of inadequacy, guilt, anger, and doubt. However, you can proceed from a basic framework that encourages you to look beyond your first thoughts or feelings to basic issues. Andrew Jameton of the Institute for Health Policy Studies at the University of California, San Francisco, presented the following process you can use to help guide you in this task (Jameton, 1984).

CLARIFY THE ETHICAL PROBLEM

In identifying the ethical problem, you will first determine what decision must be made. Then examine that decision. Consider what ethical principles might be involved. Are those principles in conflict? Who are the relevant parties to this decision? Ask yourself what your role and relationship to the problem is. Is this really someone else's decision that you should not assume, or is it one in which a collaborative decision must be made? What are the time boundaries for making this decision?

GATHER DATA

It is important to have as much information about the unique situation as possible. The facts of the situation will make a difference in what the possible options are. However, remember that most situations do not have some magic pattern of true facts. The facts are always screened through each person's background and experience. What clearly appears to be a "true fact" to one person may seem to be "opinion" to another. Therefore, seeking other viewpoints may help you to see the situation more clearly. You need to understand the relevant people in the situation and their concerns and perspectives as much as possible. Consider whether legal cases might affect decision-making in this case.

IDENTIFY OPTIONS

Most ethical problems do not have only one possible solution. If there were only one solution, there would be no ethical dilemma because there would be no choice. Usually many options exist. In some cases more than one may be satisfactory; in others, none of the options will seem satisfactory. The more options you can identify, the more likely you are to find one you can support.

THINK THROUGH THE ETHICAL PROBLEM

For each option consider its impact on each person involved. Also think about the impact on society as a whole if this option were to be chosen. Consider the ethical theories presented and ask yourself how each particular option compares with the basic principles of that theory. In this way you might determine that one option is basically a utilitarian approach (seeking the greatest good for the greatest number), whereas another is clearly supporting a deontological position of doing one's duty.

MAKE A DECISION

At some time you will have to make a decision. This is often difficult and in some instances painful. However, refusing to make a decision that is yours is not a responsible position. There will never be enough time, enough data, or enough alternatives in some situations. No matter how thorough your analysis or how carefully you weighed all competing claims, you may still be left with uncomfortable feelings.

ACT AND ASSESS

Once you have chosen a course of action, then you must carry out your decision. This may involve working with others or carrying out plans yourself. Assess the outcomes as you proceed. Unforeseen outcomes are common in ethical situations. Share your thoughts and concerns with others as you proceed and continue to seek new insights into the situation. As you assess the outcome in this particular situation, consider its relevance for a wider range of situations and concerns. Use this situation as a foundation from which to grow and develop.

Specific Ethical Issues Related to the Profession of Nursing

Some of the ethical issues of concern to nurses relate specifically to the nursing profession; others relate to bioethical issues confronting all of society. In this section we discuss the areas facing nursing through commitment to the patient, commitment to personal excellence, and commitment to the nursing profession as a whole. Bioethical issues that relate to the whole society are discussed in Chapter 7. We present a definite viewpoint regarding ethics in the nursing profession. We feel strongly about the individual's responsibility for nursing practice and place high value on personal integrity in professional relationships.

COMMITMENT TO THE PATIENT/CLIENT

Nursing has a strong history of being committed to the well-being of the patients and clients who need care. Both the ANA Code for Nurses and the International Code for Nurses clearly point out the obligation that the nurse has in fulfilling this commitment. This obligation has been used to try to persuade nurses that they must not be concerned for self, working conditions, salaries, or other aspects of the employment situation. This is not realistic and may even be counterproductive to the development of effective autonomous nurses. However, rejection of a handmaiden philosophy does not require rejection of a basic philosophy that identifies nursing as a profession focused on providing patients and their families with support for growth to maximum health and well-being. Patients/clients can never become objects for nursing but must be approached as unique individuals who deserve concern, respect, and the best we have to offer.

RECOMMENDING A CARE PROVIDER

Clients and other people of your acquaintance may ask you to recommend a physician or other type of care provider because they believe that, as a nurse, you have special expertise in such matters. In the past, nurses were admonished not to express opinions about care providers and were simply to direct clients to the yellow pages, directories, or hospitals that referred patients to staff physicians on a rotating basis. If you indeed have no personal knowledge about the requested information, then this would be a reasonable approach. But if you do have knowledge, it seems inappropriate to sidestep the issue. You could recommend several competent persons, pointing out characteristics of each that might be factors in personal choice. For example, if asked to recommend an obstetrician, you might recommend three. You could then further state that Drs. A., B., and C. are all board-certified specialists in obstetrics. You might add some information about their practices: Dr. A. is an older physician with a more traditional approach to childbirth; Dr. B. is a young and innovative physician who strongly advocates father participation and the Lamaze natural childbirth method; Dr. C. is new in the community but appears to allow patients a great deal of choice in their approach to childbirth. The client can further research these physicians and make a personal choice.

If you are specifically asked about a physician whose care you believe to be less than satisfactory, you are faced with a different dilemma. Making severely critical statements might leave you open to a legal charge of slander by the physician (see Chapter 5). However, to say nothing is ethically a problem because you are not acting to protect the client. A safe approach is to state, "I personally would not choose Dr. X. as my physician. Instead I would prefer to see Dr. N. or Dr. O." If pressed to give reasons, you are legally more secure if you indicate that you would prefer not to discuss specifics.

You do need to be careful that any recommendations are not based on hearsay or gossip. If you do not have solid information on which to base a referral, do not be drawn into making one. Being a nurse does not obligate you to be an expert on all health care questions.

CONFRONTING SUBSTANDARD CARE

The day has passed when nurses could be expected to provide unwavering support of all members of the health care team, whatever their actions or the outcomes for the patient. Concern for the welfare of patients requires that nurses acknowledge the existence of substandard care and work toward change. We see the issue in terms of the form and extent the involvement should take, rather than whether the nurse should become involved.

A Basic Pattern for Action

The first step in any situation in which you believe substandard care exists is to collect adequate, valid information. Do not make decisions based on gossip, hearsay, or a single isolated instance. If you do, you may create problems for yourself rather than solving problems for the patient. Sometimes a single incident is serious enough that you want to act, but before taking action be sure of your facts.

Your second step is to be certain you understand both the official and the unofficial systems of authority and responsibility within your facility. You need to know which people have the authority to make decisions and changes, what the official prescribed route of change is, and what the hidden priorities of the institution might be. For example, the official lines of authority may provide the physician who has been elected chief of staff with authority within the medical group. Your knowledge of the informal system may reveal that a certain respected physician who does not have an official position actually is able to exert more influence for change. Within the nursing chain of responsibility, you may be aware that the head nurse of your unit, although officially having authority, in reality refers all decision-making to the supervisor.

The most commonly recommended initial action is that you take your concerns to your immediate supervisor. If you do this, your legal responsibility, if there is one, usually is satisfied. However, in some states, laws exist that require that poor practice be reported directly to the relevant licensing board. Many people believe that reporting to a supervisor fulfills your ethical responsibility as well as your legal responsibility. If the system always worked effectively, your supervisor would carry the concern onward within the organizational structure, and each person contacted would forward the concern to the next appropriate person until it reached the individual or committee with the authority and duty to act.

Alternative Approaches for Action

However, the system does not always work. Your concern may be dropped or ignored at any one of many points. You may never learn what was done even when positive action has been taken because of the constraints of confidentiality. Occasionally results are identified only much later, when a change in procedure and policy occurs.

Sometimes an alternative initial approach is more appropriate to the situation. You may volunteer to serve on committees such as those that deal with peer review. If there are no such committees, you may work to have them established, perhaps through a bargaining unit. This route of action will require a considerable investment of your own time and effort. The cry of "Why doesn't somebody do something?" may often be answered "Because nobody takes the time." This is a real constraint on action.

Another initial approach is to use the informal system within the facility. You may discuss your concern with a trusted person who has influence within the system. You may learn that you are not alone in your concerns, that efforts toward change are being made, and that your input of data is welcomed. Be careful when using informal systems; they can backfire. If your immediate superior learns that you went over his or her head with your concerns, he or she may direct anger at you.

If your initial approach is not effective, one formal route for seeking further change would lead you through the official lines of authority within your facility. After discussing your concern with your immediate supervisor and receiving no satisfactory response, you would tell the supervisor formally that you intend to carry your concern to the next higher authority. Technically you could proceed in this manner until you reached the administrator or even the board of directors.

Another formal route for seeking further change is through designated committees or procedures within your facility. This might require a carefully written documented report explaining your concern. You might then be called to answer questions that the committee has.

You might also decide to return to the unofficial power system within the facility. You might seek out other health care professionals whom you believe would be interested and secure support for change in this way.

A final alternative to a problem in your work setting is to offer your resignation if the change is not made. Continuing to exist in an environment in which poor practice exists may place you in conflict with your ethical standards and values. If you find it necessary to do this, be careful that you do not jeopardize your own future with angry letters or intemperate remarks. Render your resignation in a polite and professional manner even when expressing dissatisfaction with the system.

Reporting directly to a state licensing board or professional organization's disciplinary committee is an avenue of action outside of the employment setting. These organizations and agencies usually deal with serious problems that represent a breach of the public trust or serious harm. They may not have the capacity or desire to pursue minor though still important problems. The same constraints apply when reporting to these organizations. Remember that their investigation and decisions may be done in a judicial or legal manner. This may involve the requirement that you provide legal testimony in regard to your complaints.

Personal Risks in Reporting

If you decide to pursue any of these routes, you need to be fully aware of the possible consequences. You may be labeled a troublemaker, or worse. You may lose the opportunity to be promoted because you are seen as being antagonistic to the system. It is even possible that you could lose your job for creating too many waves. Officially this should not happen, but in reality it can and does. We do not mean to be unduly discouraging, but we want to warn you that the role of change agent is not easy, and you should be aware of and weigh the consequences before you decide to act.

COMMITMENT TO PERSONAL EXCELLENCE

To meet the commitment to the patient/client, each individual nurse must be committed to personal excellence. Basic to moving toward personal excellence is a willingness to engage in self-evaluation and assume responsibility in the work setting.

Self-Evaluation

Self-evaluation is discussed throughout this text in relationship to personal career goals, legal concerns, and continuing education. There also exists a strong ethical responsibility for the health care professional to practice self-evaluation. You are the one who is best able to identify your weaknesses and practice deficits as well as your strengths. Your careful self-evaluation is the patient's best protection against poor or inadequate care.

Self-evaluation is not always an easy or pleasant task. If we are truly honest with ourselves, we will be likely to uncover areas we wish were not there. Remember, done informally, these do not have to be shared with anyone; that is one of the beauties of self-evaluation. On the other hand, do not hesitate to ask for assistance if you think you need it. One is seldom criticized for trying to do a better job. Many institutions are now including self-evaluation in the formal evaluation of employees. If this is the case, you may be asked to prepare a written self-evaluation that will be shared with at least your immediate supervisor.

One avenue of approach to self-evaluation is the use of the nursing process format. Begin by a thorough personal assessment. To do this you will have to gather data about your own performance. This requires a level of objectivity that is not easy. You might outline areas in which you want to gather data and actually keep notes on yourself.

After data have been collected, you will need to give yourself time to reflect on it and analyze it thoroughly. The self-assessment outline includes questions you would ask yourself; however, the criteria that you use to determine whether your answers reflect the quality of performance you want to attain are not included. Those specific criteria must be individualized to the setting in which you work and the nature of your role in that setting. The breadth of data that represent excellent practice for the nurse in the emergency department differs from what would represent excellence for the nurse working in a rehabilitation setting. The amount of decision-making in which the patient participates differs between the recovery room and the outpatient clinic.

Your analysis can reveal strengths, weaknesses, and areas for growth or improvement. Congratulate yourself on the strengths identified and then clearly delineate those areas in which you want to change. As in nursing care planning, clearly identifying and stating the problems or growth needed helps you to plan more effectively.

After you have identified your problems, it is appropriate to establish a plan of action. The plan is more helpful to you if it contains clearly defined goals. What is a realistic expectation for yourself? When is an appropriate time to reach that expectation? As part of realizing these goals, you might find it helpful to establish criteria you will use to identify your progress. Once the goals are set, you are better able to plan appropriate action to meet them. You might consider such things as requesting in-service education, taking continuing education courses, consulting with colleagues, and doing independent reading and study. Some plans would need to include specific things that you will be doing in your daily nursing care for improvement. To do this you may want to request assignments that will provide opportunities for practice of skills.

SELF-EVALUATION PLAN

Assessment of Patients

1. Do I gather enough breadth of data about patients and families, including both strengths and deficits?
2. Do I gather data in great enough depth?
3. Do I listen closely to the patient and attend to what is being said?
4. Do I regularly use all available sources for information about my patients? (patient, family, other staff, chart, Kardex, and so forth.)
5. Have I recognized problems quickly so that they did not become worse through inattention?
6. Do I recognize physiological, social, and psychological problems?

(continued)

FIGURE 6–5 Self-evaluation plan.

SELF-EVALUATION PLAN (continued)

Planning for Patient Care

1. Do I routinely seek more information on which to base decisions about patient care?
2. Do I include the patient in decision-making whenever possible?
3. Do I consult with others on the health care team when planning?
4. Are my written plans clear, concise, and reasonable to carry out?
5. Do I take into account the realities of the situation when planning care?
6. Are my plans for care sound and appropriate to the individual patient?
7. Do I employ principles from the biological and social sciences in planning?

Intervention

1. Is my work organized and finished on time?
2. Do I maintain optimum safe working habits?
3. Do I perform technical skills in an efficient and safe manner?
4. Do I communicate clearly and effectively with patients, family, and staff?
5. Do I use therapeutic communication techniques appropriately and effectively?
6. Do I use teaching approaches appropriate to the individual patient and family?
7. Do I keep accurate and complete written records?
8. Do I understand and perform any administrative tasks which are my responsibility? (ordering supplies, planning for laboratory tests, and so on.)
9. Do I make the effort to learn about new techniques and procedures?

Evaluation

1. Do I routinely evaluate the effectiveness of the nursing care I give?
2. Do I effectively assist in evaluation of the patient's response to medical care and to ordered therapies?
3. Do I encourage the patient to participate in evaluating both the process and the outcomes of care?
4. Is self-evaluation a planned part of my activities?
5. Do I use data collected during evaluation for the improvement of my own functioning and patient care?

Personal Growth and Relationships

1. Have I established a sound trust and working relationship with co-workers?
2. Do I support and assist my co-workers when possible?
3. Do I communicate effectively with others on the health care team?
4. Have I sought opportunities for learning and personal growth?
5. Is my attitude helpful and productive?
6. Do I have sound working habits? (appearing on time, limiting coffee and lunch breaks to the correct time, and so forth)
7. Is my appearance appropriate to the working environment?
8. Do I use appropriate channels of communication within the institution correctly?
9. Do I handle criticism constructively?
10. Am I doing my share in overall professional activities such as serving on committees or assisting with development projects?
11. Am I honest with myself, being neither too harsh nor too easy going?

FIGURE 6–5 (Continued)

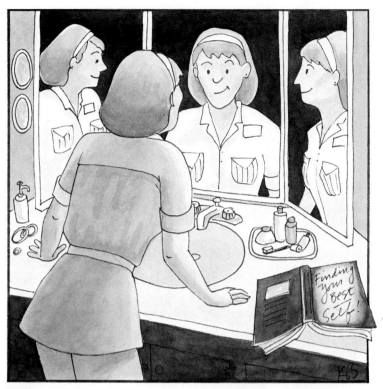

FIGURE 6–6 One of the advantages of self-evaluation is that it does not have to be shared.

All this planning must not go to waste. Implementing this plan will require you to remain focused on what you are trying to accomplish. Keeping records on yourself is often helpful.

Periodic evaluation of your progress is necessary so that you do not become discouraged. Any records you have kept will be valuable for this purpose. Sometimes it is hard to identify gradual change. You might even plan rewards for yourself for improvement that occurs. Try not to become discouraged if you do not see the improvement you desire. Remember that just as in patient care planning, a reassessment and a new or revised plan are often necessary, so may it be in the self-evaluation process. Keep in mind that your overall goal is personal excellence in nursing practice.

Responsibility for Supplies

Pilfering is stealing in small amounts or stealing objects of little value. In fact, many people who are otherwise scrupulously honest do not recognize that taking small items from a place of employment is indeed theft. Employees often take home a thermometer, adhesive bandage strips, and other such objects so routinely that they do not even consider whether this is right or wrong. With the large number of employees in modern agencies, this constant petty theft may total thousands of dollars. The cost of this must be passed on to those who pay the bills—the patients. As a leader in the care setting, the registered nurse is often in a position to clearly communicate to all employees that pilfering is unacceptable and to serve as an example of careful stewardship of the hospital supplies.

Sometimes removing supplies is an oversight rather than a planned action. To make efficient use of time, nurses commonly place many small items such as alcohol wipes, extra needles, and pens in their pockets. One hospital unit found that their yearly supply budget for black pens was almost exhausted in the first 6 months of the year. The simple action of placing a basket in the lounge into which nurses dropped everything from their pockets before leaving cut the pen costs dramatically. Perhaps you can be equally creative in helping to solve such problems in your work setting.

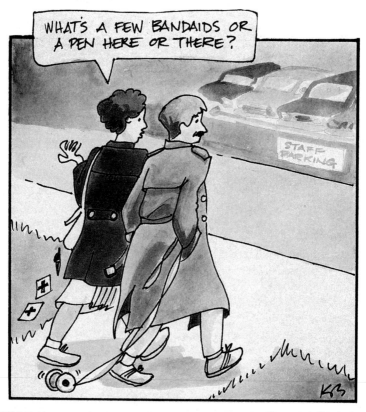

FIGURE 6-7 Many people who are otherwise scrupulously honest do not recognize that taking small items from a place of employment is theft.

COMMITMENT TO THE NURSING PROFESSION

Commitment to the nursing profession requires that each individual nurse be concerned not only about personal performance but also about how nursing is practiced. This involves participation in peer evaluation, formal evaluation of nursing care, dealing with poor care, and identifying the impaired nurse.

Evaluating Peer Performance

Nurses always have evaluated one another in both formal and informal ways. Some people think that evaluation implies noting error or deficiency. Good evaluation is much broader than this. The main purpose of peer evaluation is to maintain consistent high-quality nursing care. This is an ethical, professional obligation.

Informal Evaluation

The methods of evaluation vary. An important component of peer evaluation is actual observation of the performance of others. Often coworkers are the ones who are best able to observe a nurse's performance. Watching other nurses will also help you to grow in your own practice. When you observe coworkers, you need to strive for objectivity. A common mistake is to let personal feelings, likes, and dislikes influence our observations so that we see only what we want to see. We may view a close friend only in a positive light, whereas we see only the negative aspects of a nurse with whom we have a poor personal relationship.

Another important aspect of evaluation is examining results or outcomes of care. Two nurses may use different approaches or techniques in similar situations, but both may achieve positive results.

Evaluation is not negative. As you observe behavior and outcomes in nursing practice, you will most often see good nursing care. Do not hesitate to commend others and share your positive feelings. Everyone benefits from positive reinforcement of skill. Doing this would help nurses to create a good climate for personal growth and sharing.

An ethical dilemma arises when you observe a colleague practicing what you think is poor patient care, such as poor sterile technique. Various avenues of actions are available to you. What you choose to do depends on the seriousness of the situation you have observed. We suggest the following pattern for action as one that may assist in correcting a problem and at the same time maintaining positive working relationships.

Usually the simplest and most effective answer to any problem is to go directly to the person involved and state: "I observed this specific incident and it seemed to me that it was not in the best interest of the patient because . . .

How do you feel about it?" This does not level accusations of good and bad nursing and does allow the nurse to give rationale for the action taken. When you understand the situation more fully, you may have a different point of view also. If you disagree and the situation is not critical, you might want to simply state that you do differ. Sometimes just calling an incident to the attention of the person will result in a change in behavior, even if there is no open agreement that a change is needed.

If you observe poor care another time, you might again approach the person. State what you have seen, and note that it is the second time. If the person still disagrees that a problem exists, state that you feel obligated to discuss this with your immediate superior because it is not in the best interest of the patient. You should then follow through on this.

When you approach a supervisor, you need to give specific information with dates, situations, and the action you took. You should not indulge in generalities or sweeping statements but should stick to specific observed instances. Let the supervisor know that you have talked with the person under discussion and have informed the person that you would speak with the supervisor. It is important to specify the action you would like to see occur. You might ask the supervisor to discuss the matter with both of you to clarify the correct nursing procedure. Or you might ask that the supervisor talk about the matter with the other nurse or observe the nurse. A vague declaration of "You should do something about this!" is not helpful.

If your focus has been on enhancing the welfare of patients and you have been quick to praise the good care provided by others, your action in response to poor care will be more readily accepted. Remember that your attitude when approaching another nurse is crucial. Facial expressions and tone of voice as well as words need to be considered. If you are perceived as friendly and caring, your comments probably will be accepted in a far different manner than if you are seen as being negative and critical.

But you cannot always count on this. Many nurses feel threatened by the idea of evaluation or have had bad experiences in which evaluation only involved pointing out deficiencies. These nurses may be angry and upset with any colleague who deems evaluation to be part of the colleague role. There is a great deal of pressure in these situations to close your eyes to what is happening around you and concentrate only on your own care.

If you observe an incident that has the potential for serious danger to the patient (such as an unreported medication error) or one that has legal ramifications (such as falsifying narcotic records), you would have a legal as well as an ethical responsibility to go immediately to a supervisor with your information. In a situation that has the potential for legal involvement, it is prudent to keep an exact personal record of your observations and actions. Your record should include times and dates of the incident and of your reporting efforts (see Chapter 5).

Formal Evaluation

Formal evaluation of nursing is occurring in most settings under the title of quality assurance. Quality assurance is a planned program of evaluation that includes ongoing monitoring of the care given and of outcomes of care. It includes a mechanism for instituting change when problems or opportunities for improvement are identified. Quality assurance programs are required by the Joint Commission on the Accreditation of Healthcare Organizations and by Medicare.

The first aspect of nursing care that is usually evaluated is whether the nursing actions taken were complete and appropriate for the situations. Criteria developed to evaluate this aspect are called process criteria. One basis for developing process criteria is the "Standards of Clinical Nursing Practice" developed by the ANA (American Nurses Association, 1991). General standards refer to all settings and more specific ones for gerontologic, maternal/child, community health, psychiatric/mental health, and other specialty areas of nursing. Some specialty organizations such as the Intravenous Nurses' Society have also published standards that refer to their specific specialty.

Another basis for formal evaluation is the use of outcome criteria for patient care. Outcome criteria are specific, observable patient behaviors or clinical manifestations that are the desired result of care. They usually are established by nurses working in groups. Nursing literature is consulted so that appropriate criteria are established.

A number of methods have been used to evaluate both the process and the outcomes of nursing care. Conferences designed to discuss the matter to be evaluated are personal and flexible but may lack objectivity. Simple interviews with either patients or staff also lack objectivity, although valuable insight and direction may be gained from them. Direct observation of patients provides an excellent means of evaluation if specific criteria are set up before the observation, but it is time consuming. The method that is gaining wider acceptance in nursing is the audit based on review of the patient's record. If information does not appear in the record, then, for the purposes of the audit, the observations were not done or the action was not taken. This may come as a shock to nurses who reply, "But we always do that!"

All types of evaluation first call for establishing specific criteria to be used in the evaluation. These criteria may refer to process, to outcome, or to both. The creation of the criteria is a professional nursing responsibility. The chart review involves comparing the patient record with the criteria. Often medical records personnel may do this. The accuracy of the review depends on the adequacy of the charting. This is just one of the reasons why you must recognize the importance of your charting and make sure that you maintain a high standard in written records. If audits are being done at your institution, you should become familiar with the criteria being used. These criteria can serve as guidelines for you in evaluating your own care and in record-keeping.

This kind of review has raised some serious concern and often results in increased attention to documentation and even revision of record systems in some areas. Once the information has been gathered, nurses again take the initiative in determining the meaning of the data and what the next step should be. Because the goal is improvement of patient care, it is hoped that the audit will result in plans to enhance patient well-being. Changes in policies and procedures and in-service education classes are some of the approaches that have been used. Once remedial action has been taken, reevaluation is done to determine its effectiveness. Formal evaluation of nursing care is successful only if all nurses recognize their individual responsibility and accountability for practice and are willing to learn and grow to enhance patient care.

THE CHEMICALLY IMPAIRED PROFESSIONAL

The *chemically impaired professional* is a term used to describe that person whose practice has deteriorated because of chemical abuse, specifically the use of alcohol and drugs. There is a strong possibility that each of you, if you remain active in the profession, will at some time find yourself working with a chemically impaired colleague.

One would like to believe that nurses, who have studied the physiologic effects of alcohol and drugs on the system, would avoid the chances of such abuse. This is not the case. Statistics regarding chemical dependency in nurses are flawed owing to the social stigma and the subsequent efforts to protect the individuals involved (Sullivan, Bissell, and Williams, 1988). From September 1980 to August 1981 the National Council of State Boards of Nursing collected data on disciplinary actions from its member state boards. Of the cases reported during that period, it was determined that 67% of the disciplinary proceedings involving nurses were related to some form of chemical abuse (Sullivan, Bissell, and Williams, 1988). The state boards have not published data since that time. Several studies of alcoholic physicians and nurses have revealed that only a small percentage were ever reported to their respective state boards (Bissell and Haberman, 1984; Bissell and Skorina, 1987). In their discussion of chemical dependency in nursing, Sullivan and colleagues (1988) estimated the numbers of chemically dependent nurses based on statistics for the general population and the numbers in treatment. Although both physicians and nurses are overrepresented among those in chemical dependency treatment programs, it may be that they are more predisposed to enter treatment than is the population at large. They conclude that the percentage of chemically dependent nurses is at least as great as the percentage of chemically dependent people in the general population, and it may be that there is a greater percentage in the nursing population based on accessibility of drugs.

Why are nurses affected by this problem? Factors that lead to chemical dependency include the stress that one encounters in the nursing profession, particularly in intensive care units and emergency departments. Frequent shift changes and staffing shortages add to the situation. Unrealistic personal expectations, frustration, powerlessness, anxiety, and depression contribute to the problem. Once the problem exists, denial is a big part of the disease.

Jefferson and Ensor (1982) provide the following information about addiction:

> Addiction is an insidious process that occurs as the result of a) prolonged intake of a chemical, b) processes going on within the individual (including genetic, psychological, and chemical), and c) processes external to the individual (that is, the actions and reactions of family, friends, co-workers, supervisors, and society). . . . Addiction is present any time a chemical interferes with any aspect of a person's life and that person keeps using the chemical.

In 1981, the ANA appointed a Nursing Task Force on Addiction and Psychological Disturbance to develop guidelines for treatment and assistance for nurses whose practice was impaired by alcoholism, drug abuse, or psychological dysfunction. The guidelines were designed for use by state nurses' associations. These guidelines served as a basis for efforts by state associations in approaching chemical dependency in nursing from a treatment and rehabilitation viewpoint rather than from a punishment viewpoint. Then in 1990 the ANA developed suggested state legislation to respond to the problems of chemical dependency and drug diversion in nurses (American Nurses Association, 1990). The emphasis in this recommendation was on a voluntary treatment and monitoring program for nurses with problems rather than the traditional legal proceedings.

The concerns for the chemically impaired nurse are twofold. The first is on a personal level for the nurse who is afflicted: the illness may go undetected and untreated for years. The second concern is for the patient, whose care is jeopardized by the nurse whose judgment and skills are weakened.

Because nurses, by virtue of their education, are socialized into caring roles, they have not always dealt with the problem in a straightforward fashion. The impaired nurse was often protected, transferred, ignored, and, in some instances, promoted. None of these actions helped solve the problem.

What are some of the behaviors you will notice in a chemically impaired colleague? The following behaviors are commonly seen in alcoholic nurses:

- More irritable with patients and colleagues; withdrawn; mood swings
- Illogical and sloppy charting
- Excessive errors
- Unkempt appearance
- Social isolation; wants to work nights, lunches alone, avoids informal staff gatherings
- Elaborate excuses for behavior such as being late for work
- Blackouts: complete memory loss for events, conversations, phone

calls to colleagues; euphoric or "glossed over" recall of events on floor (ie, arguments or unpleasant events)
- Frequent use of breath purifiers, drinks high volume of "sodas"
- Flushed face, red or bleary eyes, unsteady gait, slurred speech
- Signs of withdrawal; tremors, restlessness, diaphoresis (Washington State Nurses Association, 1992, p 10)

Drug-addicted nurses commonly exhibit the following behaviors:

- Extreme and rapid mood swings, irritable with patients, and then calm again (after taking drugs)
- Wears long sleeves all of the time
- Suspicious behavior concerning controlled drugs:
  - Consistently signs out more controlled drugs than anyone else
  - Frequently breaks and spills drugs
  - Purposely waits until alone to open narcotics cabinet
  - Constantly volunteers to be the medications nurse
  - Disappears into bathroom directly after being in narcotics cabinet
  - Vials/medications appear altered
  - Incorrect narcotic count
  - Discrepancies between his/her patient reports and others' patient reports on effect of medications
  - Patient complaints that pain medications dispensed by this individual are ineffective
  - Defensive when questioned about medication errors
  - Abnormal number of syringes being used or missing
  - Frequent use of restroom by the nurse; evidence of broken syringes, bloody pieces of cotton in bathroom (Washington Health Professional Services, 1992)

Problems related to drug abuse are complicated by the fact that the nurse usually is obtaining drugs from the supply available on the hospital unit and is therefore in violation of the Controlled Substances Act.

In addition to personal behavioral changes, job performance changes also occur in those with drug and alcohol problems. These job performance changes include:

- Doing the minimum necessary
- Difficulty meeting schedules and deadlines
- Illogical and sloppy charting
- Excessive medication errors
- Excessive incidence of controlled drugs broken or spilled
- Increasing absences without adequate explanation (Washington State Nurses Association, 1992, p 11)

What should you do if you suspect that a colleague has a chemical dependency problem? First of all, you need to know what the law in your state requires of you. In many states any professional is legally obligated to report such a chemically dependent health care professional. This reporting most commonly is done through channels at the place of employment but may also be done directly to the State Board of Nursing. If you do not know the requirements, you should immediately learn what they are. In some states failure to report can result in disciplinary action toward you.

When planning to report you do not have to be sure beyond any doubt that a problem exists. You need to have enough data to represent a reasonable concern. The investigation to clearly establish the problem is the responsibility of the employing agency or the state board.

To establish reasonable concern, collect data and document it, including objective facts, dates, and times that support your concern. Do not confront or accuse the person whom you suspect. For at least several good reasons you should not confront the person whom you suspect at this time.

First, the person may become more secretive about the behavior because of the danger of being caught. This will make collection of data more difficult, if not impossible. Personal defenses and denial may become stronger. The suspected person may ask for a transfer to another shift or to a different part of the hospital, or, if truly threatened, may seek employment in another hospital.

Second, the person may feel attacked and rejected. A confrontation needs the support of a knowledgeable professional to not end in disaster. Through the support of the appropriate health care person, the individual may be be guided into appropriate choices for treatment and rehabilitation.

We have already alluded to another reason you should not confront the suspected person at this time. You are still collecting data and documenting it. You cannot be sure from a single observation that a problem exists. There are often reasons why things are not the way we initially perceived them. If the person is someone you know well who confides in you regarding personal problems, you might use that occasion to refer the individual to appropriate resources for personal assistance and counseling.

Once you feel you have data to support a realistic concern, you should report it to a supervisor to validate your observations. Usually once you have notified your supervisor, he or she will assume responsibility for the problem but may ask for your continued assistance with data collection or with confrontation.

Once adequate information has been gathered, agency administrative personnel will notify the State Board of Nursing. In addition they usually must notify the State Board of Pharmacy if drugs are involved. More investigation will be carried out; records will be examined. If a problem exists, actions appropriate to the situation will be taken. These usually include a carefully planned confrontation by an intervention team, a requirement that treatment be sought, and a presentation of the consequences of not seeking treatment.

The worst thing you can do if you suspect a problem is to ignore it or help a colleague "cover" for inadequacies. The problem will not get better if it is not recognized and treated. The longer the delay, the greater the chance that an innocent patient will be placed in jeopardy.

Fortunately help and rehabilitation are being made available to those who need it. Many states now have programs to provide support for treatment of health care professionals with chemical dependency. These programs usually provide a specific contractual agreement in regard to professional practice during the treatment and monitoring period. This is often done without formal disciplinary proceedings. Through this process the goal is restoration of the individual to effective functioning.

In some states the licensing boards may institute formal disciplinary proceedings to suspend a license or provide a license with limitations on practice and provide monitoring and supervision as the individual seeks treatment. When treatment is completed, the board may reinstate the license with temporary limitations and continued monitoring and support. The goal is the eventual full rehabilitation of the health care professional to the service of the community. Baldwin and Smith (1994) reported a much higher treatment success rate in nurses than in the general population. These researchers further identified that successful recovery was highest in those nurses who retained their employment during treatment. Therefore, reporting a chemically dependent colleague may be the most caring action you can take.

Key Concepts

▷ Ethical decision-making may be based on personal religious and philosophical viewpoints but must always be grounded in professional standards seen in the Codes for Nurses and the statements of patient rights.

▷ The basic ethical concepts of beneficence, nonmaleficence, autonomy, justice, fidelity, and veracity underlie ethical decision-making and may be in conflict in an individual situation.

▷ The ethical theories of utilitarianism, deontology, natural law, and social equity and justice may be used to examine the implications of ethical decisions.

▷ A variety of social and cultural factors including attitudes, science and technology, legislation, judicial decisions, and funding all influence ethical decision-making.

▷ The nurse's status as an employee, collective bargaining contracts, collegial relationships, the authoritarian and paternalistic backgrounds of health care, deliberations of ethics committees, and consumer involvement create pressures in regard to ethical decision-making.

▷ A basic framework for ethical decision-making emphasizes clarifying the problem, gathering data, identifying options, thinking the problem through, making a decision, acting, and assessing.

▷ Nurses have ethical obligations with regard to commitment to the patient/client, maintaining an objective stance in regard to other health care providers, and confronting substandard care. Commitment to personal excellence and to the profession of nursing also characterize the excellent nurse.

▷ The chemically impaired nurse is a concern to the profession and a danger to clients. All nurses have an obligation in regard to reporting those who demonstrate chemical impairment and in regard to assisting impaired colleagues toward treatment and rehabilitation.

CRITICAL THINKING ACTIVITIES

1. Identify four situations you might confront in nursing in which your personal religious values would be involved. If they are in conflict, how will you deal with the differences? Are there any other alternatives? What might they be?

2. Identify ways in which the concept of beneficence has shaped medical and nursing care provided to clients. Do you believe this is a concept that will have the same impact in years to come? Provide a rationale for your response.

3. Of the ethical theories provided in this chapter, select the one that most appeals to you and describe the aspects of the theory that make it most attractive.

4. Identify two sociocultural factors with which you have had personal experience that could impact ethical decision-making. How is your view of this different than it might have been five years ago? In what ways have your views remained the same? Why do you think your views have changed or remained the same?

5. Assume that you have serious concerns that a colleague is delivering poor patient care because of problems with chemical dependency. Where would you begin? What is your personal responsibility? What is your responsibility to your colleague? What is your responsibility to the patients? What steps should you take? Do you have a personal liability in the situation?

References

American Hospital Association. A Patient's Bill of Rights. Chicago, IL: AHA, 1992

American Nurses Association. Standards of Clinical Nursing Practice. Washington, DC: American Nurses Association, 1991

American Nurses Association. Suggested State Legislation: Nursing Practice Act, Nursing Disciplinary Diversion Act, Prescriptive Authority Act (Publ. No. NP-78). Washington, DC: American Nurses Association, 1990

Baldwin L, Smith V. Relapse in chemically dependent nurses: Relevance and contributing factors. Issues 15(1):1, 4–5, 1994

Bissell L, Haberman PW. Alcoholism in the professions. New York: Oxford University Press, 1984

Bissell L, Skorina J. 100 alcoholic women in medicine. JAMA 257:2939–2944, 1987

Bok S. Lying: Moral Choice in Public and Private Life. New York: Pantheon Books, 1978

Cohen MM, Cohen EN, Thomasma DC. Making treatment decisions for permanently uncon- scious patients. *In* Monagle JF, Thomasma DC: Medical Ethics: A Guide for Health Profes- sionals. Rockville, MD: Aspen Publishers, 1988

Jameton A. Nursing Practice: The Ethical Issues. Englewood Cliffs, NJ: Prentice-Hall, 1984

Jefferson LV, Ensor BE. Confronting a chemically impaired colleague. Am J Nurs 82(4):574, 1982

Kroeger-Mappes EJ. Ethical dilemmas for nurses: Physicians' orders versus patient's rights. *In* Mappes TA, Zembaty JS: Biomedical Ethics, 2nd ed. New York: McGraw-Hill, 1986:127

New encyclopedia of bioethics includes A.N.A. code. Am J Nurs 77(8):872, 1977

Sullivan E, Bissell L, Williams E. Chemical Dependency in Nursing: The Deadly Diversion. Menlo Park, CA: Addison-Wesley, 1988

Washington Health Professional Services. A Guide for Assisting Colleagues Who Demonstrate Impairment in the Workplace. Olympia, WA: Washington State Department of Health, 1992

Washington State Nurses Association. Handbook for Working With the Chemically Dependent Nurse. Seattle: Washington State Nurses Association, 1992

Further Readings

Bagwood T. Substance abuse and obligations to colleagues. Nurs Management 21(8):40–41, 1990

Conlon C. Developing Ethical Competence. Am Nurs 26(3):1, 11, 1994

Czerwinski BS. An autopsy of an ethical dilemma. J Nurs Admin 20(6):25–29, 1990

Gilfand G, Long P, McGill D, Sheerin C. Prevention of chemically impaired nursing practice. Nurs Management 21(7):76–78, 1990

Hughes TL, Smith LL. Is your colleague chemically dependent? AJN 94(9):30–35, 1994

Sherry D. Autonomy vs. beneficence. Home Healthcare Nurse 8(6):13–15, 1990

Supples JM. My colleague, my friend: The impaired nurse. Nurs Management 21(8):48I–48P, 1990

7
Bioethical Issues in Health Care

Objectives

After completing this chapter, you should be able to

1. Define bioethics and give reasons nurses need to have some understanding of bioethical concerns.

2. Discuss the history and family planning practices in the United States and identify opinions people have related to family planning practices, including abortion.

3. Discuss the arguments some people have against the Human Genome Project and its relationship to genetic screening.

4. List some of the possible ethical and legal problems associated with the practice of using a surrogate mother.

5. Discuss the problems associated with determining when death has occurred.

6. Review and examine right-to-die issues, differentiating between active euthanasia and passive euthanasia.

7. Discuss the major issues related to withholding or withdrawing treatment and patients rights with regard to informed consent and treatment.

8. Identify major concerns associated with organ transplantation.

9. Discuss reasons we have difficulty establishing firm rules regarding the treatment of the mentally ill.

10. Outline concerns related to the rationing of care.

Ellis JR, Hartley CL: NURSING IN TODAY'S WORLD:
CHALLENGES, ISSUES, AND TRENDS, 5th ed.
© 1995 J.B. Lippincott Company

Bioethics is the study of ethical issues that result from technological and scientific advances, especially as they are used in biology and medicine. This area of study may also be called biomedical ethics because of its association with medical practices. It is a subdiscipline within the larger discipline of ethics, which, as discussed in Chapter 6, is the philosophical study of morality or what is right and what is wrong. This chapter should be read, studied, and discussed within the framework of the information concerning ethical decision-making that was provided earlier. It should provide a basis on which you can look at judicial rulings, legal mandates, and social standards and how they can be used to assist in resolving some of the concerns with which we are faced in health care delivery. You have had some experience in looking at what is right or wrong with regard to your personal professional practice. This chapter examines more specifically those issues that apply to the bioethics of patient care.

Major Areas Where Bioethics Are Applied

The bioethical issues surrounding the delivery of health care are numerous and multifaceted. They are also always changing. At an earlier point in time most of the truly serious debates related to birth, death, or the processes that bring a person to either point. Today that represents just the "tip of the iceberg" as we explore such concerns as universal access to health care, rationing of health care, cost containment, where and how federal dollars should be spent with regard to the nation's health, and the obligation of others to assist the homeless.

These concerns confront us for many reasons. As a nation our population is getting older and living longer. Many persons who in earlier days would have died now grow old and infirm. Diseases such as Alzheimer's and acquired immunodeficiency syndrome (AIDS), for which no cure exists at this time, have increased in prevalence. New technologies result in treatments that were not available 15 years ago. Many of the treatments require use of technologies so expensive that they are priced beyond what an individual or family can afford without help from third-party payers. Finding new and better ways to treat life-threatening conditions challenges us.

Some would indicate that the "birth of bioethics" occurred with the publication of an article in Life Magazine titled "They Decide Who Lives, Who Dies" (November 9, 1962). This article told the story of a group of individuals in Seattle whose duty it was to select patients for a recently opened hemodialysis program in the city. Many more patients needed treatment than could be accommodated; those not selected would likely die. This event was followed several years later by an article regarding the ethics of medical research that provided impetus for developing means to examine these issues. When Christian Barnard performed his first heart transplant in 1967, the world again responded with awe and concern. Who was the donor? Where did he come from? Was he truly dead? (Jonsen, 1993).

Centers for research in bioethics emerged, most notably the Institute of Society, Ethics, and the Life Sciences, located in Hastings-on-Hudson, New York (often called The Hastings Center), and the Kennedy Institute Center for Bioethics, located at Georgetown University in Washington, DC. Journals such as the *Hastings Center Report* and the *Journal of Medicine and Philosophy* have come into being and an encyclopedia, *The Encyclopedia of Bioethics*, has been published. When Hillary Rodham Clinton established the Health Care Task Force, ten of the "special government employees" could be identified as bioethicists.

Entire textbooks have been devoted to bioethical considerations. Initially most of these were written for medical students, but now just as many are written for nursing students. This chapter will only introduce the topic and, we hope, broaden your perspective and deepen your interest. You are encouraged to do further reading and study of issues as they affect your practice as a nurse.

Most of the bioethical issues with which we wrestle were not a concern 20 or even 10 years ago. They are a product of the technological advances that have occurred in medical practice and research. Forty years ago heart–lung and other organ transplantations were not being done. There was no need for donor organs or critical decisions with regard to the life status of the possible donor. We were not able to fertilize ova outside the human body and reimplant fertilized eggs in a woman's uterus. Lifesaving machines, such as ventilators, and miracle drugs, such as some of the chemotherapeutic agents used today, were not available to offer extension of life. Technologies, such as magnetic resonance imaging (MRI), a procedure than gives us information about the structure of tissues that allows for early diagnosis and treatment, were not available. Concerns related to the quality of life were often more clear-cut. As advances occur in medical practice, we must challenge ourselves to think through our own beliefs and feelings with regard to these practices.

It is our intent in this short section to share with you some of the major bioethical issues confronting the new graduate today. You will have an opportunity to gain information, explore philosophical and religious issues, and integrate your own beliefs into your role as a nurse.

Bioethical Issues Concerning the Beginning of Life

A number of the bioethical issues with which we wrestle are focused on the process by which conception occurs, the products of conception, and the beginning of life, including whether it should occur. Much of the early debate related to family planning and conception.

FAMILY PLANNING

The modern population control movement probably can trace its beginnings to the writing of a minister in the Church of England. In 1798, Thomas Malthus, in an essay titled "On Population," expressed deep concern about a population that was growing faster than were the resources to support it. To offset this problem he advocated late marriage, no marriage, or abstinence in marriage. No forms of contraception as we know them today were available, although women may have had homemade devices that they developed in an effort to prevent pregnancy. Most commonly these devices were sponges dipped in various herbs and other substances that, when inserted in the vagina, soaked up semen.

In the United States another approach was taken that undoubtedly led to some of the controversy related to the issue of birth control. In 1873, Congress passed the Comstock Act prohibiting the sale, mailing, or importing of any drug or article that prevented conception. This resulted in the illegal importation and distribution of contraceptive devices. You may have read about Margaret Sanger (1883–1966), a nurse who championed for contraceptive practices at a time when such activities and viewpoints were extremely unpopular and illegal. Although charged and sentenced for disseminating information on birth control, she went on to establish the National Committee on Federal Legislation for Birth Control, the forerunner of the Planned Parenthood Federation.

It was not until 1965 that a clear, legal concept of planned parenthood was developed, when the Supreme Court of the United States established the right of the individual to obtain medical contraceptive advice and counseling in the case of *Griswold and Buxton v. the State of Connecticut* (Hayt, 1977).

Additional controversy over birth control is related to theological teachings of some religious groups, who believe interference with procreative powers is wrong. Encyclicals from popes of the Roman Catholic Church from early times to the present have forbidden the use of artificial birth control. The Catholic Church strongly advocates the natural use of reproductive powers to ensure the propagation of the human race. Anything that impedes attainment of the purpose for which these organs were created (ie, reproduction) is considered immoral. We see high birth rates in countries that are predominantly Catholic. Orthodox Judaism has specific rules about when sexual intercourse may or may not occur; these rules are geared toward increasing the Jewish population. The Orthodox Jewish population is so small, proportionately, to other groups that the impact is not significant. The members of the Church of Jesus Christ of Latter Day Saints (Mormons), although less adamant in their teachings, also discourage the use of artificial birth control under normal circumstances. Some conservative Protestant Christians also advocate allowing God to plan families and do not use birth control methods.

When caring for patients whose personal beliefs prohibit the use of artificial birth control, you must be knowledgeable about natural methods of family spacing that will meet the patient's needs. Your personal views regarding contraception must be set aside as you focus on meeting the patient's needs.

Among the methods of birth control available to those who have no religious sanction against their use, not all methods are acceptable to all people. For example, some find the intrauterine device unacceptable because they believe that interfering with a fertilized egg should be viewed as abortion. (Researchers are not entirely sure how the intrauterine device works, but some suggest that it prevents the fertilized egg from implanting in the wall of the uterus.) The other extreme is represented by those who find abortion an acceptable method of family spacing. During your career as a nurse you will care for patients who represent many viewpoints.

Central to all discussions of contraception is the issue of freedom to control one's body. This immediately raises a second question: who has that right? Is it the woman's right because it is her body? Avid feminists would answer with a resounding "yes." What if the partners disagree about family planning practices? Does one have more say than the other? What if one partner wants to have a family and the other does not? It is not within the scope of this chapter to explore the ramifications of all these concerns, but nurses working in this area need to be aware of the many issues that are present.

Largely because of personal values, there is disagreement over how contraception should be practiced, by whom, and at what age. In general, it is assumed that adults are capable of giving free and informed consent. The ability to procreate precedes what is generally considered legal age, however, and we find ourselves grappling with problems related to age of consent and its definition.

PROBLEMS OF CONSENT AND FAMILY PLANNING

In legal terms, the *age of consent* is "the age at which one is capable of giving deliberate and voluntary agreement, especially to marriage or to unlawful sexual intercourse" (Thomas, 1993). This implies physical and mental ability and the freedom to act and make decisions. Before reaching the age of consent, parents are required to give consent for care of their children. Implicit in this is the assumption that the parents have the best interests of the child at heart and that they are better qualified than the child to make decisions in the child's best interest. (Do you see how this generates the concept of "paternalism" that has been discussed in other parts of the book?) The authority to give consent goes along with the understanding that the parents are responsible for the care and education of the minor, including medical costs. However, trends of today cloud the issue, and legislators and concerned citizens continue to struggle with legislating "rights" through arbitrary criteria such as age. In former times the age of 7 was believed to be an appropriate age at which to give consent because by age 7 children were expected to know right from wrong and to have reached the age of reason. Although few of us would think that this is an age at which a child should be responsible to give consent for medical treatment, guidelines of the Department of Health and Human Services have allowed that it is sufficient to refuse consent, despite parental opinion (Hellegers, 1975).

The trend recently has been toward the concept of the "emancipated minor." Although *emancipation of a minor* legally means "the entire surrender by the parents of the right to care, custody, and earnings of such a child as well as renunciation of parental duties," it is done with the agreement of the parents. Both parents and child agree that the child is able to care for self, may leave home, may earn a living, and may pay for cost of health care. This usually does not occur before the age of 16, but it may. Most states recognize some form of emancipation of minors (Mancini, 1978).

Another term we often hear is *mature minor*, a relatively new concept. This term is applied to "youths who are sufficiently mature and intelligent to understand the nature and consequences of a treatment that is for their benefit" (Mancini, 1978, p 126). Under this definition, a minor who wants birth control devices because he or she is sexually active demonstrates ability to make a mature decision, although the parents may not agree with the decision. This definition also allows minors to consent to therapy for venereal disease and drug abuse as well as pregnancy care.

Health care workers have no legal obligation to inform parents of this treatment. The most liberal legislation applies to the treatment of venereal disease and is endorsed by most states. Minors of any age can consent to diagnosis and care for venereal disease.

Many parents strongly oppose this position. They believe that this undermines their parental role and sanctions sexual activity between young people. To illustrate this viewpoint, let us consider the case of an 11-year-old girl who sought treatment for gonorrhea. At her insistence the physician promised to honor her legal right to confidential health care and not to inform her parents. Later a public health nurse who was working with the girl learned that the child was being repeatedly sexually assaulted after school by a 16-year-old neighbor while her parents were still at work. The nurse also felt bound to a pledge of confidentiality but was able, with modest encouragement, to get the child to discuss this with her parents and enlist their support.

In this instance the statute that protected the "rights" of the child may have led health care professionals to become involved in activities that did not serve the best interests of the child.

In 1973, the American Academy of Pediatrics developed the Model Act, which addresses the issue of consent of minors for health care. This act recommends that minors be allowed to give consent for health services when they are pregnant or afflicted with reportable communicable disease, including venereal diseases, or drug and substance abuse, including alcohol and nicotine. It is generally accepted that the age of the patient is not to be considered for some treatments, but that parental consent is automatically required for other treatments if the patient is younger than 18. Certainly there will be times when physicians' ethical and moral convictions will prevent them from complying with adolescents' requests for care. This occurs most commonly with requests for contraceptive pills and abortions. In such cases, physicians often discuss their beliefs with the adolescent and frequently refer the patient to a medical colleague for assistance.

A major controversy exists around the role of the school in the sex education of high school students and the dispensing of contraceptives. Those who are concerned about the rising incidence of teenage pregnancies and sexually transmitted diseases argue that the information must be disseminated, regardless of who does it. Conservatives think that this is an erosion of the role of the family, and worry that the indiscriminate dispensing of contraceptives encourages promiscuity among teenagers. Concern about the spread of AIDS has done much to liberalize thinking regarding the dispensing of condoms in particular.

ABORTION

What has been said about contraception becomes an even greater issue when related to abortion. In medical terms, abortion is the termination of the pregnancy before viability of the fetus, that is, any time before the end of the sixth month of gestation. An abortion may occur spontaneously as a result of natural causes (*spontaneous abortion*). The pregnancy may be interrupted deliberately for medical reasons (*therapeutic abortion*), or for personal reasons (*elective abortion*). It is these last two classifications, especially the latter, that induce bioethical debate. Ethically, the entire debate revolves around the definition of human life and when the fetus should be considered a human being. There exist two schools of thought about the nature of the fetus. One supports the belief that new life occurs at the moment of conception. The other contends that human life does not exist until the fetus is sufficiently developed biologically to sustain itself outside the uterus.

The legal aspects of abortion were clarified on January 22, 1973, when the U.S. Supreme Court ruled that any state laws that prohibited or restricted a woman's right to obtain an abortion during the first 3 months of pregnancy were unconstitutional. In the case of *Roe v. Wade* the Supreme Court recognized that during the first trimester of pregnancy a privacy right exists that allows the individual woman to make the final decision with regard to what happens to her own body (*Roe v. Wade*, 1973). "Jane Roe" was the fictitious name Norma McCorvey used when two young attorneys, both women, filed her lawsuit. A pregnant, divorced waitress, a victim of a gang rape and beating, Jane Roe sued the State of Texas because she could not obtain a legal abortion in that state and was too poor to travel to New York or California where abortion was legal. Without access to abortion, she had the baby, whom she placed for adoption. Four years later the Supreme Court struck down the laws that prevented her seeking abortion. It was also determined that some time limitations as to when an abortion can be performed were necessary because of the states's interest in protecting potential life. At the period of viability the state's interest took precedence over the mother's desire for an abortion. Supreme Court Justice Blackmun, in writing an opinion that met with agreement from six other justices, decided that a woman's decision to terminate a pregnancy was encompassed by the right to privacy, up to a certain point in the development of the fetus (Blackmun, 1981). It was established that this lasted until the end of the first trimester. Thus, the courts ruled that the state could not prevent abortions during the first trimester but could regulate abortions in the second and third trimesters of pregnancy, at which point the interests of the fetus took precedence over those of the mother.

Despite these rulings the issue of abortion versus right to life continues to surface with new legislation and rulings being considered each year. The legal positions also do little to help us deal with the bioethical concerns. Many people view termination of life at any point after conception as murder. The position of the Roman Catholic Church remains firm on the church's position on abortion. Many conservative Protestant Christian groups are also active in opposing abortion.

Others believe that although abortion is not desirable, under certain circumstances it would be justifiable, for example, in the cases of rape or incest or in instances where amniocentesis indicates that a fetus would be born retarded or genetically defective. Still others think that early termination of the pregnancy could be acceptable, but any termination after the fourth month would not be appropriate.

Those supporting abortion without restriction usually do so because they believe that women should have control over their own bodies. They further argue that the quality of life of a child who will be born as "unwanted" or with a deformity or genetic defect may be minimal. Interesting and challenging cases have emerged with respect to this concept. These are generally known as "wrongful birth" cases and are based on the principle that it is wrong to give birth to a child whose life will not have the same quality as that of other children, as in the case of children with birth defects or limitations that can be diagnosed or anticipated before birth.

As a nurse, these issues may present some difficult questions you will need to answer. To what extent do you believe you can personally participate in the abortion procedure? You may find it easier to assist with an abortion done as a dilation and curettage at 10 weeks' gestation in a doctor's office or clinic than to assist with a saline abortion carried out at $5\frac{1}{2}$ months' gestation in a hospital labor room. The products of conception aborted at 10 weeks have little that is lifelike in their appearance. The fetus aborted at $5\frac{1}{2}$ months appears much like a premature infant. Certainly, as a nurse, you have the right to refuse to be involved in abortion procedures or the care of patients seeking abortion. However, employment in a given area, for example, labor and delivery room, may rest on the nurse's willingness and ability to assist with abortions and to give conscientious care to the patient who has had the abortion. Some religiously affiliated hospitals have elected to close their labor and delivery suites rather than perform abortions.

Attention has been focused on events in which an abortion was attempted toward the end of the fifth or sixth month of gestation and the fetus was born showing signs of life. Is the doctor or nurse obligated to try to keep the infant alive? Is the doctor or nurse guilty of malpractice, or even murder, if he or she does anything to hasten the infant's death? Should this infant be considered a human being? Does the infant have "rights"? Does the mother have legal possession of and responsibility for the child if, in fact, she attempted to abort the fetus? This issue, like so many others, probably will be settled in a court of law while we continue to debate it ethically.

The abortion issue is also complicated by consent problems. Many states have recognized the special problems related to parental consent for teenagers and to health care involving pregnancy and have legislated special exceptions.

Recently the abortion issue has been made more complex by research that would use the fetal tissue resulting from the abortion for therapeutic purposes. Research has suggested that implantation of fetal brain tissue recovered at the time of abortion may be helpful in the treatment of Parkinson's disease if implanted in the brain of the patient with that diagnosis. The ramifications of this type of research and treatment are so great that a special committee has been appointed to develop guidelines to govern future research and treatment activities that require the use of fetal tissue.

As a society it seems likely that we will continue to debate the issue of abortion. Ultimately the decision rests with the individual who is having to make the choice. Certainly the legal entanglements become more complex with each court ruling and seem to be limited only by someone's willingness to challenge another aspect of the question.

AMNIOCENTESIS, PRENATAL DIAGNOSIS, AND GENETIC SCREENING

A major breakthrough in our ability to detect genetic abnormalities before birth occurred in the 1970s with the development of techniques to carry out amniocentesis. An amniocentesis is done between 14 and 20 weeks after the last menstrual period. With this test, a 4-inch needle is inserted through the pregnant woman's abdomen and uterus, and about 20 mL of amniotic fluid is removed and analyzed. From these cells a number of genetic problems can be diagnosed prenatally, among them such conditions as Down syndrome (which accounts for about one third of the cases of mental retardation in western countries), hemophilia, Duchenne's muscular dystrophy, Tay-Sachs disease, and problems related to the brain and spinal column (eg, anencephaly and spina bifida).

Down syndrome, a condition occurring with higher frequency in mothers in their early 40s and older, is the most common reason for seeking amniocentesis. When genetic screening reveals a genetic disease, the woman will often choose to have an abortion. Rothstein (1990, p 39) reports that "termination rates for muscular dystrophy, cystic fibrosis, and alpha and beta thalassemia are nearly 100%; they are 60% for hemophilia; and 50% for sickle cell anemia." Some couples request amniocentesis if they are in an "at-risk" group but state that under no circumstances would they abort the fetus. They believe that the additional 5 months will give them time to adjust to the fact before the baby is born. Usually doctors are reluctant to do an amniocentesis under these circumstances because the risk, although small, does not seem justified.

Some people are concerned about this procedure because of where it might end. Is mass genetic screening a possibility? Ethicists have expressed concern about the government's making diagnostic amniocentesis and abortion of all defective fetuses mandatory. Still others argue against genetic counseling and amniocentesis because of the stress it places on the marriage of the couple and, in cases in which it can be determined, the guilt placed on the partner carrying the defective gene. Their argument is that there are some things we are better off not knowing. Genetic screening also may result in at least one of the partners, often the carrier, seeking voluntary sterilization to prevent pregnancies with less than favorable outcomes.

Amniocentesis does have some positive aspects. Prenatal diagnosis, for example, may save more fetal lives than it terminates. Many women carrying fetuses at high genetic risk might resort to abortion if the diagnostic techniques were not available. Such women, unwilling to take a chance, would rather abort a healthy fetus than risk bearing a defective one.

The advent of amniocentesis has heralded the development of yet another medical specialty, that of prenatal surgery. Although the specialty is still new, some corrective surgery is being done on infants while they are in their intrauterine environment.

As a nurse you may care for patients with any one of many viewpoints regarding amniocentesis and abortion and you will also have your own values to consider. Will your values conflict with those of your patient? Are you obligated to advocate for the patient if the patient's request is squarely in opposition to what you believe to be right? Should you try to sway a woman who is indecisive toward either decision?

STERILIZATION

For years surgical operations that have resulted in permanent sterilization of the patient have been performed for purposes of therapy. Examples of this could include removal of reproductive organs to halt the spread of cancer or other pathologic processes. Although problems may arise for the patient and family as a result of such surgeries, usually they are resolved without serious ethical debate, depending on the family's religious values, the patient's body concept, family plans, and personal values.

With increasing frequency, voluntary sterilizations have been requested by couples for purposes of terminating reproductive ability. These surgical procedures, performed on either the man or woman, should, for all intents and purposes, be considered permanent and irreversible. For those who are satisfied with the size of their family, sterilization may pose few problems. In most cases, full and informed consent generally is obtained from both partners, and the surgery is performed. (Questions have been raised whether the man or woman is free to make an independent decision regarding sterilization without consultation with the partner.) Although many people see this as the prerogative of the couple, others find any type of sterilization in conflict with their religious and moral beliefs. A few states still have laws forbidding voluntary sterilization for contraceptive purposes, although these laws may not be enforced.

EUGENICS

Of greatest controversy is any type of sterilization performed for eugenic purposes, especially if there is any question about the procedure being voluntary. Eugenics is the movement devoted to improving the human species through genetic control. The practice of eugenics is not new. The idea of improving the quality of the human race is at least as old as Plato, who wrote on the topic in his *Republic*. The modern eugenic movement is thought to have started in the 19th century. Charles Darwin's theory of evolution was advanced by his cousin Francis Galton, who created the term *eugenics*. Keyed to this were philosophical beliefs of certain 18th century thinkers about the notion of human perfectibility. When Mendel's law provided an explanatory framework about the transmission and distribution of traits from one generation to another, the eugenics movement took hold. Organizations focusing on eugenics were created around the world.

The center of the eugenics movement in the United States was the Eugenics Record Office at Cold Spring Harbor, New York, and its leader was geneticist Charles Davenport. Until the early 1930s the eugenic movement grew. Eugenicists presented a two-part policy. Negative eugenics advocated the elimination of unwanted characteristics from the nation by discouraging "unworthy" parents. This movement included a variety of approaches such as marriage restriction, sterilization, and permanent custody of "defectives." Many eugenicists were actively involved in other issues of the day including such timely causes as prohibition, birth control, and legislation that would outlaw miscegenation (marriage between two persons of different races, especially between white and black in the United States). During this time states passed compulsory sterilization bills. By 1929, California, for example, had sterilized approximately 6250 people, almost twice as many as had all other states combined (Kevles, 1993).

Also passed at this time was the Immigration Restriction Act of 1924, which dramatically limited the immigration of people from southern and eastern Europe on the grounds that they were "biologically inferior."

Positive eugenics encouraged the increase of desirable traits in the population by urging "worthy" parents. "Superior" couples were encouraged to have more children.

The eugenics movement grew in Germany as well as in the United States. In 1933, Hitler sanctioned as law the Hereditary Health Law, or the Eugenic Sterilization Law, which ensured that the "less worthy" members of the Third Reich did not pass on their genes. It resulted in the sterilization of several hundred thousand people and helped lead to the death camps.

By the late 1930s, eugenics in the United States began a tremendous decline. Americans became concerned about the concept of a "master race." At the same time, psychologists and anthropologists were conducting research that indicated that culture and environment also had great influence over human development.

When the eugenic movement was rekindled in the 1960s, it had a different focus—one related to genetic counseling and genetic research. Today a couple who gives birth to a child with a congenital anomaly or who realizes that one of them is carrying a genetic trait that could result in an anomaly in the child might voluntarily seek genetic counseling and possibly opt for sterilization of one of the partners. Again, this approach may offend the religious and moral values of some, but generally it is viewed as the couple's prerogative.

Problems are created when the concept of eugenics is applied to minors or to institutionalized people. Problems also arise in the language of laws in certain states that would include "epileptics, habitual criminals, and moral degenerates" among those eligible for compulsory sterilization. Some states have expanded compulsory sterilization to include those who might become wards of the state (Hayt, 1977). In the case of epilepsy, modern medical advances have changed our understanding of the role of heredity in disease and our attitudes toward people who are affected. The trend in recent years has been for states to either modify or repeal their eugenic sterilization laws.

In states that still permit compulsory eugenic sterilization, questions can be raised as to who would request the sterilization, who would sign the consent, and who would fund the procedure. As the result of a court decision, federal monies may not be used for this purpose (Hellegers, 1975). However, the taxpayer contributes to the costs of institutionalization for people who are not capable of existing independently in today's society and for the care of those with severe illnesses and disabilities. Therefore, it is not only a personal concern but also society's concern.

THE HUMAN GENOME PROJECT

Genome may be defined as all the genetic material in the chromosomes of a particular organism. You will remember from your biology classes that the human genome consists of 46 chromosomes: 22 pairs of autosomes and a pair of sex chromosomes. Genomes have been studied for many reasons, including disease prevention, determination of the effects of radiation and chemicals on living species, and more recently, genetic therapy.

The Human Genome Project was first proposed by Nobel prize-winning virologist Renato Dulbecco in 1986. The actual project officially started in 1990. Its cost is estimated at $3 billion and it is planned to last for 15 years. The project has two goals: to develop detailed maps of the human genome (genetic makeup), and other well studied organisms and to determine the order (sequence) of the individual nucleotides in the DNA of these genomes (Rossiter and Caskey, 1993).

This research is inspired by the discovery that an estimated 4000 disease genes are thought to reside with the human genome. Identification and isolation of the defective gene and its replacement with a functional gene (gene therapy) could result in elimination of diseases that have plagued society for years. Several significant conditions currently under study are cystic fibrosis, Huntington's disease, myotonic dystrophy, gout, and adult polycystic kidney disease.

Gene therapy can be divided into two categories. The first relates to an alteration in germ cells (sperm or ova) that results in a permanent genetic change for the whole organism and subsequent generations. For ethical reasons this is not currently being considered for human beings. The second is called "somatic cell gene therapy" and is similar to an organ transplant. Several cases of somatic cell gene therapy have been initiated, most relating to treatment of cancers and blood disorders (Rossiter and Caskey, 1993).

The Human Genome Project brings the promise of improved diagnosis and the possible development of treatment measures for many inherited diseases. Most people are initially excited at the possibility of preventing such diseases as diabetes or cystic fibrosis. Then they begin to think about other ramifications. What would be the effects of manipulating stature, intelligence, or sex? Do we run the risk of creating "super-babies?" What might be the advantages and disadvantages of knowing the diseases to which you are susceptible? With whom should that information be shared? Employers? Insurance companies? The government? Does this project represent eugenics revisited? Thus, this project carries with it vast and controversial bioethical challenges. How can its misuse be prevented? Should couples with a family history of a certain disease conditions be required to participate in genetic screening? If the screening is done and the results indicate a one-in-four chance of bearing a child who will have the disease, what next? These and many other questions are yet to be answered. Students interested in having more extensive knowledge of this project are encouraged to do research in their school or local library.

IN VITRO FERTILIZATION

Another interesting bioethical issue relates to the creation of life or, more correctly, the conditions under which it may occur. In 1978 in England, attention was directed at the birth of a child who was conceived in a test tube, a process we refer to as *in vitro fertilization* (IVF). Owing to a blockage in the mother's fallopian tubes, conception in her tubes was impossible. The ovum was removed from the mother, united with the father's sperm in a laboratory test tube, and then implanted into the mother's uterus, where it grew to term and was delivered by cesarean section.

Many heralded this as one of medical science's great advances. Others thought that this was going too far, that there are already too many risks involved in the birth process, and that we are only asking for more complications. Others expressed concern about the ethics of using tax dollars to fund this type of research.

Despite the objections raised against IVF, it is now recognized as a viable alternative for many couples who would otherwise be childless (at least as far as natural parenting is concerned). Reproductive problems often stem from blocked fallopian tubes. By means of a laparoscope, mature eggs are obtained from the woman. These are then fertilized with the man's sperm. A number of fertilized ova are then allowed to develop. Three to five of the fertilized ova are then implanted in the woman's uterus in the hope that at least one will survive the procedure (a process that has resulted in some multiple births). The remainder of the fertilized ova are discarded. In some instances when more of the implanted fertilized ova continue to develop within the uterus

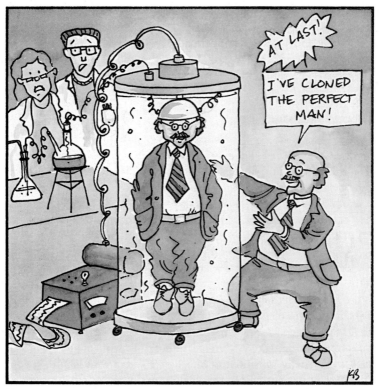

FIGURE 7–1 Another interesting issue involves the creation of life or, more correctly, the circumstances under which it may occur.

than was anticipated, several of the embryos will be aborted to allow one or two the opportunity to reach viability. Once again a serious bioethical concern is raised if one believes that life begins at conception.

In 1990, British researchers announced that they had identified the sex of human embryos just 3 days after they were conceived through IVF. This medical discovery would allow a mother to be implanted with only female embryos and could be used to prevent the birth of boys in situations where the mother was at risk of passing on a severe genetic disease that occurs only in males (there are about 200 known sex-linked genetic diseases). It also provides the opportunity to identify severe genetic problems from a single cell and raises the question of whether couples would seek the "test tube baby" procedure to be ensured of genetically perfect children or even to select a child's gender.

Recently concern has been raised regarding another use of IVF. In Italy a 62-year-old woman became pregnant using donated eggs and IVF before implantation in the woman's uterus. She gave birth by cesarean section in 1994. This also occurred in England to a 59-year-old woman who delivered twins.

Situations such as this prompted the French Senate in January 1994 to prohibit the use of reproductive options in certain cases (Capron, 1994). One can readily identify some of the disadvantages of starting the mothering process at age 59 or 62, not the least of which would be living long enough to see the child reach adulthood.

ARTIFICIAL INSEMINATION

Other discussions revolve around the topic of artificial insemination, which is the planting of sperm in the woman's body to facilitate conception. Although we tend to think of this as a fairly new procedure, the first time artificial insemination is said to have been used was in Philadelphia in 1884 (Fromer, 1981). There are two different kinds of artificial insemination: homologous, in which the husband's sperm is used, and heterologous, in which a donor's sperm is used. Using the husband's sperm is by far the most common and creates the fewest problems legally, ethically, and morally. In some instances the sperm from the husband and the sperm from a donor with similar physical characteristics are mixed together. As a result, if conception occurs, the couple could easily believe it was the husband's sperm that was accepted by the ovum.

Although some religious groups may have objections, few concerns arise if the husband's sperm is used. That is not true with donor sperm. If the woman is artificially inseminated with donor sperm without the knowledge and consent of her partner, the problems are multiplied. One of the major questions raised is that of adultery, which is considered a criminal act in most states. If conception occurs and the child is not biologically that of the husband, can one say that adultery has occurred? In at least one instance the wife was found guilty of adultery after being artificially inseminated with donor sperm (Hayt, 1977). Others question whether the child should be legally adopted by the husband, an act that, to some extent, helps to clarify issues of inheritance, child support (if the couple should later divorce), and the legal status of the child.

SINGLE PARENTS

Another ethical issue has arisen as our society has granted greater acceptance to single-parent families. More single women are trying to adopt children, and some see artificial insemination as a logical solution. In some instances these women have also professed to being lesbians. One of the couple will seek artificial insemination with a donor sperm. The child is then raised as family in the lesbian relationship. Providing a parenting option to lesbians is totally unacceptable to many people. Aside from the additional emotion that the issue of a lesbian life-style may introduce, there is the argument against artificial insemination of any single woman on the basis that the traditional two-parent family composed of a man and woman is in the best interest of all children.

SURROGATE MOTHERS

Unique problems arise with surrogate mothers, a practice by which a woman agrees to bear a child conceived through artificial insemination and to relinquish the baby at birth to others for rearing. This practice has occurred with increasing frequency and in a variety of relationships.

In one instance a 47-year-old woman agreed to serve as gestational surrogate for her own daughter whose uterus had been removed. The daughter's eggs were inseminated with her husband's sperm and the embryos were then implanted in the mother who gave birth to triplets when she was 48. Thus, this woman became the gestational mother and the genetic grandmother to triplets.

Surrogate mothering within the larger family group has had fewer problems than have been seen when a stranger serves as the surrogate mother. The majority of the serious problems have occurred in situations in which a woman has been paid to serve as a surrogate mother. A formal, contractual relationship is usually established. The couple who wish to have the child agree to pay all expenses associated with the pregnancy and additionally pay the surrogate mother an agreed on sum for her time and involvement. The contract must be carefully drawn up because it is illegal in all states to sell a child.

What happens if the child is born with an anomaly, as occurred with a New York couple in 1982? The man who paid a woman to be artificially inseminated with his sperm and carry his child rejected the infant, who was born with microcephaly, stating that he could not be the father. The surrogate mother and her husband also did not want to accept the responsibility for parenting the child. How are these dilemmas to be solved? What will eventually become of the child?

More recently problems associated with surrogate mothering have centered around the surrogate mother's unwillingness to give up the child after birth, as in the case of "Baby M," as the court calls her. This baby was born to a surrogate mother after she was impregnated with the sperm of a man for whom she agreed to bear the child. This man's wife, a pediatrician, believed that she could not bear a child because she had multiple sclerosis. Although signed agreements existed, the surrogate mother broke the contract within days of the baby's birth and asked for custody of the child

These artificial means of reproduction have complicated even the language that we are accustomed to using. The term *biological* is no longer adequate for making some critical conceptual distinctions. Macklin (1991, p 6) states, "The techniques of egg retrieval, in vitro fertilization (IVF), and ga-

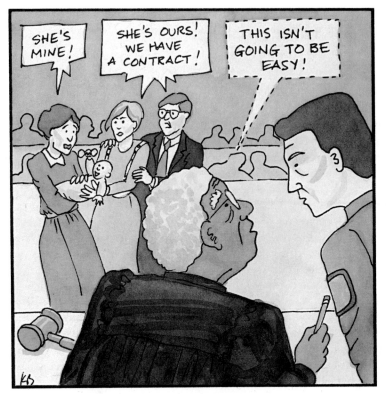

FIGURE 7–2 Complexities arise when surrogate mothers are unwilling to relinquish the infant after birth.

mete intrafallopian transfer (GIFT), now make it possible for two different women to make a biological contribution to the creation of a new life." Macklin further believes that the woman who contributes her womb during gestation is also a biological mother. We find terms such as *genetic mother* used to refer to the individual contributing the ovum and the term *gestational mother* being used to refer to the individual who provides the uterus in which the child developed. In some instances the surrogate mother is both.

SPERM BANKS

Another aspect of the artificial insemination issue is that of sperm banks. Sperm banks have been established in different parts of the United States for various reasons. Men who want to have a vasectomy may contribute to a sperm bank "just in case" they change their minds at some future time. Men who are to be exposed to high levels of radiation or other harmful substances that might result in sterility or mutation of genes also have had sperm stored. In most cases the sperm banks are established by the medical community so that sperm is available for artificial inseminations. In California a sperm bank was started that contains sperm of only outstanding and brilliant men. The idea was to create children with this sperm who will be genetically endowed with greater intelligence and creativity. Many find this unacceptable because it brings up the issue of creating a super race. Concerns regarding the possible number of offspring in a single community who might be genetically related without knowing it have been raised.

THE RIGHT TO GENETIC INFORMATION

All the issues of artificial insemination with donor sperm, surrogate mothering, single parenting, and sperm banks are further complicated by a recent trend toward providing individuals with information regarding their genetic background, makeup, and history. You can readily anticipate the problems that would be created if donor sperm were used for insemination. In some instances no record has been maintained with regard to who donated the sperm.

How many individuals would be willing to donate sperm if it were to include a detailed genetic background? What might be the ultimate legal involvement? On the other hand, what are the rights of the child with regard to knowing what genetic factors he or she carries? Whose rights should take precedence?

Bioethical Issues Concerning Death

One of the most important areas of ethical debate involves the topic of death and dying. As mentioned earlier, the advent of lifesaving procedures and mechanical devices has required redefinition of the term *death*, has caused us to examine the meaning of "quality of life," and has created debates about "death with dignity."

Also associated with the issue of death are a number of companion concerns that did not exist before we had some of the technological advances that have occurred within the past 10 years. Some of these concerns relate to euthanasia, the right to refuse treatment, and the right to die. Other concerns relate to organs retrieved from the dying because of the scarcity of these medical resources. Generally, the demand for donated organs far exceeds the numbers of organs to meet the needs. Superimposed on all these issues is that of informed consent.

DEATH DEFINED

Until recently the most widely accepted definition of death was from *Black's Law Dictionary*, which defines death as the irreversible cessation of the vital functions of respiration, circulation, and pulsation (Rothman and Rothman, 1977). This traditional view of death served us well until the development of ventilators, pacemakers, and other advances in medical science made it possible to sustain these functions indefinitely. We also have learned that various parts of the body die at different times. The central nervous system is one of the most vulnerable areas, and brain cells can be irreversibly damaged if deprived of oxygen, whereas other parts of the body will continue to function.

Newer definitions of death have been built around the concept of human potential, in other words, the potential of the human body to interact with the environment and with other people, to respond to stimuli, and to communicate. When these abilities are lacking, there is said to be no potential. Because this potential is directly related to brain function, the method most generally used to assess capability is electroencephalography. Brain activity, with few exceptions, is said to be nonexistent when flat electroencephalographic tracings are obtained over a given period of time, often 48 hours (Rothman and Rothman, 1977). At this point the person may be considered dead, although machines may be supporting the vital functions of respiration and circulation. Many institutions now accept this definition of cerebral death and use it as a basis for turning off respirators and stopping other treatments.

PLANNING FOR END-OF-LIFE ISSUES

Increasing emphasis is being placed on prior planning for end-of-life issues. One aspect of this is identifying futile treatments. Another important consideration relates to patient self-determination in regard to these issues. Many hope that the use of such planning will decrease the ethical dilemmas present in end-of-life situations.

Futile Treatments

Futile treatments are those that "cannot, within a reasonable possibility, cure, ameliorate, improve or restore a quality of life that would be satisfactory to the patient" (Hudson, 1994b). For example, when an individual is dying of terminal cancer, treatment for a respiratory infection may be deemed futile because it will not alter the fact that the person is dying and will not restore a satisfactory quality of life. Identifying whether further treatment is futile may be extremely difficult. However, Schneiderman and Jecker (1993) suggest that if in the last 100 cases of the same nature, there was no change in the outcome based on the treatment, it can be considered futile. Others take a position that treatment never can be declared futile. In their thinking the future cannot be predicted accurately and if there cannot be absolute certainty about the outcome, then futility cannot be clearly identified.

Another problem may arise if futility is declared. Does a patient have a right to treatment even if it has been identified as futile? What about cost considerations? Should insurance companies be required to pay for treatment that has been classified as futile? What about Medicare or Medicaid? Should there be differences in decisions based on age or quality of life?

Patient Self-Determination

When end-of-life concerns do arise, the patient is often unconscious or not able to participate in decision-making. This raises the questions of obtaining consent. Does the responsibility for action, or the lack of action, then fall to the family, the physician, or the nurse? The law in each state specifies who may give consent when an individual is incapacitated and there is no directive as to the patient's choice for a surrogate decision-maker. Would the ethical answer to this question be the same as the legal answer? Who is to decide?

In an attempt to gain greater control over the area of dying, many people are now completing a variety of documents that have been titled *advance directives*. An advance directive is a legal document that indicates the wishes of an individual in regard to end-of-life issues.

In the fall of 1990, Congress took a major step regarding this issue by passing legislation that requires all Medicare and Medicaid providers to inform patients, on admission, of their right to refuse treatment. In December 1991, this federal Patient Self-Determination Act (PSDA) went into effect. The intent of this legislation was to enhance an individual's control over medical treatment decisions by promoting the use of advance directives. The PSDA requires individual institutions to inform patients of state law regarding directives, document the existence of directives in their medical records, and educate the community. An "interim final rule" gave considerable latitude to institutions in the way that requirements could be met. Many institutions have used this as an opportunity to promote patient decision-making. The entire process has not been without its problems. The time of admission to a health care facility is often filled with anxiety, making it almost impossible to consider such matters. Most patients indicate that they prefer that this discussion occur with a doctor or nurse who is involved in their care, but in some settings this task is delegated to an admissions clerk (Hudson, 1994a).

A living will is a document that has been widely used as an advance directive. In a living will the person requests that, if he or she becomes terminally ill, no extraordinary measures be implemented to sustain life. Although the living will is not necessarily considered legal consent, it does reveal the desires of the person receiving care. It may help families to more confidently make decisions. Another approach that is being used with increasing frequency is the signing of a *durable power of attorney for health care*. In entering into this type of an agreement, an individual (referred to as the "principal") may designate another person who is given the power and authority to make health care decisions for the principal should the principal be unable to make those decisions for himself or herself. The durable power of attorney does not go into effect until after the principal is no longer capable of making decisions. These forms can be purchased in most office supply stores and become effective if signed before a notary public. However, it is best to consult an attorney before entering into such an arrangement.

**TO MY FAMILY, MY PHYSICIAN, MY LAWYER, MY CLERGYMAN
TO ANY MEDICAL FACILITY IN WHOSE CARE I HAPPEN TO BE
TO ANY INDIVIDUAL WHO MAY BECOME RESPONSIBLE FOR MY
HEALTH, WELFARE OR AFFAIRS**

Death is as much a reality as birth, growth, maturity and old age—it is the one certainty of life. If the time comes when I, _____
can no longer take part in decisions for my own future, let this statement stand as an expression of my wishes, while I am still of sound mind.

If the situation should arise in which there is no reasonable expectation of my recovery from physical or mental disability, I request that I be allowed to die and not be kept alive by artificial means or "heroic measures". I do not fear death itself as much as the indignities of deterioration, dependence and hopeless pain. I therefore, ask that medication be mercifully administered to me to alleviate suffering even though this may hasten the moment of death.

This request is made after careful consideration. I hope you who care for me will feel morally bound to follow its mandate. I recognize that this appears to place a heavy responsibility upon you, but it is with the intention of relieving you of such responsibility and of placing it upon myself in accordance with my strong convictions, that this statement is made.

Signed _____

Date _____

Witness _____

Witness _____

Copies of this request have been given to _____

_____

_____

_____

FIGURE 7–3 The Living Will.

[PLEASE NOTE: This is a standardized legal document that may not be appropriate for a person in your particular situation. You should consult your attorney before signing this or any legal document.]

DURABLE POWER OF ATTORNEY FOR HEALTH CARE DECISIONS

I, _____ as principal, domiciled and residing in the State of Washington, hereby enter into a Durable Power of Attorney to provide informed consent for health care decisions pursuant to the laws of the State of Washington.

1. **Designation.** I designate _____ , if living, able and willing to serve, as my attorney-in-fact. If he or she is not living, able and willing to so serve, then I designate _____ , if living, able and willing to serve, as my attorney-in-fact.

2. **Powers.** The attorney-in-fact, as fiduciary, shall have all powers to provide informed consent for health care decisions on principal's behalf.

3. **Effectiveness.** This power of attorney shall become effective upon the disability or incompetence of the principal. Disability shall include the inability to make health care decisions effectively for reasons such as mental illness, mental deficiency, physical illness or disability, advanced age, chronic use of drugs, chronic intoxication, confinement, detention by a foreign power or disappearance. Disability may be evidenced by a written statement of a qualified physician regularly attending me. Incompetence may be established by a finding of a Court having jurisdiction over me.

4. **Duration.** This power of attorney shall remain in effect to the extent permitted by RCW 11.94 notwithstanding any uncertainty as to whether the principal is dead or alive.

5. **Revocation.** This power of attorney may be revoked in writing by notice mailed or delivered to my attorney-in-fact, and by recording the written instrument of revocation in the office of recorder or auditor of the county of my residence.

6. **Termination.**
   a. By Appointment of Guardian. The appointment of a guardian of the person of the principal terminates this power of attorney. The appointment of a guardian of the property only does not terminate this power of attorney.
   b. By Death of Principal. The death of the principal shall be deemed to revoke this power of attorney upon proof of death being received by the attorney-in-fact.

7. **Reliance.** The designated and acting attorney-in-fact and all persons dealing with the attorney-in-fact shall be entitled to rely upon this power of attorney so long as neither the attorney-in-fact nor person with whom they were dealing at the time of any act taken pursuant to this power of attorney had received actual knowledge or actual notice of the revocation or termination of the power of attorney by death or otherwise, and any action so taken, unless otherwise invalid or unenforceable, shall

FIGURE 7–4 Durable Power of Attorney.

be binding on the heirs, devisees, legatees, or personal representatives of the principal.

8. **Indemnity.** The estate of the principal shall hold harmless and indemnify the attorney-in-fact from all liability for acts done in good faith and not in fraud on behalf of the principal.

9. **Applicable Law.** The laws of the State of Washington shall govern this power of attorney.

10. **Execution.** This power of attorney is signed on this _____ day of _____, 199 _____ , to become effective as provided in Paragraph 3.

> Signature: _____
> Print name: _____

STATE OF WASHINGTON)
) ss.
COUNTY OF KING   )

I certify that I know or have satisfactory evidence that _____ is the person who appeared before me, and said person acknowledged that _____he signed this instrument and acknowledged it to be h_____ free and voluntary act for the uses and purposes mentioned in the instrument.

DATED: _____

> NOTARY PUBLIC in and for the State
> of Washington residing at _____ .
> My commission expires: _____

FIGURE 7–4 *(Continued)*

Since 1985, New York has had a Task Force on Life and the Law, which has dealt with issues related to organ procurement and distribution, the determination of death, and surrogate motherhood. The group has also worked on the issue of appointing a surrogate to make health care decisions for an incapacitated adult patient who lacks a precise advance directive or a previously appointed health care agent.

EUTHANASIA

Euthanasia, meaning "good death," may be classified as either negative or positive. The word, as it is generally applied, refers to the act or method of causing death painlessly so as to end suffering.

Negative Euthanasia

Negative, or passive, euthanasia refers to a situation in which no extraordinary or heroic measures would be undertaken to sustain life. The concept of negative euthanasia has resulted in what are called "no codes" (also designated as DNR—do not resuscitate) in hospital environments, a situation in which hospital personnel do not attempt to revive or bring back to life persons on this status whose vital processes have ceased to function on their own.

It is difficult to describe what constitutes extraordinary measures and on whom they should or should not be used. Is it one thing to defibrillate a 39-year-old man who is admitted to an emergency department suffering from an acute heart attack and quite another to defibrillate a 90-year-old man whose body is riddled with terminal cancer and whose heart has stopped? Often people who are involved in giving medical and emergency care develop an almost automatic response to lifesaving procedures and have difficulty accepting dying as an inevitable part of the life process. It is difficult to know when it is permissible to omit certain life-supporting efforts, or which efforts should be omitted. If the 90-year-old man who is dying of terminal cancer were to also develop pneumonia, should the physician prescribe antibiotics? This brings us to a distinction between stopping a particular life-supporting treatment or machine, or withdrawing treatment, and not starting a procedure in the first place, that is, withholding treatment.

Positive Euthanasia

Positive, or active, euthanasia occurs in a situation in which the physician would prescribe, supply, or administer an agent that would result in death. In the case cited later in this chapter in which the parents chose to let a newborn with Down syndrome and an intestinal blockage die, positive euthanasia would have been used if the doctors had hastened the infant's death with medication. There may well be more instances of positive euthanasia than we know about publicly.

The issue of positive euthanasia is cloudy. On some occasions the physician will prescribe strong narcotics for a terminally ill patient and will request that the medication be given frequently enough to "keep the patient comfortable." Nurses often are reluctant to administer a medication that they realize has a potentially fatal effect when given in that dosage. In such cases the ethical intent of the action is often considered. Medications given for the comfort of the dying patient may be ethically justifiable even if they hasten death to some extent. When nursing staff have difficulty with this issue, a patient conference with an oncology specialist or with a nurse skilled in the area of death and dying will help the staff to clarify values and deal with individual feelings.

RIGHT-TO-DIE ISSUES

Right-to-die issues are gaining much more attention than in previous years. Kass (1993, p 37) identifies four reasons for such a right being asserted:

- fear of prolongation of dying due to medical interventions; hence, a right to refuse treatment or hospitalization, even if death occurs as a result;
- fear of living too long, without fatal illness to carry one off; hence, a right to assisted suicide;
- fear of the degradations of senility and dependence; hence, a right to death with dignity;
- fear of loss of control; hence, a right to choose the time and manner of one's death.

Much debate currently rages around the issue of maintaining the lives of persons considered to be in a persistent vegetative state. Some of the issues that arise are the patient's rights, the family's wishes, and the cost to society. In most cases the problems emerge when the life of a family member is being maintained through support measures that might be considered extraordinary.

In 1991, St. Francis-St. George Hospital in Cincinnati was sued in one of the first cases of its kind. The suit charged that the nurses should not have resuscitated an 82-year-old man when he suffered a heart attack. In so doing they disregarded a "no code" status of the patient (Hospital Sued, 1991).

Withholding Treatment

Withholding treatment could be considered as negative euthanasia. A historic case occurred in 1963 when a couple on the East Coast gave birth to a premature infant who was diagnosed as having Down syndrome, with the added complication of an intestinal blockage. The intestinal blockage could be corrected by surgery with minimal risk; without the surgery the child could not be fed and would die. The Down syndrome, however, would result in some degree of permanent mental retardation. The severity of the retardation could not be determined at birth but would usually run from very low mentality to borderline subnormal intelligence.

The parents (the mother was a nurse, the father was an attorney) had two normal children at home. They believed that it would be unfair to the other children to raise them with a child with Down syndrome and refused permission for the corrective operation on the intestinal blockage. Although it was an option, the hospital staff did not seek a court order to override the decision, believing that it was unlikely that the court would sustain an order to operate on the child against the parents' wishes because the child had a known mental handicap and could be a burden to the parents financially and emotionally, and perhaps to society. The child was put in a side room (an interesting action) and was allowed to die, a process that took 11 days. When confronted with the possibility of giving medication to hasten the infant's death, both doctors and nurses were convinced that it was clearly illegal (Gustafson, 1973). Certainly this case represents an extreme of withholding treatment.

The situation above stimulates both ethical and legal questions. Would the approach have been the same if the infant had not been mentally retarded? Would the staff have been guilty of murder if the infant had been given medication to hasten death? If a court decision had been requested and granted to proceed with the surgery, who would have been responsible for the costs incurred? What are the rights of the child? Who advocates for those rights if the child is unable to do so?

Withdrawing Treatment

In some instances the family has sought court orders to have extraordinary life-support measures discontinued. A landmark case is that of Karen Quinlan, a young woman left in a vegetative state after suffering severe brain damage as a result of chemical abuse. She was placed on a respirator, and her physicians thought that she would live only a short time if it were to be removed. Her parents requested that the respirator be discontinued, but because she continued to manifest a minor amount of brain activity, their request was refused. After previous petitions to the Supreme Court of New Jersey had been rejected, the courts ruled on March 31, 1976, that her parents could exercise her privacy right on her behalf and the respirator was discontinued. Much to everyone's surprise, Karen continued to live after the respirator was stopped, although she never emerged from her comatose condition; she died in 1986.

A more recent case has attracted equal publicity. In March 1988, Joe and Joyce Cruzan requested through the Jasper County Probate Court they be allowed to remove the gastrostomy tube that kept their daughter Nancy alive. Nancy had been in a persistent vegetative state since an automobile accident in 1983. Although the request was granted, Missouri's attorney general appealed the decision, asking for a clear precedent from a higher court. In June 1990, the U.S. Supreme Court effectively denied the request in asking for "clear and convincing" evidence of the patient's view. In reaching this point, a fine line was drawn between initially withholding medical treatment and later withdrawing it. In Missouri, once the family gives initial consent for treatment they forfeit all power to undo that consent or to stop treatment. No other state has such a law (Colby, 1990). Treatment can be stopped only two ways: if it can be demonstrated that it causes pain or if the patient left behind clear and convincing evidence of his or her wishes prior to incompetency. The first was not an option because of Nancy Cruzan's persistent vegetative state. Therefore, her parents presented a state court with testimony from her physician and three friends that Nancy would not have wished to continue existing with irreversible brain damage. The Circuit Court judge ruled that this met the test and Nancy's feeding tube was removed on December 14, 1990. She died on December 26.

Both the Quinlan and the Cruzan cases represent examples of situations in which treatment was withdrawn although the treatment was not futile and the individual was not considered immediately terminal. Such cases represent hard decisions for all involved and evoke legal, moral, and ethical questions in almost all instances.

Other cases have reached the headlines as individuals and families strive to have more voice in determining issues related to the right to die. In all cases, much conflict exists in the arguments put forth by those supporting the right-to-die and those supporting right-to-life movements. In the fall of 1990, Congress took a major step regarding this issue by passing legislation that requires all Medicare and Medicaid providers to inform patients, on admission, of their right to refuse treatment. The matter is far from settled and is discussed in greater detail later in this chapter.

Of particular concern to nurses are their own feelings when a decision is reached to remove life-supporting measures, whether they are tube feedings or ventilators. Over the years of caring for the patient, strong emotional attachments often are formed between nurses and patients, even when the patient is in a vegetative state. Nurses who have worked to preserve the patient's dignity have great difficulty "letting go." In some instances, patients have been transferred to other facilities to be allowed to die in an environment where the nurses are not so emotionally involved with the patient.

Positions on Withholding and Withdrawing Treatment

Several organizations or groups have issued guidelines for use of their members and others who would find them useful with regard to the issue of withholding or withdrawing treatment. Key to all of these guidelines is whether the patient is able to make decisions for herself or himself or whether someone else must make those decisions, which is referred to in legal terms as *competent* and *incompetent*.

In 1983, the President's Commission Report, "Deciding to Forego Life-Sustaining Treatment," focused on the ethical, medical, and legal issues in treatment decisions, especially as applied to individuals who could not make those decisions for themselves. The report distinguished between withholding and withdrawing treatment, referring to "withholding" as not starting treatment, while "withdrawing" meant stopping treatment after it was started. The commission did not make a moral distinction between the two but suggested that more justification may be needed for withholding treatment because the decision would be made without knowledge of the positive effects of treatment. On the other hand, withdrawing treatment is always initiated after it has been determined that the treatment has not helped the patient. The commission concluded that there was not a morally significant difference between decisions to withdraw or withhold treatment (Fry, 1990).

In May 1986, the American Medical Association issued a "Statement on Withholding or Withdrawing Life Prolonging Medical Treatment." This document stated that life-prolonging medical treatment and artificially or technologically maintained respiration, as well as nutrition and hydration, could be withheld from a patient in an irreversible coma even when death is not imminent.

In 1987, the Office of Technology Assessment of the U.S. Congress issued the results of its study of the use of life-sustaining technologies on elderly persons. This report noted that the most controversial of the technologies was that of nutritional support and pointed out that this issue was emotionally highly charged. They identified that the most troublesome part of nutritional support is whether it is intravenous feeding and hydration or a tube feeding (Fry, 1990).

The Hastings Center issued "Guidelines on the Termination of Life-Sustaining Treatment" in 1987, which provide clear definitions of key terms and a general guideline for making decisions regarding treatment. They view nutrition and hydration as medical interventions that may be forgone in some cases much as other life-sustaining measures (ie, ventilators) can be forgone in some instances. The guidelines place emphasis on the patient's ability to make decisions and would require careful assessment on a case-by-case basis (Fry, 1990).

In January 1988, the American Nurses Association issued its "Guidelines on Withdrawing or Withholding Food and Fluid." In general, these guidelines indicate that there are few instances under which it would be permissible for nurses to withdraw food or fluid from their patients. Neither the American Nurses Association nor American Medical Association guidelines make a distinction between withholding treatment or withdrawing treatment.

Assisted Death

The activities of a Michigan physician, who is alleged to have assisted patients in their suicide, have received much media attention in the past year. Although charged on several cases, to date, he has not been found guilty. The first case involving an Oregon woman, who was said to be suffering from Alzheimer's disease, drew national attention. She sought the assistance of the physician, who assembled intravenous equipment and medication in the back of his Volkswagen van. He set up the medication and started the intravenous solution. She initiated the administration of the solution that would allow her to end her own life. The courts decided the woman's death was a suicide. Michigan has since passed legislation outlawing assisted suicide.

In 1991, the Washington legislature wrestled with a referendum initiative sponsored by the Washington Citizens for Death with Dignity that would allow patients who are in a medically terminal condition to request and receive "physician aid-in-dying." The initiative permitted a medical procedure to be performed by a physician that would end the life of a "qualified" patient and changed Washington State's Natural Death Act to the Death with Dignity Act. Both this bill, and a similar one in California, were narrowly defeated, in part because they were badly drafted laws.

The Right to Refuse Treatment

This issue is closely aligned to the right to die but carries some special implications that require separate consideration. Although we discussed some of the parameters of this issue in the previous section on the right to die, other aspects can create even bigger problems for the nurse.

The moral, if not legal, precedent for refusing treatment occurred in 1971. Carmen Martinez was dying of hemolytic anemia, a disease that destroys the body's red blood cells. Her life could be maintained by transfusions, but her veins were such that a "cut-down" (a surgical opening made into the vein) was necessary to accomplish the transfusions. Finally Martinez pleaded to have the cut-downs stopped and to be "tortured" no more. The physician, fearful of being charged with aiding in her suicide, asked for a court decision. The court ruled that Martinez was not competent to make such a decision and appointed her daughter as her guardian. When the daughter also asked that no more cut-downs be performed, the compassionate judge honored the daughter's request. He decided that although Martinez did not have the right to commit suicide, she did have the "right not to be tortured." She died the next day (Veatch, 1976).

People working in the health care professions are frequently confronted by such dilemmas. Cases in which a patient refuses to have a leg amputated, although it is evident that not performing the surgery will undoubtedly result in death, frequently make the news. When children are involved, it is even more newsworthy. In such cases the courts usually are involved. A case in Illinois in 1952 is typical. Eight-day-old Cheryl suffered from erythroblastosis fetalis (Rh incompatibility). Her parents, who were Jehovah's Witnesses, refused to authorize the administration of blood necessary to save her life. The judge in the case ruled that Cheryl was a neglected dependent and overrode the parent's refusal. In such instances the child is usually made a temporary ward of the court and legal documents are attached to the record authorizing the needed treatment. Such court decisions usually have been based on the premise that the right to freedom of religion does not give parents the right to risk the lives of their children or to make martyrs of them (Veatch, 1976).

In some cases in which time is not a factor, the court will recommend that treatment be delayed until the child is aged 15 or 16 and can make a decision for himself or herself as an older minor. Other judges will rule just the opposite, deciding that it is cruel to place the burden of the decision on this older minor. Such was the case of Kevin, whose parent's refusal of a blood transfusion made the surgery to correct a deformity of his face and neck too risky to consider. The family court judge ruled against the delay and against letting Kevin participate in the decision on the basis that it would cause him psychological harm if he had to choose between his parents' wishes and his own (Veatch, 1976).

Situations like the above are always difficult for those involved. Because nurses have the most contact with the patient, they must examine their own feelings and attitudes. Nurses must recognize that patients also have the right to attitudes and beliefs. If the nurse decides that his or her own feelings are so strong that those feelings may interfere with the ability to give compassionate care, it would be wise for the nurse to ask to be assigned to other patients.

The right to refuse treatment can take on additional implications when the patient, by refusing one type of treatment, is essentially demanding alternative medical management. Our support of the right to refuse treatment is based on basic beliefs and respect for the autonomy of the patient. When the refusal of medical intervention means that the individual is no longer a patient, it is known as a *negative right simpliciter* by bioethicists. In these cases the

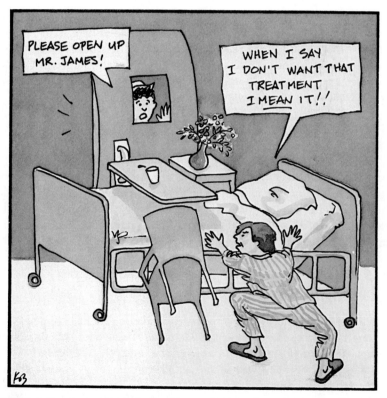

FIGURE 7–5 People working in the health care field are frequently confronted with the dilemma of patients who may wish to refuse treatment.

patient's physician need only do nothing, as in cases in which the patient discharges himself or herself from the hospital. When the patient refuses treatment but does not withdraw from the role of being the patient, the matter becomes more complex. An example would be the patient who refuses to have a gangrenous toe surgically removed and demands to have it treated otherwise. These are referred to as positive rights. In the treatment of a gangrenous toe, one form of treatment may be more accepted than the other but both may be successful. A case occurring in late 1993 in Chicago attracted national attention when a mother, a Pentecostal Christian, refused to have a cesarean section when physicians recommended the procedure because the fetus was being deprived of oxygen and would die if delivered vaginally. The courts upheld the patient's right to refuse the surgery. She later gave birth to an apparently healthy boy.

Additional Bioethical Concerns

Most of you will probably find the area of bioethics interesting. Although many topics are central to the area of bioethics, such as right to die, right to refuse treatment, and all the issues related to conception, a number of less well defined concerns are encountered in our health care delivery system. We cannot discuss all of these without creating a separate bioethics textbook; however, several deserve some review.

ORGAN TRANSPLANTATION

Developments in the area of organ transplantation have created a number of issues deserving consideration. In many ways it has necessitated a clearer definition of death. The supply of organs that can be used for transplantation has not been able to keep up with the demand. This is due to the larger number of organs that can be transplanted today. It is also due to the decreased availability of organs as a result of modern technology being used to save more lives.

Concerns About Procurement

Conflicts between the interest of the potential donor and the person receiving the donor organ are easy to anticipate. Certainly no one would want to remove an organ from a donor as long as that person had any potential for recovery. On the other hand, it is imperative that donor organs be removed soon after the death of the host, before the organ to be removed is rendered unusable.

Although there is lack of uniformity in the definition of death throughout the 50 states, it is generally accepted that organs can be removed from donors who have a flat electroencephalogram. This action is based on the 1975 definition of death, which states: "For all legal purposes, a human body with irreversible cessation of total brain function, according to usual and customary standards of medical practice, shall be considered dead" (Capron, 1978, p 300).

The idea of consent again becomes important when we talk about organ transplantation. It is preferable to have the consent obtained from the donor. This has been facilitated in many states by the Uniform Anatomical Gift Act, which was drafted by a committee of the National Conference of the Commissions of Uniform State Laws in July 1968 and adopted in all American jurisdictions in 1971 (Hayt, 1977). People who are willing to donate parts of their bodies after death may indicate the desire to do so in a will or other written documents or by carrying a donor's card. Many states now provide a space on driver's licenses where an individual can authorize permission for organ donations.

The spouse or the next-of-kin can also grant permission for the removal of organs after death. However, the time factor is crucial; the deaths are often accidental, and the relatives are often so emotionally distressed at the time that the process of obtaining permission may be difficult. Most medical personnel have at least some initial hesitancy in requesting permission for donor organs at this critical time. As we gain more experience in this process, we also have developed better ways to deal with delicate issues. It is generally recommended that two groups of personnel be involved in requesting organs. The first group are those who help the family realize that death has occurred or is imminent, usually nurses or medical personnel. This allows the family to grasp the reality of the situation. The second group, often referred to as the procurement team, are those who request the organ donation; persons skilled in recognizing the stress being felt by the family and experienced in providing information that will be important to them. A form, typical of those that the family would be requested to complete is provided in the accompanying display. A Spanish translation is also provided.

Some states have regulations that will allow donation of organs from an unidentified donor. Once a diligent search has been completed for next-of-kin, organs can be harvested. A coroner's consent is required in cases of accidental death, homicide, suicide, or any questionable cause of death.

In response to the inadequate supply of organs to meet societal needs—a situation labeled scarce medical resources—some states have passed legislation that requires that donor organs must be requested of the family when it is apparent that the patient has no chance for survival. This brings forth other problems. Who is to be responsible for approaching the family and requesting the organs? Must it be the family's physician? Would critical time be saved if it were the emergency department nurse or hospital social worker? An increasing number of hospitals are designating a nurse as transplantation coordinator to facilitate this process.

Consent for Removal of Organs from the Deceased

I, _____ , next of kin (_____)
             Name   *Relationship*

of _____
                          Name of Donor

for humanitarian reasons hereby give consent for removal of _____

_____ from
                 Names of Organs and Tissues

_____
                 Name of Donor

after his or her death for the purpose of transplantation, or for the retention of such organs and tissues for any other scientific or therapeutic purposes.

I understand that some of the procedures necessary for determination of suitability for transplantation will include testing for HBsAg (hepatitis B virus) and human immuno-deficiency virus (AIDS virus antibody). I further authorize the release of medical information gathered in this process to the physicians involved in transplanting the above stated organs and tissues.

_____
                 Signature

_____
                 Date

_____
      Witness

_____
      Witness

An interesting and controversial case occurred in California in 1990. An 18-year-old woman, an only child, was diagnosed as having chronic myelogenous leukemia. Although this form of leukemia responds favorably to bone marrow transplants, no compatible donor could be found after testing the girl's family and contacting the National Marrow Donor Program. In desperation the parents decided to have another child in hopes that the new baby would genetically have matching tissue type. This required that the father have a vasectomy reversed and that the mother, aged 43, go through another pregnancy that terminated in a cesarean section. The baby provided a good match and was able to provide donor tissue for her sister. The case drew considerable attention as medical ethicists voiced concern about creating one child to save another. Citing Immanuel Kant, they argued that the baby was

Consentimiento para Remover los Órganos de la Personal Fallecida

Yo, _____ , familiar (_____)
         Nombre   *Relación*

de _____
                              Nombre del donador

consiento por razones humanitarias, la extracción de _____

_____ de
                         Nombrar órganos y tejidos

_____
                         Nombre del donador

posterior a su muerte para el propósito de trasplantes, o para la retención de dichos órganos y tejidos para cualquier otro propósito científico o terapéutico.

Entiendo que se requieren ciertos procedimientos para determinar si el trasplante es adecuado, estos incluyen las pruebas de HBsAg (virus de la hepatitis B) y del virus de immunodeficiencia humana (anticuerpo del virus del SIDA). También autorizo que los médicos que van a trasplantar los órganos y tejidos antes mencionados, tengan toda la información médica obtenida en este proceso.

_____
                                      Firma

_____
                                      Fecha

_____
                    Testigo/a

_____
                    Testigo/a

Source: Certified as a correct Spanish translation of all relevant information from the English original by Sarina Cats Frank, Notary Public.

conceived, not as an end in itself, but for utilitarian purposes. Some medical ethicists argue the rights of the individuals involved, saying that it is not the concern of biomedical ethicists to intrude into matters affecting private citizens, especially when that intrusion approaches "intruding into a couple's bedroom." Still others say that striking cases must be brought before the public because an obligation to inform society exists.

The critical need for human organs also causes us to challenge previous decisions. A good example is that raised when considering organs removed from an anencephalic infant. An anencephalic infant is one born with only

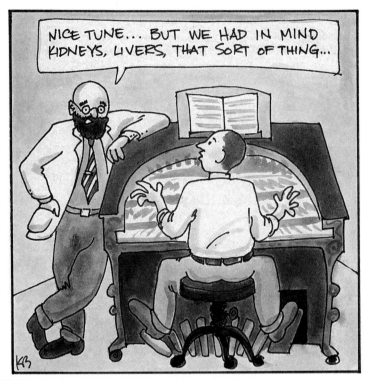

FIGURE 7–6 The need for organs that can be used for transplant has become greater, and obtaining these organs has become more difficult.

enough brain to support such vital functions as heartbeat and respiration. It has been estimated that about 60% of these infants are stillborn and of those born alive only about 5% will live more than 3 days. Because anencephaly affects only the brain, other organs can be used for transplantation if the infant is kept alive on a respirator until a donor is located. This would challenge our definitions of death. How can current definitions of "brain" death be applied to a condition in which there is no brain as we normally recognize it?

Other problems arise with regard to organ transplantations, especially because there are more people who need organs than there are organs available. The skill of modern technology resulted in the development and implantation of artificial organs such as the heart. Such technological advances were once viewed as science fiction. As a result, historic cases received a great deal of publicity, such as the implantation of an artificial heart in Barney Clark. Over the years the use of artificial organs has not proven effective, and the practice of implanting artificial organs is not common today. This is not true of artificial parts. The use of artificial joints, heart values, and other prostheses continues to grow.

Concerns About Allocation

How will it be determined who will receive a donated organ? Is there any "elitism'" in their distribution; that is, does a white-collar worker have a better chance to receive an organ than does a blue-collar worker? Most insurance policies and Medicaid refuse to pay for the cost of many organ transplants, although the costs of corneal transplants and kidney transplants are usually covered by Medicare. Transplants are expensive procedures, often running into several hundreds of thousands of dollars. If money is required "up front," as it sometimes is, where can the needy person procure such funds? Other questions involve both donor and recipient. Should the donor or the donor's family be able to say who will receive the organ? How can one "get in line" for an organ, and how can that need be made known?

Much has been written about the problem of selecting recipients for organ transplantation when the number of applicants exceeds the number of available organs. Many criteria have been suggested, and as one might anticipate, these criteria have received arguments both pro and con. The criterion requiring medical acceptability is probably the only exception. Many transplants require that compatibility exist in the tissue and blood type of donor and recipient. It would not be logical to give a much needed organ to a person whose body would automatically reject it.

The criterion of the recipient's social worth is probably one of the hardest to defend, although it was used in the Pacific Northwest in the early 1960s to decide who should be allowed to live by kidney dialysis. Social worth, both of past and future potential, was considered, and even such factors as church membership and participation in community endeavors were considered.

Others suggest some type of random selection once the criterion of medical acceptability has been met. This could be either a natural random selection of the first come, first served variety or an artificial selection process such as a lottery. A criticism of this method is that it removes rational decision-making from the process.

We offer no suggestions to solve this problem but merely demonstrate the difficulty it presents. Even the issue of who should serve on the decision-making committee can be touchy. The problem of personal biases is one big concern.

In an effort to gather donations and disseminate information about people who need various organs, an Organ Procurement Program was started in Pittsburgh, Pennsylvania. This program was established to facilitate the matching of donor with recipient and provide a central listing agency for those in need of transplants. Today organ procurement agencies are located in many regions of the country. These groups carry out many activities related to organ procurement, including establishing groups for individuals who have received donated organs and their families, publishing newsletters and developing educational materials, increasing public awareness of the need for organs, as well as serving as a clearinghouse for organ procurement and matching. They are connected through the federally funded United Network for Organ Sharing.

Concerns About Individual Property Rights

Concern for an individual's property rights in regard to human tissues has also attracted attention. Biotechnological developments allow profit-oriented companies to use human tissue to generate lucrative products such as drugs, diagnostic tests, and other medically related materials. The modern legal system has consistently held that no property rights are attached to the human body (Swain and Marusyk, 1990). In 1990, a Seattle man sued the University of California, two researchers, and two biotechnology and drug companies. In 1976, he had sought treatment for hairy cell leukemia and subsequently had his spleen removed, which is the standard treatment. It was later discovered that the removed spleen contained unique blood cells that produced a rare blood protein used experimentally in the treatment of certain cancers and possibly AIDS. The patient was never told that his cells had great potential value, although he was brought from Seattle to Los Angeles frequently for blood and other tests. His cells were then developed into a self-perpetuating cell line to mass produce the rare blood protein. The patient's suit claimed that the defendants wrongfully converted to their own use his personal property (ie, the blood cells) and that this was done without his consent.

TRUTH-TELLING AND HEALTH CARE PROVIDERS

The issue of "to tell" or "not to tell" may not carry the emotional and bioethical impact that one experiences with concerns such as euthanasia, but it is one that is frequently encountered in the hospital environment. Although informed consent has forced a more straightforward approach between physician and client, the problem of having the patient fully understand the outcome of care still exists. Sometimes the question about telling the patient the expected outcome of care results from a request made by a close relative, but most of the time it results from the persistence of past medical practices.

In such instances the physician operates in a paternalistic role in relation to the patient. Under this model of care, the locus of decision-making is moved away from the patient and is now with the physician. "Benefit and do no harm to the patient" is the dictum often cited as the ethical basis for this approach. It rationalizes that complete knowledge of his or her condition would place greater stress on the patient. More recent discussions of medical ethics explore the rights of patients, particularly their right to make their own medical decisions. These discussions emphasize that in our pluralistic society, which has also fostered medical specialization to keep up with advances in knowledge and technology, physicians may be unable to perceive the "best interests" of their patients and act accordingly.

Physicians do not agree on how much patients should know about their condition. We usually experience the major controversy relating to this issue when the patient has a terminal diagnosis such as cancer. Because, ideally at least, physicians are committed to protecting their patients from potential harm, both physical and mental, many have difficulty sharing bad news that will result in unhappiness, anxiety, depression, and fear. These physicians are concerned that if the patients know they are suffering from a terminal illness, they will give up. After all, medical science might be wrong, or research may develop new cures that would change the course of the disease.

Physicians who argue the other side of the issue state that there exists a common moral obligation to tell the truth. They believe that the anxiety of not knowing the accurate diagnosis is at least as great as knowing the truth, especially if the truth is shared in a humane manner. These physicians also argue that one needs to have control over one's life and, if the news is bad, to have time to get personal affairs in order.

Although to tell or not to tell is a problem that exists between patient and physician, nurses often become involved in it. First of all, the nurse may have definite personal feelings one way or the other. For example, if the physician has decided not to tell the patient, or to delay sharing this information until later, and the nurse believes that the patient has the right to be informed, the nurse may be in a frustrating situation and may even be angry with the physician. Because the nurse is in contact with the patient for a more extended period of time, he or she may be put on the spot by the patient's questions. The nurse may feel that by hedging on a response there is a compromise of the ethics of nursing practice. In such instances a conference, whether formal or impromptu, that would involve the physician, nurses, and other appropriate members of the health team, may help everyone deal with the situation. The nurse who is a novice in the health care system should realize that anyone can initiate a patient care conference, although appropriate channels of communication should be followed in organizing it.

Thus far we have discussed situations in which information regarding a terminal illness may be shared with the patient and family. At least one other circumstance that involves telling the truth is worth mentioning, although many examples could be included. One that we often see in the obstetric area of the hospital deals with sharing information with the parents of a newborn who is critical or who has a malformation. Sometimes physicians may want to spare the mother unpleasant news until she is stronger. This occurs frequently enough for obstetric nurses to have labeled it the *spare-the-mother syndrome*. In other instances the physician may want to delay giving information until suspicions can be validated. If the doctor is waiting for the return of laboratory tests to confirm suspicions of genetic abnormalities, several days may be required. If good communication exists between nurse and physician, so that the nurse is well informed, the nurse can provide emotional support and meet the patient's need for information. Once again, a team approach usually is most effective.

ETHICAL CONCERNS AND BEHAVIOR CONTROL

Before leaving this discussion of bioethical issues, we should say a few words in relation to behavior control. Many people experience extreme discomfort when contemplating research into human behavior. Although it may be one thing to work with atoms, molecules, and genes, it seems quite another to look at the science of human behavior.

Some of the problem seems to center around the fact that people define "acceptable behavior" in different and sometimes conflicting ways. When is behavior deviant? When is the patient mentally ill? An excellent example is that of homosexuality, which at one time was listed by the American Psychiatric Association as a mental illness. Although many people may not approve of homosexuality, they would not classify all homosexuals as being mentally ill. Increasingly, society looks on sexual orientation as a personal matter.

The world has benefited from the work of many people whose behavior might not be looked on as being normal. Van Gogh cut off his ear; Tchaikovsky had terrible periods of depression; Beethoven was known for his uncontrollable rages. Some have suggested that Florence Nightingale's flights into fantasy could better be described as neurosis. Should this behavior have been changed and by what methods?

We can now change behavior by a variety of methods. Certainly one of the most common methods in which nurses will be involved is the administration of pharmacologic agents. Tranquilizers are now one of the largest classifications of drugs in the United States. Other chemicals, such as alcohol, marijuana, cocaine, and lysergic acid diethylamide (LSD), also change behavior. Some of these are considered socially acceptable, whereas others are not. Some are socially acceptable to some people or to some whole cultures, yet unacceptable to others.

Electroconvulsive therapy, known earlier as electric shock therapy, has been used for years to treat severe depression. Although antidepressant drugs are more commonly used today, electric shock therapy is still used in many areas of the country for depression that does not respond to drugs. Opponents of this form of therapy, who see it as inhumane, are becoming an organized political force. Proponents point out that with the current safeguards, it can be an effective therapy.

Psychosurgery, for example, frontal lobotomy (portrayed in *One Flew Over the Cuckoo's Nest*), was used in the 1930s. This is undoubtedly one of the most criticized of treatment modalities because of its effect on the person. It is rarely used today although another type of brain surgery is now being suggested for obsessive compulsive disorder.

Psychotherapy can change other behavior. This technique includes verbal and nonverbal communication between the patient and the therapist. Although psychotherapy requires considerable time, it is widely used.

When are any of these methods justified? Who makes the decision? What behavior is beyond the realm of acceptability? Who determines this? How does behavior control mesh with our beliefs about the autonomy of the individual or with concepts of self-respect and dignity? The issues of power and coercion pose a concern at this point. Problems related to involuntary commitment have moved this from the arena of ethics to that of legal determinants.

Halleck (1981, p 268) has defined behavior control as treatment "imposed on or offered to the patient that, to a large extent, is designed to satisfy the wishes of others. Such treatment may lead to the patient's behaving in a manner which satisfies his community or his society." Halleck goes on to point out that the question of behavior control has become more critical because newer drugs and new behavior therapy (such as aversive therapy and desensitization) make it possible to change specific behavior more rapidly and effectively. Traditional psychotherapy, which works slowly, offered the patient time in which to contemplate the change and reject it if it was unacceptable.

Dworkin (1981, p 278) has proposed a set of guidelines that preserve autonomy in behavior control, as briefly stated here.

> We should favor those methods of influencing behavior that support the self-respect and dignity of those who are being influenced.
>
> Methods of influence that destroy or decrease a person's ability to think rationally and in his or her own interest should not be used.
>
> Methods of influence that fundamentally affect the personal identity of the person should not be used.
>
> Methods of influence that deceive or keep relevant facts from the person should not be used.
>
> Modes of influence that are not physically intrusive are preferable to those that are (such as drugs, psychosurgery, and electricity).
>
> A person should be able to resist the method of influence if he or she so desires, and changes of behavior that are reversible are preferable to those that are not.
>
> Methods that work through the cognitive and affective structure of a person are preferable to those that "short-circuit" his beliefs and desires and cause him to be passively receptive to the will of others.

RATIONING OF HEALTH CARE

As we move into the 21st century perhaps no issue in health care will receive more attention than that which deals with the rationing of health care. Technology has allowed people to live longer and longer. New treatment modalities have become more and more expensive. Dollars do not exist within our current social system to make all forms of health care available to all who may wish to receive it. What should be treated and what should not? Who should receive the treatment and who should not? Should age be a factor? Mental status? Ability to contribute to society?

A number of states have begun to address these issues. In 1989, the Oregon legislature passed several statues that, among other things, created a process by which health care priorities would be established so that Medicaid and state-encouraged private coverage could provide the most cost-effective and beneficial forms of care for the largest number of persons. Implicit in this legislation was the involvement of the public in the process of building consensus on the values to be used to guide health resource allocation decisions. Oregon as continued to lead the nation in health care reform, especially at the consumer involvement level.

In Vermont a statewide public education and discussion project was initiated that was designed to explore public attitudes and values that underlie health care and the public's priorities in the allocation of health resources. The project focused on the need for individuals to make known their preferences with regard to personal treatment.

In New Jersey a Citizens' Committee on Biomedical Ethics has taken the position that citizens have the right and responsibility to insist that their preferences and values influence the development of health care policies and the allocation of medical resources. They have launched into a community health program to clarify the ethical and social issues surrounding the provision of health care in that state.

Other states are following the examples set. Citizens are being asked to make informed decisions regarding health care. As a nurse you have a vital role to play in the sharing of information regarding the delivery of services. It is critical that you have anticipated some of the questions you may be asked and have analyzed your own values.

Key Concepts

⬦ Bioethics is the study of ethical issues that result from technological and scientific advances, especially in biology and medicine. The bioethical issues surrounding the delivery of health care are ever increasing.

⬦ The leading bioethical issues can be divided into two major categories: those related to the beginning of life and those related to the end of life.

⬦ Issues related to the beginning of life include the use of family planning and the associated concern regarding age of consent.

⬦ Abortion, amniocentesis, prenatal diagnosis, genetic screening, sterilization, the concept of eugenics, the Human Genome Project, in vitro fertilization, artificial insemination, surrogate mothers, single parents, sperm banks, and the right to genetic information are additional topics presenting concerns.

▷ Bioethical issues concerning death start with changing definitions of death, essentially when it occurs.

▷ End-of-life issues include identifying futile treatment and establishing patient self-determination.

▷ The concept of euthanasia, both negative and positive, and whether it should be practiced has been discussed for many years.

▷ Of more recent concern are the many right-to-die issues, including those related to withholding treatment, withdrawing treatment, assisted death, and the right to refuse treatment.

▷ Additional bioethical concerns include the problems associated with organ transplantation, including procurement of organs, allocation or organs, and individual property rights.

▷ Determining the degree of information that should be shared with patients and their families has long been a subject of debate and controversy.

▷ The area of behavior control is subject to bioethical review and guidelines have been established to preserve autonomy in behavior control.

▷ Receiving major attention at the present time is the matter of rationing of health care. Many states have begun to establish citizen committees to respond to this concern.

CRITICAL THINKING ACTIVITIES

1. Select one of the positions taken regarding abortion. Defend your position, providing a strong rationale for your thinking. Discuss this with a classmate who holds a different position.

2. What do you see as the major issues associated with the Human Genome Project? What do you see as the major benefits to come from it? Weigh the issues against the benefits and take a position with regard to how far it should be developed.

3. What safeguards would you recommend with regard to in vitro fertilization, artificial insemination and surrogate mothers to ensure sanctity of human life?

4. Have you signed an organ donation card? If not, discuss the reasons why you have chosen not to. If you have, discuss the reasons why you have. Is there a possibility you will change your mind? Why or why not?

5. What do you see as the major issues regarding the rationing of care? Develop a list of the major health conditions you believe should be funded. Identify those that should receive partial funding. List those that you believe should not be funded. Give a rationale for placing the various conditions on one of the three lists.

References

Blackmun H. Majority opinion in Roe vs Wade. In Mappes TA, Zembaty JS: Biomedical Ethics, 2nd ed. New York: McGraw-Hill, 1981:478–482

Capron AM. Death, definition and determination of: Legal aspects. In Reich WT: Encyclopedia of Bioethics, vol 1. New York: Free Press, 1978:300

Capron AM. Grandma? No, I'm the Mother! Hastings Cent Rep 24(2):24–25, 1994

Colby WH. Missouri stands alone. Hastings Cent Rep 20(5):5–6, 1990

Dworkin G. Autonomy and behavior control. In Mappes TA, Zembaty JS: Biomedical Ethics, 2nd ed. New York: McGraw-Hill, 1981:273–280

Fromer MJ. Ethical Issues in Health Care. St. Louis: CV Mosby, 1981

Fry ST. New ANA guidelines on withdrawing or withholding food and fluid from patients. In Lindeman CA, McAthie M: Readings: Nursing Trends and Issues. Springhouse, PA: Springhouse, 1990:499–507

Gustafson JJ. Mongolism, parental desires, and the right to life. Perspect Biomed, Summer 1973:529

Halleck SL. Legal and ethical aspects of behavior control. In Mappes TA, Zembaty JS: Biomedical Ethics, 2nd ed. New York: McGraw-Hill, 1981:267–273

Hayt LR. Medicolegal Aspects of Hospital Records, 2nd ed. Berwyn, IL: Physicians' Record Company, 1977:397

Hellegers AE. Bioethical debates in gynecology and obstetrics. In Romney SL, et al: Gynecology and Obstetrics: The Health Care of Women. New York: McGraw-Hill, 1975:36

Hospital sued for "wrongful life." Am J Nurs 91(5):111, 1991

Hudson T. Advance directives: Still problematic for providers. Hospitals and Health Networks 68(6):46, 48, 50, March 20, 1994

Hudson T. Are futile-care policies the answer? Hospitals and Health Networks 68(4):26-32, February 20, 1994

Jonsen AR. The Birth of Bioethics. Special Supplement to Hastings Cent Rep 23(6):S1–S4, 1993

Kass LR. Is there a right to die? Hastings Cent Rep 23(1):34–43, 1993

Kevles DJ. Social and ethical issues in the Human Genome Project. National Forum LXXIII(2): 18–21, Spring, 1993

Macklin R. Artificial means of reproduction and our understanding of the family. Hastings Cent Rep 21(1):5–11, 1991

Mancini M. Nursing, minors, and the law. Am J Nurs 78(1):124–127, 1978

Roe v. Wade, 410 U.S. 113 (1973)

Rossiter BJF, Caskey CT. Medical consequences of the Human Genome Project. National Forum LXXIII(2):12–14, Spring, 1993

Rothman DA, Rothman NL. The Professional Nurse and the Law. Boston: Little, Brown, 1977

Rothstein MA. The challenge of the new genetics. National Forum 69(4):39–40, 1990

Thomas CL. Taber's Cyclopedic Medical Dictionary, 17th ed. Philadelphia: FA Davis, 1993

Schneiderman LF, Jecker N. Futility in practice. Arch Intern Med 153:437–440, 1993

Swain MS, Marusyk RW. An alternative to property rights in human tissue. Hastings Cent Rep 20(5):12–15, 1990

Veatch RM. Death, Dying and the Biological Revolution. New Haven, CT: Yale University Press, 1976

Further Readings

Arras GJ. Crazy making: Embryos and gestational mothers. Hastings Cent Rep 21(1):35–38, 1991

Arras JD. Anencephalic newborns as organ donors: A critique. JAMA 259:2284–2286, 1988

Bailey LL. Organ transplantation: A paradigm of medical progress. Hastings Cent Rep 20(1):24–28, 1990

Battin MP. The least worst death: Biotechnology and the right to die. National Forum 69(4): 36–38, 1989

Callahan D. Medical futility, medical necessity: The problem without a name. Hastings Cent Rep 21(4):30–35, 1991

Chervenak FA, McCollough LB. Justified limits on refusing intervention. Hastings Cent Rep 21(2):12–18, 1991

Colbert T. Public input into health care policy: Controversy and contribution in California. Hastings Cent Rep 20(5):21, 1990

Cranford RE. A hostage to technology. Hastings Cent Rep 20(5):9–10, 1990

Crawshaw R. A vision of the health decisions movement. Hastings Cent Rep 20(5):21–22, 1990

Daniels N. Duty to treat or right to refuse? Hastings Cent Rep 21(2):36–46, 1991

Ellman IM. Can others exercise an incapacitated patient's right to die? Hastings Cent Rep 20(1): 47–50, 1990

Fowler MD. The role of the clinical ethicist. Heart Lung 15(5):318–319, 1989

Garland MJ, Hasnain R. Health care in common: Setting priorities in Oregon. Hastings Cent Rep 20(5):16–18, 1990

Gaylin W. Fooling with mother nature. Hastings Cent Rep 20(1):17–21, 1990

Guido GW. Legal Issues in Nursing: A Source Book for Practice. Norwalk, CT: Appleton & Lange, 1992

HHS stands by "Baby Doe" policy despite court's ruling on regs. Am J Nurs 83(6):851, 868–869, 1983

Hill TP. Giving voice to the pragmatic majority in New Jersey. Hastings Cent Rep 20(5):20, 1990

How far should we push Mother Nature? Newsweek 17:54–57, January 1994

Jecker NS, ed. Aging and Ethics: Philosophical Problems in Gerontology. Clifton, NJ: Humana Press, 1991

Lauritzen P. What price parenthood? Hastings Cent Rep 20(2): 38–46, 1990

Lippman H. After Cruzan: The right to die. RN 54(1):65–68, 73, 1991

Lynn J, Glover J. Cruzan and caring for others. Hastings Cent Rep 20(5):10–11, 1990

Moody HR. Ethics in an Aging Society. Baltimore/London: Johns Hopkins University Press, 1992

Moss RJ, La Puma J. The ethics of mechanical restraints. Hastings Cent Rep 21(1):22–25, 1991

Nurses seek a voice in right-to-die cases. Am J Nurs 91(3):26, 1991

Overall C. Selective termination of pregnancy and women's reproductive autonomy. Hastings Cent Rep 20(3):6–11, 1990

Pence T. Ethics in Nursing: An Annotated Bibliography, pt 2. Publication No. 20-1989. New York: National League for Nursing, 1986

Powledge TM. Capital report—springtime for fetal tissue research? Hastings Cent Rep 21(2):5–6, 1991

Reich WT (ed). Encyclopedia of Bioethics. New York: Macmillan, 1982

Robertson JA. Cruzan: No rights violated. Hastings Cent Rep 20(5):8–9, 1990

Rothman, DJ. Strangers at the Bedside: A History of How Law and Bioethics Transformed Medical Decision Making. New York: Basic, 1991

Rousseau PC. How fluid deprivation affects the terminally ill. RN 54(1):73–74, 1991

Veatch RM. Bioethics discovers the bill of rights. National Forum 69(4):11–13, 1989

Vernale C, Packard SA. Organ donation as gift exchange. Image 22(4):239–242, 1990

Wendling EM. Anencephalics as organ donors. Imprint April/May 1990:47–48

Wurzbach ME, The dilemma of withholding or withdrawing nutrition. Image 22(4):226–230, 1990

III Economic and Political Aspects of Health Care Delivery

Health care in the United States is part of the overall economic and political life of the nation. It reflects much of what is best about life in the United States but also serves to point out those areas where serious problems exist.

In this unit we try to help you understand the health care delivery system in a basic way. The complexity of the system as it exists cannot be completely explained in one short chapter, but we have tried to focus on the aspects that will best help you put health care issues into context. From an overview of the system, we move to the issue of collective bargaining and how it affects nursing. The political process and how that relates to health care is the final chapter in this unit. Our hope is that you will find an understanding of the political process relevant to your professional life.

8

The Health Care Delivery System

Objectives

After completing this chapter, you should be able to

1. Explain the role of the primary health care provider and identify the individuals who fulfill this role.

2. Describe the roles of the various allied health care workers.

3. Discuss the ways in which alternative health care resources meet health care needs.

4. Describe the different mechanisms of health care financing.

5. Explain how regulatory agencies, payers, providers, and consumers demonstrate power in the health care system.

6. Describe economic influences on health care delivery.

Ellis JR, Hartley CL: NURSING IN TODAY'S WORLD:
CHALLENGES, ISSUES, AND TRENDS, 5th ed.
© 1995 J.B. Lippincott Company

We refer to the health care system as if it were an organized entity, with each part relating to another in a systematic way. In reality the current situation is more like a nonsystem of many diverse people and organizations, each going in its own direction. There has been no central authority in the U.S. health care system, no setting of overall priorities, and no general planning for the use of resources. There are private components and governmental components, nonprofit sectors and profit-making sectors, and individuals and groups all operating independently.

Although this nonsystem has been chaotic, it has produced some of the most significant advances in medicine and health care ever seen. At the same time there is a maldistribution of the benefits of those advances, as attested to by such factors as the high infant mortality rate in the United States, which exceeds that of many other major industrialized nations (Hughes et al., 1989). Some people receive outstanding health care in the most modern of settings. Others receive no health care. Health insurance grows ever more expensive, and many working people are unable to afford coverage for their families. Society appears to stagger under the increasing costs of governmental programs such as Medicare and Medicaid (Kenkel, 1990)

The United States is on the brink of a major change in health care de-

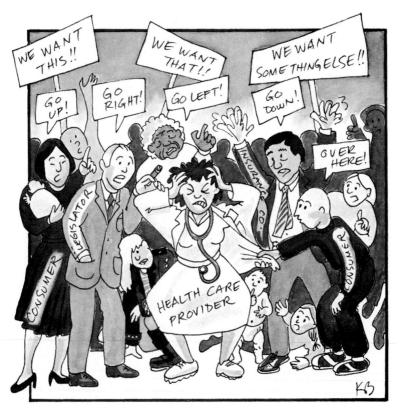

FIGURE 8–1 The impetus for change in health care delivery has been growing.

livery. The impetus for change has been growing. Several states have already instituted efforts to create a more coordinated system for their citizens. Multiple bills for health care reform are being considered by the U.S. Congress. President Clinton has established health care reform as a major priority for his administration. The details of the future system are still not established, but we will try to point out the major changes likely to be part of the new health care system.

Colleagues in Health Care

Many different groups of individuals deliver health care. These providers exist because they meet the needs of our society in some way. Some of these groups are believed to provide a valuable service; the services of others are of questionable benefit. There are problems with the supply of qualified individuals in some of these areas. In other areas there are enough qualified providers, but the providers tend all to be of a single gender or ethnic background. This may pose difficulties for both the client and the care provider when they are unable to communicate effectively. Many programs are in place that are striving to increase the diversity among health care providers to better meet the needs of all clients. As the health care workforce has changed, some clients must adapt their perceptions to accept a wider diversity in their health care providers.

More than 230 types of health care workers have been identified within the United States. It is not within the scope of this book to discuss each of these occupations individually, but we do attempt to outline the general categories of health care providers with whom you may be working.

PRIMARY HEALTH CARE PROVIDERS

The primary health care provider furnishes entry into the health care system. This person is consulted by the patient for routine health maintenance, as well as for care of episodic illness. This health care provider has traditionally been a medical doctor, osteopathic physician, or dentist. These professionals are licensed in all states and are authorized to treat illness, including the prescribing of drugs.

The planned cornerstone of health care reform is the increase in number of primary health care providers and the focus on the primary care provider as the "gatekeeper" for the system. The primary provider will implement those health maintenance activities that prevent the need for more expensive care. This is the individual who will provide referral to more specialized care when that is needed. One of the problems for those in rural areas, economically disadvantaged areas of large cities, and those on welfare programs has been the lack of access to primary care. The lack of access often has resulted in delaying care until the problem is more complex and requires greater resources to re-

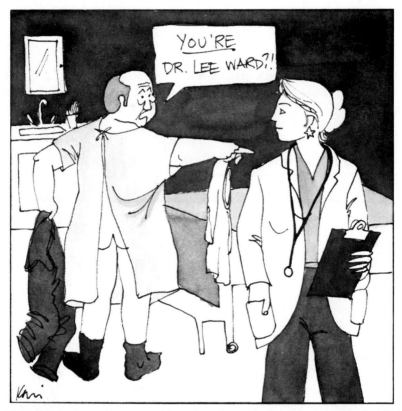

FIGURE 8–2 As the health care workforce has changed, some clients must adapt their perceptions.

solve. To meet the needs of society, some nurses are moving into this area of practice as *nurse practitioners*.

Physicians

The differences between traditional (allopathic) medicine and osteopathic medicine are becoming less distinct. Historically, the philosophy of care and remedial techniques of osteopathic physicians included more treatments such as back manipulation and nutritional counseling, while fewer drugs were prescribed and less surgery was performed. Osteopathic physicians and allopathic physicians practiced entirely independently of each other and used separate hospitals; a visible antagonism between the two groups was often apparent. Recently the move has been toward greater cooperation, with physicians from both traditions practicing side by side in hospitals. The osteopathic group is considerably smaller, has far fewer specialists, has fewer resources for research, and is less well known. However, the educational patterns for both are the same.

Undergraduate medical education may vary in focus, but a strong science background is required. This is followed by 4 years of medical school. During this time formal education is stressed, with patient contact occurring most often at the latter part of the program. Some medical schools are beginning to provide patient contact earlier in the educational process. After completion of medical school, licensing examinations are taken.

Once individuals are licensed as physicians, they participate in a residency program. These programs are developed by hospitals and primarily focus on patient care. Their length varies depending on the specialty. The resident is paid a salary by the hospital. In state, county, and city hospitals the resident physician may serve as the primary physician for some patients. For patients who are responsible for their own medical bills (either directly or through insurance), the admitting personal physician usually remains in charge and the resident serves a supporting role in the patient's medical care. At the end of the residency, the physician is able to practice independently.

After residency training is completed, the physician is prepared to write examinations to become certified in the specialty. The person who successfully passes the specialty examination is termed *board certified*. It is not legally required that a physician be board certified to practice in a specialty area. Certification in family practice is increasingly being considered the basic requirement for primary practice.

Subspecialty training occurs after specialty training is completed. Given this pattern of education and training, a physician may have a total of 10 or more years of postsecondary education and training before beginning to work independently.

Podiatrists

Podiatrists (formerly called chiropodists) are educated in the care and surgery of the foot. They care for corns, bunions, and toenails; prescribe and fit corrective shoes and arch supports; and perform surgery on the feet, such as correction of deformities, removal of bunions, and removal of small tumors. A podiatrist does not prescribe systemic medication or care for any generalized disease condition.

Nurse Practitioners

As demands on the system have increased, additional people have been added to the group of primary care providers. Nurses working in specialized roles as primary care nurses or nurse practitioners are one example. These nurses have obtained education in addition to that required for basic licensure and have earned certification in a particular specialty. Nurse practitioners may work with a physician in an office or clinic, or they may function independently in a nurse clinic. Some states grant nurse practitioners who meet special guidelines the authority to write prescriptions. This type of authority is the subject of heated debate in other states.

Some suggest that the increased utilization of the nurse practitioner as a primary care provider is one of the major thrusts of health care reform. They point to the geographic availability and cost savings as critical elements. In keeping with this approach, the majority of federal money available for nursing education has been allocated to advanced preparation (see Chapter 10).

Physician's Assistants

Another primary caregiver is the physician's assistant. This person, sometimes called the *medex*, often has medical and emergency training, such as from the military service or other health occupations, and has completed a university program. Physician's assistant programs vary from 1-year to 4-year baccalaureate programs. Physician's assistants must work under the direction of a physician at all times.

Physician's assistants usually see patients with commonly recurring health problems such as colds, flu, and minor trauma, such as cuts needing suturing. Physician's assistants may also provide some primary health care such as routine physical examinations. If the patient needs referral to a specialist or hospital admission, the physician's assistant first refers the patient to the physician with whom he or she works. In some instances the physician's assistant may work with a specialty physician such as an orthopedic physician and have different responsibilities, such as applying and removing casts.

The use of physician's assistants is sometimes controversial. Some patients believe that they are receiving less than quality care if they are treated by a physician's assistant instead of seeing the physician. Within the health care team, the appropriateness of physician's assistants writing prescriptions and orders on the charts of hospitalized patients has been questioned. Nurses have been concerned because their own licensure laws state that they can administer medications only on the order of a licensed physician, osteopath, or dentist, and in some instances they have been asked to give medications on the order of a physician's assistant. In Washington State a court decision stated that nurses should not give medications ordered by a physician's assistant until those orders are countersigned by a physician.

Another area of concern has been whether nurses working in expanded roles should be classified as physician's assistants and be governed by the Board of Medicine rather than the Board of Nursing. Some nurses have enrolled in and completed the regular physician's assistant programs and are working in this capacity. Other nurses believe strongly that the role of the nurse is an independent one and that the nurse in primary care should not be considered a physician's assistant but rather an independent nurse. The American Nurses Association (ANA) has supported the view that the nurse in primary care is more than a physician's assistant and should not be included in that classification.

Other Primary Care Providers

Social workers and *clinical psychologists* have historically performed a primary care role by providing a person's entry into the mental health care system, serving as the supervisors of care, and furnishing referral as needed. Because they are not able to treat physical problems, they often work in cooperation with physicians or nurse practitioners who are able to manage this aspect of care. Whether they will be able to provide care as primary providers or will be limited to providing care on referral only is one of the subjects being debated as part of health care reform.

Optometrists provide vision testing and prescribe glasses, contact lenses, and corrective exercises for eye problems. They have a general background in assessment of eye disease so that they can screen and refer patients to an *ophthalmologist* (a physician who specializes in eye disease) when diagnosis and treatment are needed. Because ophthalmologists offer some of the same services as optometrists there is some disagreement between the two groups over scope of practice. Whether eye examinations and corrective lenses for vision should be part of basic health care is another area of debate in the health care reform legislation.

Dentists provide for primary care of the teeth and mouth. Many dentists are beginning to include general health screening, such as examining the mouth and throat for tumors or disease and taking blood pressure in their basic examination. The patient is referred to a physician if an abnormality is noted. Dentists have an educational background similar in length to that of the physician—4 years of baccalaureate education followed by dental school. There is no residency period, and dentists begin independent practice after passing state licensing examinations. Dentists are empowered to prescribe medications in addition to providing care for the mouth and teeth. There are specialty areas in dentistry, such as orthodontics (the application of devices to change the occlusion of the teeth), just as there are in medicine. Education for specialties occurs in universities that have dental schools. After the student has graduated, the diploma indicates competence in the specialty. There is no legal requirement for advanced education to practice a dental specialty, although strong professional constraints exist.

Dental care is another concern as basic health care is being debated. Certainly dental health is a part of overall health. However, some voices suggest that health care reform must limit demands and not try to cover every aspect of health for all individuals to be economically viable.

Issues Related to Primary Health Care

One of the problems in U.S. health care is maldistribution of primary care providers. Urban areas have proportionately more health workers of every kind than do rural areas. Within large cities, care providers are concentrated in more affluent areas. Many programs that would provide an incentive to establish a practice in an area that is insufficiently served have been attempted. Some of these programs include educational loans that are forgiven or canceled if the person works in an underserved area after completion of the course of study. In other instances schools have tried to recruit students from underserved areas, hoping that after graduation the student would return home to practice. Some schools incorporate into their programs learning experiences in rural or poorly served areas in the hope that graduates may be attracted to the area and return later to work.

Despite these efforts, the problem still exists for several reasons. Physicians prefer to practice where there is access to specialized medical centers and where opportunities for consultation are readily available. Another factor that deters physicians from practicing in rural areas is the tremendous physical strain involved in being the only care provider. The rural physician often receives little respite from 24-hours-a-day, 7-days-a-week availability to the community. Incomes of rural physicians also tend to be less than incomes of physicians in urban areas. Nurse practitioners increasingly are providing health care to underserved populations and have been more willing to relocate to rural or poverty areas.

Another major concern is the relative distribution of physicians prepared as specialists and those who act as primary care providers. In the United States approximately 60% of the physicians practice in specialties and 40% practice in some area of primary care such as general practice, family practice, pediatrics, and obstetrics/gynecology. The result in the system is too few primary care providers and excess numbers of specialists in some areas. Part of the health care reform legislation being introduced provides for incentives and support for those entering primary care practice.

The trend in private medical practice is toward group practices. Several specialties may be represented within the group. Although patients may have a private physician, they may easily receive care from other members of the group. Group practice ensures the individual physician of more time for personal and family life.

Care in private practice usually is based on fee for service. Although some physicians may attempt to make adjustments for those with less ability to pay, one of the serious health care problems of our day is the cost of health care for even middle-class individuals. Insurance may pay for some outpatient care, and it funds most of the care given during hospitalization, but increasing numbers of people have inadequate or no insurance.

ALLIED HEALTH CARE WORKERS

Allied health care workers are categorized in many ways. Frequently the term *technologist* is used to refer to those with baccalaureate preparation and *technician* is used to identify those with 2 years of education or less. The term *thera-*

pist usually denotes more advanced functioning than *therapy technician*. Most of the allied health care professions provide diagnostic and treatment services for patients. Some, such as those who work with records, serve in roles to support the system.

Laboratory and Diagnostic Services

Included in the category of laboratory and diagnostic occupations are those who work in the clinical laboratory, such as the medical technologist and medical laboratory technician, as well as those who work in all the specialized diagnostics fields, such as nuclear medicine technician, electroencephalograph (EEG) technician, and radiologic technician. They assist with all of the tests that are now used to diagnose and monitor progress in illness. As new sophisticated diagnostic technology is introduced, new technicians are created to operate and monitor the equipment. Some occupations, such as the medical technologist, require a baccalaureate degree. Others, such as the radiology technician and medical laboratory technician, usually have 2-year associate degrees. Still others, such as the electrocardiographic (ECG) technician, may be trained on the job.

Administrative and Business Personnel

As health care facilities have become more complex, the administrative and business aspects have similarly become more demanding. Many people are needed to maintain and retrieve information from the medical record. These workers include the health information administrator, the medical record technician, and the medical secretary. The positions of hospital administrator and assistant administrator are changing. In the past these appointments may have been filled by a physician, an attorney, or a businessman. Because the health care system now has such specialized demands, the administrative positions are increasingly being filled by those with a baccalaureate or master's degree in health care administration. A special certification is required for those who administer nursing homes.

Community Health Care Workers

As a growing field, community health has required an increasing number of workers. The major focus of community health care is the promotion of health rather than care of illness. Some workers, such as the health educator and community health visitor, work directly with individual clients. Others, such as the sanitarian, are engaged in assisting the community as a whole toward better health through maintenance of standards related to cleanliness and infectious disease control.

Other community health care workers are those who help individuals with health and personal care after discharge from the hospital. Although some of these positions are held by registered nurses who provide skilled care, many more are held by home health aides who assist with nontechnical aspects of care and may even help with household tasks and shopping. Education for home health aides which in the past was conducted as on-the-job training now takes place in courses leading to certification.

Makers of Prosthetic and Assistive Devices

With technological advances, the number of different types of prostheses and assistive devices increases. Those who make and fit devices such as eyeglasses, braces, and artificial limbs need specialized education. They do not usually have licenses. Most are employed by health care institutions, although some (eg, dispensing opticians who make eyeglasses) may be in private business.

Dietary Services

The nutritionist or dietitian spends a large percentage of time planning for the special dietary needs of patients as a group, that is, determining the menu for those on a diabetic diet, a low-salt diet, or any other special diet ordered by the physician and provided by the facility. In addition, dietitians work with individual patients in planning appropriate diets and teaching nutrition. Registered dietitians have 4 years of college plus an internship. Dietetic technicians have a 2-year associate degree education.

Respiratory Care

Those who provide direct care related to respiratory treatments and the use of respiratory devices are called respiratory technicians and respiratory therapists (RT). Many are educated in associate degree programs; others have baccalaureate degrees. They are employed by hospitals, long-term care facilities, and home health care agencies. They may provide patient teaching, as well as specific treatments in respiratory care.

Pharmacy Services

The pharmacist has a baccalaureate or higher degree in pharmacy. In many universities a pharmacy program includes clinical work in a hospital or other patient care setting. Although pharmacists are principally involved with dispensing medications, they also provide drug therapy consultation to physicians and nurses and directly teach patients how to comply with their drug regimens. Many pharmacies also employ pharmacy technicians trained on the job to complete certain routine tasks in the pharmacy. Programs to prepare pharmacy technicians are beginning to appear in many community colleges.

Physical Therapy

The physical therapist (PT) is educated in a master's degree program or a 5-year baccalaureate program. The focus of physical therapy is the restoration of normal function of large muscle groups, bones, and joints. Treatment includes exercise, heat and cold therapy, electrical stimulation, and the use of other physical agents. The physical therapist also teaches the patient to use crutches, prostheses, and other assistive devices. There is a strong movement within the profession that advocates the master's degree as the requirement for practice as a physical therapist. Physical therapy assistants (PTA) are educated in 2-year associate degree programs and work with registered physical therapists in carrying out planned therapeutic regimens.

Occupational Therapist

The occupational therapist (OT) assists the client to restore fine motor skills and perform activities of daily living. Treatment includes exercise, the making of splints and assistive devices, and identifying ways to modify the environment to make the performance of daily living activities possible. Meaningful activities such as crafts and games are often used to provide needed exercise. Occupational therapists also provide diversional activities appropriate to the patient's strength, ability, and interest or designed to achieve physical or psychosocial goals for the patient. The occupational therapist has a baccalaureate degree and a 1-year internship. Occupational therapy assistants (OTA) have associate degrees and carry out plans for therapy that have been established by the registered occupational therapist.

Other Specific Therapies

Many health occupations involve the provision of specific types of therapy. The speech pathologist and radiation therapy technician are among these. Also included in this group, but more rarely seen, are the music therapist, the bibliotherapist, and the art therapist.

Only a few of the many different health occupations have been mentioned here. Table 8–1 outlines some common health occupations and identifies the educational level and credentialing of each.

Institutions Providing Care

Many different institutions are involved in providing various types of health care within our communities. It has been estimated that there are more than 7000 hospitals, 26,000 long-term care facilities, and 4000 community health

(*text continues on page 297*)

TABLE 8–1 Occupations in Health Care With Corresponding Level of Education and Type of Credential

Occupational Group	Educational Requirement					Credentialing		
	Less Than 1 Year	1 Year	Associate Degree	Baccalaureate	Post Baccalaureate	Professional Certification or Registration	Legal License	None
Primary Care Providers								
Clinical psychologist					4 y plus		X*	
Dentist				4 y		X	X	
Doctor of medicine					5 y plus		X	
Doctor of osteopathy					5 y plus	X	X	
Doctor of podiatry					3–4 y	X	X	
Nurse practitioner			X		1 y		X	
Optometrist			X		4 y		X	
Physician's assistant	X			plus X		X	X*	
Administrative and Business								
Hospital administrator					1–2 y			
Medical records administrator				X	1–2 y	X		
Medical records technician			X			X		
Medical transcriptionist	X		X			X		
Medical secretary		X					X	
Medical assistant	X					X		
Ward manager	X		X				X	

(continued)

Laboratory and Diagnostic Services

EEG technician	X		X			X	
ECG technician	X		X			X	
Cytology technician			X			X	
Medical technologist				X			
Medical laboratory technician			X	X		X	
Radiologic technologist			X	X		X	

Direct Care Services

Registered nurse			X	X		X	
Practical nurse							
Nursing assistant	X	X					
Dietitian		X				X	
Dietetic technician			X		1 y	X	
Emergency medical technician	X					X	
Paramedic		X	X			X	

Specific Therapies

Child life worker (play therapist)							X
Occupational therapist				X		X	X
Occupational therapy technician				X			X
Pharmacist	X		X	X		X	X
Pharmacy technician						X	

(continued)

TABLE 8–1 Occupations in Health Care With Corresponding Level of Education and Type of Credential *(Continued)*

Occupational Group	Educational Requirement					Credentialing		
	Less Than 1 Year	1 Year	Associate Degree	Baccalaureate	Post Baccalaureate	Professional Certification or Registration	Legal License	None
Specific Therapies (continued)								
Physical therapist				X	——1 y	X		
Physical therapy technician			X			X		
Speech pathologist				X		X		
Radiation therapy technician		X	X	X		X		
Recreation therapist				X			X	
Respiratory therapist			X			X		
Makers of Prosthetic and Assistive Devices								
Prosthetist				X				
Prosthetics technician			X					
Optician	X		X			X	X*	
Community Health								
Health educator				X			X	
Community health worker	X		'	X			X	
Environmental technologist							X	
Environmental technician			X				X	

X   X indicates that preparation varies between categories marked.
*Licensure in some states, not all.

agencies in the United States. Changes in these agencies and organizations are a fundamental part of the reformation of the health care system. These institutions will be discussed more fully in Chapter 12.

Alternative Health Care

Professionals in health care often ignore the many alternative avenues of health care that people use, such as health foods, vitamins, chiropractors, and faith healers. When professionals consider these alternatives at all, they often dismiss them as quackery, with little recognition of why people turn to these resources.

One of the reasons for the appeal of these alternative health care routes is the caring and personalized response that clients often receive. To the person who has felt intimidated by a businesslike clinic and who was made to feel unimportant by an impersonal professional, the warm, concerned, accepting atmosphere of the nonconventional setting may meet many personal needs. If you understand the major role that stress and anxiety play in any health problem, you may understand why many people are helped by therapies that may or may not be based on sound scientific knowledge.

THE HEALTH FOOD MOVEMENT

The health food movement in the United States is popular. Countless books are written and innumerable products are produced for this market. One of the appeals of this approach to health care is that it focuses on the normal and natural, as opposed to science and technology. Many people are helped by paying attention to good nutrition. In addition, medicine is beginning to identify that some may benefit from using food and vitamins in therapeutic ways. Often it is possible to work with clients who rely on this approach to health care by accepting what they believe helps them, as long as it is not detrimental to their well-being. When you are willing to acknowledge their philosophy and values, they may be willing to consider what you have to say about health care.

CHIROPRACTIC CARE

Many people seek medical help from chiropractors. Chiropractic care is a method of treatment based on the theory that disease is caused by interference with nerve function. It uses manipulation of the body joints, especially the spinal vertebrae, in seeking to restore normal function. The chiropractor may also use a variety of other treatments commonly associated with physical therapy, such as massage and exercise. There are definite differences among chiropractors. One group recognizes that there are illnesses that they are not competent to treat and do recommend that clients seek medical care. Another group believes that all illnesses may be treated by chiropractic methods and do not refer clients for medical care. Many people with joint and muscle strain and tension find that chiropractic treatments relieve discomfort. The major concern is for those who have more serious illnesses that may be missed altogether or not recognized in time to be given optimal medical attention.

NATUROPATHY

Naturopathy gets its name from the natural agents used in treating disease, such as air, water, and sunshine. The naturopath treats people by recommending changes in life-style, diet, exercise, and the use of vitamins. For many this is successful. The danger lies in the possibility of delaying treatment of more serious disorders. Naturopathy is licensed in some states.

HERBAL MEDICINE

The herbalist treats illness by prescribing a wide variety of natural herbs. Many of the herbs are imported from around the world. Herein lies one of the difficulties. Rules and regulations regarding labeling and content purity may not be as strict in some countries as in the United States. This means that herbs sold may contain contaminants. We know that plants often may have active ingredients that affect the human body. Digitalis, for example, was originally a dried leaf of the foxglove plant. It was indeed a potent and effective medication when used as an herb, but dosage was not accurate and there was little scientific information regarding its effects at that time. It is wise to recognize the potential problems inherent in the use of herbal medicines. Patients taking such products should be encouraged to share this information with their physician.

ETHNIC HEALTH CARE TRADITIONS

Native Americans, Hispanic Americans, Asian Americans, and many other ethnic groups have traditional health care resources that are still used by many. Often termed *folk medicine*, these traditions usually are handed down by word of mouth and relate to treating common health problems. Treatment often involves the use of herbs and foods as well as traditional ceremonies. Little is understood about many of the herbs used, but some have demonstrated therapeutic effects. Within an ethnic group there may be people who are designated as healers or people with special knowledge and ability in regard to illness. The advice of such a person may be sought instead of consulting a physician.

Those who support the conventional, official methods of health care have long ignored or repudiated the value of these nonorthodox health care traditions. We must recognize that the traditions have persisted because people have found them to be valuable. Acknowledging these health care methods and working cooperatively usually is much more productive than trying to oppose them. Currently, the federal government is supporting research in regard to alternative health care methods.

Financing Health Care

Many different approaches to financing health care are used in the United States. Insurance companies, health maintenance organizations (HMOs), preferred providers organizations (PPOs), and governmental agencies all affect how health care is delivered. Some of the proposals for health care reform will be discussed in Chapter 10. Here is a review of the current approaches to health care financing.

INSURANCE COMPANIES

The majority of insurance companies are private profit-making companies owned by stockholders. They are managed to provide profit to stockholders as well as to provide service to policy holders. Although the "Blues" (Blue Cross and Blue Shield companies) were originally seen as not-for-profit, the distinctions between the two groups have diminished.

The basic framework of insurance coverage is that of shared risk. Individuals pay for coverage whether they have health care costs or not. Then those with health care needs receive reimbursement for the costs of needed care. At the heart of determining insurance costs and coverages is the process of identifying the health risks for groups of individuals and determining what costs for care would be. Limitations on coverage protect insurance companies from the potential for excessive risk.

As costs of health care have increased, premiums for insurance have increased greatly. One of the concerns of the public is that health insurance is unobtainable for those with existing health problems and often economically out of reach for those who are not insured as part of employee groups.

Although originally focused on paying for health care, insurance companies are now involved in establishing standards for care, evaluating care, and negotiating charges. They are active participants in all of health care and because of the economic power they wield, they have great influence. Insurance companies often determine to whom they will provide payment and by determining what procedures will be reimbursed, limit health care decisions.

PREFERRED PROVIDERS

In an attempt to contain costs, insurance companies have negotiated with individual and organizational providers of health care to provide certain kinds of care at an agreed-on, usually lower, price. The insurance company then provides an incentive for clients to use these "preferred providers." This incentive may involve the waiver of co-payments by the insured or coverage of additional conditions or situations. Preferred provider organizations (PPOs) may include corporations employing care providers or groups of care providers who have joined together to negotiate more successfully with insurance companies for these special contracts. The advantage to the provider is the assurance that all bills will be paid in full and that the size of the practice is ensured. In a time of competition in health care, this may be a significant advantage. Each PPO operates independently and is not regulated by the government; therefore, the exact structure and contractual arrangements are individual.

HEALTH MAINTENANCE ORGANIZATIONS

The HMOs have been in existence in the United States for more than 50 years, but their growth in numbers was slow until the federal government provided the impetus to start new HMOs through legislation passed in 1972 and 1974. Although HMOs differ from one another in the extent of care provided, they have many similarities. Fees are a flat rate per month. This fee usually covers routine preventive health care, care for illness, and hospitalization and, in some instances, is designed to cover prescription costs, outpatient care, and other items. Primary health care providers are often employees of the organization and receive a salary that is not related to the number of patients seen or procedures performed. In other instances a group of primary health care providers contracts with the HMO to provide services for a preset fee per individual in the program. HMOs also employ many other health care workers, including nurses. In some HMOs clients have a choice of care providers; in others they do not. Because the HMO receives the same income regardless of whether the client requires extensive care or very little care, there is a built-in incentive to emphasize preventive care and avoid costly hospitalization.

The HMOs have a variety of organizational patterns. Some are operated by insurance companies, some are private profit-making organizations, and still others are consumer owned and operated. The Kaiser Permanente Health

Care organization in California and Oregon is one type of HMO. This organization owns and operates its own hospitals. The physicians are members of a group that contracts with the organization to provide medical services. The fee for membership provides for almost all health care costs, including both outpatient and inpatient costs.

Group Health Cooperative of Puget Sound, located in Washington State, is a consumer-owned and operated cooperative that owns and operates its own hospitals and clinics and employs physicians and other health care providers. People who join the cooperative as members pay a monthly fee for comprehensive health care, which includes both outpatient and inpatient services. The governing board is elected by the membership, members serve on policy-making committees, and some issues are determined by a vote of the entire membership. In addition, Group Health Cooperative contracts with employers to provide comprehensive, prepaid coverage for employee groups. Members of the employment groups are not members of the cooperative. Their monthly fees may be paid by the employer or the employee.

MANAGED CARE SYSTEMS

Managed care refers to any system in which the care of an individual from the time of contact with the health care system to discharge is carefully planned and monitored to ensure that standards are followed and costs are minimized. A managed care plan can include both payers and providers. Some HMOs have always acted in a managed care approach. The Clinton plan for health care reform relies on "managed competition" to effectively control costs while providing more universal coverage. This plan calls for large umbrella organizations that will provide all aspects of care in a managed system and will compete for the business of the health care consumer. Choice will occur only between managed care organizations and not between individual providers. In insurance companies that are already moving into managed care, nurses frequently serve as case managers. In this role, the nurse monitors the care as it is occurring, ensures that appropriate referrals are made, and ascertains that the care follows the established standards.

MEDICARE AND MEDICAID

In 1965, after years of effort and testimony by many health-related groups, (including the ANA) and with widespread public support, an amendment of the Social Security Act was passed. Title XVIII of the act, which was termed *Medicare*, provided payment for hospitalization and insurance that could be purchased for meeting physicians' fees for people over age 65. Title IX of the act, which was termed *Medicaid*, provided funds for health care for those dependent on public assistance. Medicaid is administered by the states, which determine eligibility and level of coverage.

Medicare and Medicaid have supplied an important health care resource but have not been without problems. Costs have been much larger and have risen faster than anticipated. There has been a great deal of publicity over instances of abuse and even fraud that have occurred in connection with these two programs. The goals of providing adequate health care for elders and the indigent through these programs has yet to be achieved.

The Medicare bill contained many provisions that have made a significant impact on nursing. A definition of skilled nursing care in the original bill was narrow and excluded many important aspects of care needed to maintain health. Through later efforts and testimony, nursing organizations were instrumental in getting legislators to recognize that the definition of skilled nursing was a critical matter, and through a Senate subcommittee the ANA was asked to study skilled nursing care to provide background data for the Senate. Amendments to the Medicare/Medicaid Act of 1972 encouraged increased study of alternative ways of providing health care to contain costs. These alternatives included innovation in the use of nurses in expanded roles as well as the use of HMOs.

Amendments to this act were also responsible for mandating review and evaluation of health care. This was done in the interests of cost containment. Within institutions, records of Medicare/Medicaid patients must be reviewed and compared with specific criteria for care.

In 1982, Medicare was revised by the 97th Congress to prevent the predicted bankruptcy of the system owing to rapidly escalating costs. The premium for Part B of Medicare (the optional portion that provides for out-of-hospital and physician care) and the deductible that the individual must pay for covered service were increased. The system of payment was changed to prospective payment based on diagnosis-related groups (DRGs). Many items that were previously funded separately were included in the one prospective rate. A mechanism for reimbursing hospice care was included.

Access to Health Care

As the United States examines the need for health care reform, one of the key concerns is access to health care for all citizens. Lack of access may result from economic barriers, problems with the distribution or location of services, and sociocultural barriers between providers and potential recipients of care (Center for Health Economics Research, 1993).

Key indicators of effective use of health care resources have been identified as use of family planning resources, prenatal care, child health statistics, adult health statistics, and dental health information. These key indicators have shown a lack of improvement in access in most areas and in some areas an actually worsening of access in the last 10 years.

Contraceptive use by sexually active women in general has increased between 1982 and 1988, but public spending for contraceptive services fell by 40% during the 1980s. This has resulted in teenagers and poor women being less likely to participate in family planning visits in 1988 than in 1982. This demonstrates an economic barrier to access to health care services (Center for Health Economics Research, 1993).

In 1990, despite widespread publicity regarding the effectiveness of prenatal care in improving birth outcomes, less than 65% of black and Hispanic women received early prenatal care. There are approximately one-fourth fewer obstetric care providers in low-income than in higher-income areas. Pregnant teens and pregnant black women are more likely to have low birth weight babies and the white–black infant mortality gap has widened since 1990. These indicators appear to represent an access problem created by distribution of resources and may also be exacerbated by cultural barriers (Center for Health Economics Research, 1993).

Child health is examined by looking at physician visits, immunization rates, and hospitalization for preventable problems. Whereas privately insured children had an average of 3.4 physician visits per year, those on Medicaid averaged 6.0 visits per year, and those without insurance averaged 2.8 visits. For those on Medicaid, many of these visits are to hospitals or clinics rather than primary care providers. There appears to be a concern about appropriate use of resources for those on Medicaid and a lack of resources for the uninsured. Low-income areas have 44% fewer physicians who care for children and low immunization rates. This health outcome may be related to geographical access (Center for Health Economics Research, 1993).

For adults, concern about access focuses on such health services as cancer screening (Pap smears, mammography, and rectal examinations) and availability of ambulatory care. Whereas 5% of cervical cancer in nonpoor women is diagnosed late, 14% of cervical cancer in poor women is diagnosed late. Elderly adults in poor neighborhoods have increased hospitalization for asthma, congestive heart failure, and pneumonia, conditions that could be treated with effective ambulatory care (Center for Health Economics Research, 1993).

Dental problems respond very well to health promotion and disease prevention strategies. Community water supply fluoridation, fluoride toothpaste, dental sealants, and regular oral care all make a significant difference in dental health. However, dental visits for the purpose of education and establishing appropriate dental care habits vary by income—53% of those who are poor receive these services, whereas 83% of the nonpoor had a dental visit. This has resulted in differences in overall dental health. The pattern of dental care is even more pronounced for poor adults compared to nonpoor adults (Center for Health Economics Research, 1993).

Power in the Health Care System

In trying to understand any system you need to examine some of the unique sources of power and authority within it. Smith (1994) states that as health services and educational preparation for health professions undergo systems change, we must give attention to the allocation of power within services and education systems. Some sources of power unique to health care are the authority to decide who may enter and leave the system, the authority to decide who may practice within the system, and the ability to control funding. These sources of power present problems for the client because the client is excluded from them. Clearly the client determines only the most basic entry into the system. The client cannot enter any institution without the express approval of a physician. Additionally, the client has no control over who practices and with the advent of HMOs and PPOs may have little choice of physician. Funding is usually controlled by third-party payers, and the client is often powerless to determine who will be paid, how much, or when.

REGULATORY AGENCIES

The primary regulatory agencies in health care are governmental bodies. These agencies administer licensing laws that govern who is allowed to practice. There are also agencies that approve or accredit institutions that educate personnel for health care and those that provide services. Through regulation these agencies have a profound effect on how institutions operate.

Nongovernmental agencies such as the JCAHO have a great deal of power. For example, although nursing experts had taught for years that individualized nursing care plans were important for patients, they were often not written. When the presence of nursing care plans was required by JCAHO standards, hospitals began putting time, energy, and money into systems for keeping care plans up to date. With the removal of this standard, practice may change.

THIRD-PARTY PAYERS

Because they represent the financial interests of large groups of people and control payments for services, third-party payers have the power to demand changes in the system. When initially established, these agencies did not see their role as anything beyond a financial relationship. As health care costs rose, these agencies began to look for ways of controlling costs to maintain their competitive place in the insurance market. They have set increasingly rigid criteria for payment for services. The standard rates set for payment for procedures have tended to place some restraints on charges (although actual fees often are slightly ahead of payment schedules). By determining whom they will pay for services, insurance companies reduce the choices available to those who carry insurance and do not wish to find their care outside of that program where reimbursement would not be available. Third-party payers thus have more power with institutions and with care providers than an individual has.

PHYSICIANS

Physicians have historically had almost unlimited power within the health care system. They determined who entered and when, decided if and when all other services and personnel would be used, and determined when someone would leave the system. Where other agencies and individuals have obtained some power or independence, the overall power of the physician has often diminished. As a whole, physicians have opposed changes that would disperse power in health care, arguing that they are the most educated and knowledgeable of all health care providers and that their professional judgment should be accepted. Those favoring increased distribution of power have argued that increased competition, increased choice for consumers, and judgments of others will make the system more balanced and more responsive to the individual consumers. Despite changes, physicians are still very powerful in the health care system as a whole. For example, although the consumer through a third-party payer may pay the costs of health care, the physician is the "customer" whom the facility tries to please by providing those services, supplies, and schedules preferred by the physician.

However, constraints are increasingly being placed on physician practice. Payers are reviewing plans for care and refusing reimbursement when care does not follow their established guidelines. Many hospitals routinely review costs associated with care ordered by physicians and may restrict their ability to order certain high-cost drugs and procedures because payers provide only a flat daily fee that does not extend to cover high-cost items. Care pathways may demand that physicians provide for standardized care that leads to quick discharge. These constraints on practice have been disturbing to many physicians. Most health care reform proposals include limitations on the power of physicians in the system.

CONSUMERS

Consumers do have rights in the health care system. These are stated in different ways by different institutions and groups but all revolve around the recognition of the health care consumer as an adult with the ability and right to be self-determining. As a general rule, consumers are not aware of these rights and even when aware may be reluctant to demand them. Consumers are in a particularly vulnerable place in the health care system. Because they depend on those within the system for life itself, they are often reluctant to complain or request changes for fear of offending those on whom they depend. When consumers try to exert power within the system, they may be met with resistance and comments such as "Well, you really do not have the background to understand this issue." Consumers are most often effective in exerting power in the system by working in groups and through established committees and agencies.

One of the concerns in health care reform is the lessening of consumer choice in providers and the inability of the individual to influence the larger system. Although coverage is expected to be more universal, individual coverage may not include some types of more expensive or experimental care. This is of particular concern in regard to those who are diagnosed with hard-to-treat types of cancer. Often new treatments continue to be designated as experimental when they are the only alternative available. Consumers are becoming vocal in their demands for care they perceive to be of benefit.

NURSES

Nurses have historically had limited power in the health care system, a situation that has roots in many aspects of nursing. Most nurses were women, employees of institutions, and economically unable to take risks. In addition, nursing education did not prepare nurses to try to change the system, but rather to function within it.

As changes leading to health care reform are occurring, nurses sometimes feel that their power is decreasing. When economics are the driving force, as they are in health care reform, those who argue in favor of quality of care may feel that they are not heard. The public in general and politicians in particular may have little understanding of the scope of nursing practice and its value to the patient or client. The focus has sometimes been on the providing the cheapest care from the cheapest provider, not providing for optimum care.

Nevertheless, things are changing in nursing. Nursing education programs try increasingly to educate nurses into a role as patient/consumer advocate and agent of change. Nursing organizations are working to provide nurses with a voice at higher decision-making levels in health care. Collective bargaining has provided nurses with a mechanism for demanding recognition of the importance of their role and for being participants in the decision-making processes.

Change may not occur as rapidly as desired and nurses are often frustrated because of their inability to influence the system. Many new graduates are especially distressed to learn that, as individuals, they cannot affect the system. Somehow they expected that if they spoke with a voice of reason and acted in the patient's best interests, others would respond positively. By understanding the political realities and the ways in which decisions are made, and by working together to speak with a united voice, nurses may increase their power within the system.

Economic Influences in Health Care

The cost of health care for the nation as a whole has risen at a faster rate than has the general inflation. A wide variety of factors has been responsible for this phenomenon. Much effort and attention have been given to cost containment.

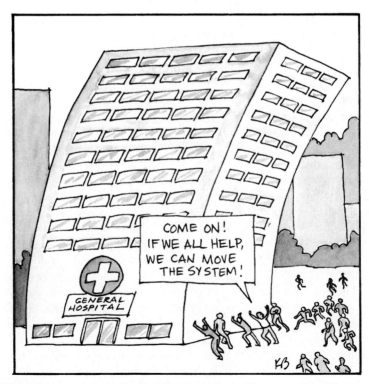

FIGURE 8–3 To have power and exert influence in the health care system, it is essential that nurses develop effective group action.

CAUSES OF COST INCREASES

One important factor in cost increase is the cost of new technology. New and more sophisticated diagnostic and treatment devices are being invented each year. This type of cost is found in every area of the health care field from the cardiac care unit to the laboratory.

The construction of new care facilities also contributes to rising costs. An increasing population needs additional facilities, but in addition the nature of facilities has changed. More space is needed for the various technologies both at the bedside and in the many other hospital departments. More offices and conference rooms are needed. The regulations governing hospital construction have also become more stringent, requiring more fire safety, infection control measures, and protection against environmental hazards. All of these factors combine to make the "per bed" cost of new hospital construction enormously high.

The average hospital stay for standard diagnoses has been steadily decreasing. The typical patient in today's hospital is rapidly discharged to convalesce at home or in a long-term care facility, leaving behind only the very acutely ill. Many patients who would have died quickly in years past are saved but require long and intensive care. All of these factors make the acuity level of a patient today much greater. This in turn requires more intensive observation and care and the use of more specialized equipment.

The population as a whole is growing older and, statistically, the elderly have an increased incidence of all chronic illnesses. A greater percentage of the population requires health care on a regular basis and may depend on medications, treatments, and therapies for continued functioning.

Salaries of health care workers (except physicians) were far below those of the general society. To remedy this, for a time health care salaries rose more rapidly than the general inflation rate. Physicians have also had an increase in income greater than the relative inflation rate.

Companies that manufacture health-related devices and drugs have reportedly some of the highest profits in industry. This has been justified by these manufacturers as being appropriate to the relative risk and cost involved in their research and development activities; however, some critics think that they have taken advantage of the public's dependence on their products.

Lack of competition in the health care field is a factor that has been included in some discussions as contributing to higher costs. Physicians have remained primary gatekeepers in the system. The advent of other primary care providers, such as nurse practitioners, has offered alternate and less costly care for many routine problems or normal life processes, such as pregnancy and childbirth. There has been opposition to allowing these practitioners to operate in collaborative rather than dependent or subsidiary roles.

One attempt to increase the availability of alternative care has been the movement to obtain legislation requiring that government agencies and third-party payers (eg, insurance companies) pay the nonphysician, such as the nurse practitioner, who provides service. The current pattern requires that payment always be directed to a physician, who then pays the provider. Although some progress has been made in regard to third-party reimbursement for nurses in primary care, in most areas physicians are still the only ones with access to third-party payment for primary care.

COST CONTAINMENT

In an attempt to slow the rapidly increasing costs of health care, the various governmental agencies have established rules, regulations, and procedures aimed at decreasing the rate of inflation in health care. There has been no expectation of cost reductions or even of cost maintenance, but rather the aim has been to control the rate of increase. This effort is termed *cost containment*.

To add new high-cost equipment or additional patient care facilities, a health care institution may be required to apply for a certificate of need. This establishes that there will not be unnecessary duplication of services in an area and that a need for them exists. For example, if each hospital were to purchase magnetic resonance imaging equipment and it was used to only one fourth or one third of capacity, the cost per use would have to be higher to cover the investment and maintenance costs than if the device were used to capacity.

In many states nonprofit hospitals must make application for rate increases. In their applications, they must document all the factors contributing to the increase. Hearings are held, and permission for rate increases is given only when the evidence indicates that all possible economies are being taken. Private, profit-making hospitals are not held to these rules. Controls are also placed on hospitals by Medicare and Medicaid, which limit the amount they will pay for care.

Within facilities, personnel are being asked to become cost conscious. This includes such ordinary things as being conservative with telephone use, canceling meal trays when patients are discharged, and using expensive supplies with care. Physicians are being asked to carefully judge the necessity of diagnostic studies and costly procedures. In some hospitals physicians are asked to consult with pharmacists before prescribing certain high-cost drugs to determine whether a low-cost alternative exists. Many physicians are upset about these cost-containment measures because they may interfere with the physician's independent decision-making. Hospitals with a high population of extra-risk patients (eg, the very elderly or poor) have expressed concern that discharging a patient for convalescence in a home with a caring family, good food, and a clean environment is very different from discharging a person to a poverty environment and that this should be considered in the regulations for length of stay. The proponents point out that these cost-containment measures have contributed to shortening hospital stays and thus to containing costs and that health care should not be used to solve social problems.

The federal government has sought to control costs for Medicare and Medicaid by establishing higher deductibles that the person must pay and by limiting the fees that the government will pay. Because the elderly or the poor are often unable to pay these deductible amounts, they become liabilities that health care providers must meet from higher fees collected from those who do pay their bills. Medicaid costs have also been limited by tightening eligibility requirements. This shuts more people out of the health care system altogether.

Statistically, HMOs have shown lower costs for health care than the conventional fee-for-service systems; therefore, the federal government has subsidized the creation of new HMOs and has encouraged employers to offer an HMO as an alternative to a traditional health insurance plan. This has speeded the development of new HMOs. Another purpose in subsidizing HMOs is to help contain costs in all health plans as a result of the competition.

All of these efforts at cost containment certainly have had effects on the health care system in many areas beyond costs. They have affected decision-making processes, power structures, the kind of care provided, and the practice of individual health care providers. It is important to recognize the impact that cost containment has had.

DIAGNOSIS-RELATED GROUPS AND PROSPECTIVE PAYMENT

A major change in the method of payment for health care services began at the end of 1983, when the federal government introduced a prospective payment system for Medicare using DRGs to determine the payment level. This change was designed to stop the spiraling costs of Medicare and to correct the inequities in which the costs of care in one facility were very different from the costs in another facility.

A prospective payment is a reimbursement amount for a procedure or illness that has been determined in advance of the provision of the service. This predetermined amount is paid without regard to costs in the individual situation. If the costs were less than the prospective reimbursement, the hospital will make a profit, and if they are more, the hospital will lose money. This is designed to be an incentive for hospitals to control costs. Hospitals had previously been paid by Medicare on a retrospective system, in which they were able to bill for each item of care independently; thus, there had been a reverse incentive—the more care items, the more the hospital received.

The method chosen to determine the rates to be paid in the prospective system—DRGs—resulted from a computerized analysis of the costs that had been billed in the past. Categories of medical diagnosis were formed. In addition, a decision was made to increase the payment if other illnesses or conditions, called *comorbidities*, were present. These were factors such as heart failure in the person with a fracture. Hospitals also receive an additional amount for cases that are determined to be "outliers." An outlier is a case in which the patient stay significantly exceeds the average. The number of days that qualify a case to be considered an outlier is predetermined. For example, if an average stay is 6 days, the stay might have to reach 35 days for the case to be considered an outlier.

Most hospital costs are included in the DRG reimbursement. Some costs are still being reimbursed separately. These include costs for nursing education, medical education, and research. These areas will be reevaluated in the future. The goal is to include all aspects of cost in one reimbursement figure. Physician costs are also being paid separately, and some suggestions have been made that eventually these should be included in the single rate.

Most of the controversy surrounding DRGs has not been an argument with the basic aim of providing an incentive for cost control, or even with the prospective reimbursement system itself, but with how the payment amount is determined and how the system is being administered. There are conflicting studies regarding whether the DRGs adequately reflect the intensity of nursing care required (Halloran et al., 1985; McKibbin et al., 1985). Another concern is that patients are reported to be discharged after much shorter stays and needing more care (the "quicker and sicker" concern). It is expected that some alterations and modifications of the system will continue to be made but that the basic prospective plan will remain in place.

There are a variety of implications for nurses in the current DRG system. Documentation that reflects the acuity level and multiple problems of the patient when records are audited for compliance is essential. The need for discharge planning is always present but is more critical as the length of stay becomes shorter. Added length of stay is a crucial component in increasing the costs to the hospital; therefore, nursing actions that prevent complications, that avoid inappropriate scheduling, and that facilitate early discharge are important. Nurses in home health agencies and long-term care facilities have identified that they are caring for patients with complex nursing needs. A major concern is whether the DRG reimbursement provides adequate funds for quality nursing care to be delivered and whether hospitals, in their attempt to cut costs, will cut quality of care as well.

In addition to the patients currently covered by Medicare, many states are considering systems similar to DRGs, and some private insurance carriers are looking at ways the basic concepts could be used in their cost-control efforts. Therefore, this will continue to be an issue of concern to nursing.

PATIENT ACUITY SYSTEMS FOR MONITORING COSTS

Patient acuity describes the relative severity of a person's current health problem. Various ways of measuring acuity in both general hospitals and psychiatric settings have been devised. Most consist of categories that reflect the kind of care needed. These categories are then assigned numerical values. All applicable category values are then summed and compared with a standard. For example, an acuity measuring system might have one category reflecting the need for assistance in personal hygiene. As the person needs more assistance, more points are assigned. Another category might reflect the amount of time needed for monitoring vital signs. The more time required, the more points are assigned. Each category is assigned appropriate points, and the total is computed. The points identified for the individual patient are then compared with a standard and the patient is assigned an acuity level. Those with the least points are level 1 and require the least care. Those with the most points are level 4 and require the most care. Each system in use has its own scale for determining acuity. These measures are also called "intensity measures" because they reflect the intensity of care needed.

In some settings acuity levels or intensity measures are being used as a mechanism for determining the staffing needs of a patient care unit. Acuity levels have also been used as a means of billing for the level of nursing care needed, rather than have nursing be a constant part of the room charge for the patient. It has also been suggested that prospective reimbursement might be based on acuity level rather than on medical diagnosis because acuity level more closely reflects the real impact on resources than the medical diagnosis does (DRG's Reflect Nursing Resources, 1985).

The state of New Jersey pioneered in the use of relative intensity measures (RIMs) as a mechanism for determining the cost of providing care (Joel, 1984). In long-term care settings similar systems have been used for determining costs for billing. In New York a system called resource utilization groups (RUGs) has been developed for this purpose (Mitty, 1987).

Continuing Concerns in the Health Care System

Throughout this chapter we have referred to changes occurring as part of the health care reform process. Some of the specific changes being debated in the political arena are discussed in Chapter 10. In whatever way the system is changed and restructured, nurses have some continuing concerns.

The most essential concern is for patient/client well-being in the midst of a powerful system. As pressures to change increase, nurses continue to speak out for consumers. Who will help them as they cope with their health problems and those of their families? Who will assist them to negotiate through the various parts of the system? Will their individual identity and unique needs be addressed or will everyone be treated as some mythical "standard patient?"

Another concern central to nurses is whether that aspect of health care that we call "nursing," with its focus on the individual, will be able to be

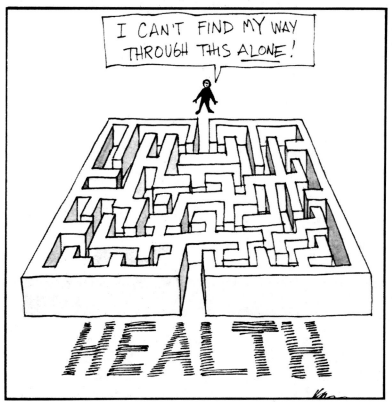

FIGURE 8–4 Clients often need assistance in finding their way through the modern health care system.

maintained. Will the pressures for demonstrating cost effectiveness result in a loss of caring because it is not always quantifiable? Will the system recognize the critical thinking skills and abilities of nurses as well as their technical skills? There are many unanswered questions in the future!

Key Concepts

▷ Primary health care providers such as physicians, nurse practitioners, physician's assistants, dentists, and optometrists provide supervision for health promotion, care for common health problems, and entry into the health care system.

▷ Allied health care workers provide for the many supportive, therapeutic, and rehabilitative services that are part of modern health care.

▷ Acute care hospitals provide for skilled care for those with complex, short-term health care needs.

▷ Long-term care facilities include nursing homes, rehabilitation centers, and a variety of residential settings; they are designed to provide some specialized health services in a living environment.

▷ Alternative health care resources provide a different approach to health care that may address many psychosocial needs.

▷ Financing of health care is a complex composed of insurance companies, health maintenance organizations, preferred providers, and governmental systems. Controlling reimbursement has been used to modify patterns of care.

▷ Power is exerted within the health care system by those who control finances and those who control resources. Nurses and consumers are working to gain power in the system.

▷ Cost increases have created stress in the health care system and resulted in a variety of approaches to cost containment.

CRITICAL THINKING ACTIVITIES

1. Identify patients you have encountered from a variety of social, cultural, and economic backgrounds. Given these patients needs and backgrounds, what type of practitioner would best meet their needs for primary care? What barriers might they meet in trying to gain access to primary care? What might you do to assist these individuals?

2. Long-term care facilities are providing more subacute care. Based on the long-term care facilities with which you are familiar, identify the problems they might encounter in caring for patients with higher levels of acuity. As a nurse in such a facility, how would you address these concerns to the administrator?

3. What cost-control measures have you seen in places where you have had clinical practice? Analyze the effects of these cost-control measures on patient care.

References

Center for Health Economics Research. Access to Health Care: Key Indicators for Policy. Princeton, NJ: The Robert Wood Johnson Foundation, 1993

DRGs reflect nursing resources. Hospitals 59(19):56, 1985

Hughes D, et al. The Health of America's Children: Maternal and Child Health Data Book. Washington, DC: Children's Defense Fund, 1989

Halloran E, Halloran DC. Exploring the DRG equation. Am J Nurs 85(10):1093–1095, 1985

Kenkel PJ. Pointing the finger: Who's to blame for high health care costs? Modern Healthcare 20(48):22–25, 1990

Joel LA. Relative intensity measures (RIMs) and the state of the art of reimbursement for nursing service. *In* Shaffer FA: DRGs: Changes and Challenges. New York: National League for Nursing, 1984

McKibbon RC, Bimmer PF, Galliher JM, and Hartley SS. Nursing Costs and DRG payments. Am J Nurs 85(12):1353–1355, 1985

Mitty E. Prospective payment and long-term care: Linking payments to resource use. Nurs Health Care 8(1):14–21, 1987

Smith GR. Power and health care reform. J Nurs Educ 33(5): 194–197, 1994

Further Readings

Baker CB. School health policy issues in the 1990s. Nurs Health Care 15(4):178–184, 1994

Brazda J. Little-noticed law should bring hospitals good cheer. Modern Healthcare 20(5):37–38, 1990

Breo DL. Severe allied health shortage cause for concern. Am Med News 31(47):10, 1989

Buerhaus PI. Managed competition and critical issues facing nurses. Nurs & Health Care 15(1):22–27, 1994

Foegelle WE, Couch GC Jr. A study of passage rates: Hospital vs. college programs. Radiol Technol 61(5):393–395, 1990

Hassanein SA. On the shortage of registered nurses: An economic analysis of the RN market. Nurs Health Care 12(3):152–156, 1991

Ketter J. ANA: Protecting nurses and patient care in the face of restructuring. Am Nurse 26(5): 1, 14, 1994

Mathews LR. The future? The respiratory therapist in the year 2000. Can J Respir Ther 26(2):18–19, 1990

Mitchell PH, Krueger JC, Moody LE. The crisis of the health care nonsystem. Nurs Outlook 38(5):214–217, 1990

Porter-O'Grady T. Building partnerships in health care: Creating whole systems change. Nurs & Health Care 15(1):34–38, 1994

Smith GR. Power and health care reform. Jrnl Nurs Ed 33(5):194–197, 1994

9

Collective Bargaining

Objectives

After completing this chapter, you should be able to

1. Define and use appropriately the terms most commonly associated with collective bargaining.

2. Discuss the history of collective bargaining as it applies to nursing.

3. Explain the concept of arbitration.

4. Identify at least four items that should be included in a contract for nurses.

5. Explain the grievance process.

6. Discuss the concerns nurses have regarding membership in a collective bargaining group.

7. Outline the advantages and disadvantages of having the state nurses' association serve as the bargaining agent for nurses.

8. Identify some of the ways shared governance may affect collective bargaining.

Ellis JR, Hartley CL: NURSING IN TODAY'S WORLD: CHALLENGES, ISSUES, AND TRENDS, 5th ed.
© 1995 J.B. Lippincott Company

Collective bargaining provides the opportunity for employees who are members of the union to participate in decisions of the management (organization) with regard to terms of employment, salaries, benefits, and similar conditions. It involves a formal negotiation process. This was first mandated in 1974 by amendments to the National Labor Relations Act (NLRA) that required nonprofit and voluntary health care employers to bargain collectively with their employees. This means that all health care workers have the right to establish and be represented by a union and have a voice in determining certain employment conditions such as salaries, working conditions, and benefits. Before this time certain nonprofit employers were excluded by law from requirements to negotiate collectively with their employees. Health care, which has come to be regarded as a fundamental right, was seen as an essential service—one that could not be disrupted. Some governmental health care institutions were compelled by law to negotiate with their employees and, although not legally required, certain nonprofit health care institutions chose to engage in collective bargaining.

Because of nursing's long history as a profession of dedication, altruism, and service, initially collective bargaining was a controversial issue within nursing. Some saw this process as detracting from the professional role of the nurse. Today, however, nurses are vitally concerned about contracts, services, third-party payers, comparable worth, patients' rights, shared governance, and a host of issues that can be discussed at the bargaining table. Nurses believe that people who choose nursing as a career should have the opportunity to have some voice in patient care assignments, length of the working day and week, fringe benefits, and wages without losing face with the public at large, members of the medical profession, or other colleagues. This thinking was succinctly outlined in a statement by Janet Muff (1988, p 245):

> We are not in this business out of charity, as altruists and nightingalists would have us believe. We are here to make money, to use our minds and our skills, to provide services to patients on our own terms. We need no longer apologize and feel guilty.

In this chapter we provide some information that is basic to collective bargaining, in the hope that as a new graduate you will have a better understanding on which to base decisions and actions. Having some knowledge of the history that surrounds the collective bargaining process in this country will be helpful in applying the process to the health care professions.

History of Collective Bargaining

As early as the 1850s, Horace Greeley, a reformer, publisher, and politician, was generating interest in and giving impetus to collective bargaining issues in his editorial columns of the *New York Tribune*. During the early part of the

20th century, efforts by workers to organize were met with opposition from employers, governmental officials, and some members of the public. After the Great Depression that immobilized the United States in the late 1920s and early 1930s, several laws were enacted to help improve workers' conditions. Franklin D. Roosevelt was elected president in 1932, and his New Deal administration saw the passage of the National Industrial Recovery Act. Among the activities that resulted from this act was the creation of the National Recovery Administration, whose purpose it was to administer codes of fair practice within given industries. The nation was called on to accept an interim blanket code that established for workers a 35- to 40-hour work week, minimum pay of 30 to 40 cents an hour, and prohibition of child labor.

On July 5, 1935, the National Labor Relations Act (NLRA) became the national labor policy of the United States. Also known as the Wagner Act, for Senator Robert F. Wagner who introduced the legislation, the NLRA gave workers federal protection in their efforts to form unions and organize for better working conditions. It listed as unfair practices any actions on the part of employers that would interfere with this process. Senator Wagner wanted management and labor to resolve their mutual problems through a system of self-government. This act also created the National Labor Relations Board (NLRB), a quasi-judicial body that was to ensure that the conditions of that legislation were properly enforced.

The NLRB has the responsibility for administering the NLRA. In addition, it has two primary functions: to conduct secret-ballot elections that will determine that the majority of employees of a unit desire the representation of a given union in collective bargaining procedures and to prevent and rectify unfair labor practices committed by employers or unions. It also has the responsibility for determining into which of the eight bargaining units established for health care workers in acute care facilities various employees will be assigned. This is important to nurses because it enables them to have a separate unit and, therefore, deal with issues important to their role in health care delivery. Although challenged by the American Hospital Association, this role of the NLRB was upheld by the Supreme Court in 1991 (Supreme Court, 1991).

The original NLRA used the term *labor organization*, which was defined in language that could be interpreted to exclude nursing and several other professions, such as teaching and medicine, that were organized through professional organizations. These early labor unions often were viewed negatively by the public, an image that was reinforced in movies, in newspapers, and on radio. Often portrayed as rowdy, aggressive, and hostile, unions did not seem to fit well in nursing.

In 1947, the original NLRA was amended through the Taft-Hartley Act (also known as the Labor Management Relations Act). Because of heavy lobbying on the part of hospital management, the act was written in such a way as to specifically exclude nonprofit hospitals from the legal obligation of bargaining with their employees. Although the administration of some hospitals chose to negotiate salaries and working conditions with their employees, many did not and no legal action could be taken to force the process.

By 1931, the American Nurses Association (ANA) was publicly recognizing its obligation with regard to the general welfare of its members and developed, within their organization, a legislative policy speaking to this concern. Some suggest that this effort was spurred by the fact that other groups, particularly the Service Employees International Union (SEIU), an affiliate of the American Federation of Labor/Congress of Industrial Organizations (AFL/CIO), was actively working to organize health care workers. Other factors also were important. Before 1930, most nurses were employed in public health, visiting nurse, or private duty positions. Much of the care within hospitals was delivered by students, aides, and orderlies under the direction of a head nurse. As more and more care was delivered in the hospital setting, the number of nurses employed by these facilities increased. The existing working conditions affected more people.

In 1945, a committee was appointed by the ANA to study employment conditions. This study culminated in 1946 in the creation of an ANA Economic Security Program. This action was followed by the enactment of a resolution that would encourage state nurses' associations to act as exclusive bargaining agents for their respective memberships in the important areas of economic security and collective bargaining. Also in 1946, the SEIU formed its first RN Guild in New York City.

The concept of professional collectivism, which emphasizes that good care is dependent on satisfactory working conditions and satisfaction with nursing itself, began to take shape. However, concern for the image of the nurse and nursing prompted a no-strike policy to be officially adopted by the ANA in 1950, and it remained in effect until it was rescinded in 1968.

By 1947, with the impetus provided by the Economic Security Program of ANA, collective bargaining between nurses and hospital administrations had been implemented in several states and negotiated contracts were in effect. Many hospital employers were voluntarily developing contracts with employees and were showing genuine concern about working conditions. Some states were mandating that state hospitals negotiate with all employees. But there was no federal requirement that this process would occur.

Federal legislation passed in 1962 enabled employees of federal health care institutions to participate in collective bargaining. In 1967, investor-owned hospitals and nursing homes were also included, and the ANA was identified as the bargaining agent for the nurses of the Veterans Administration hospitals. Legislation passed in 1970 saw the inclusion of nonprofit nursing homes in the collective bargaining process. Concurrently, SEIU and other labor-related organizations were also bargaining for nurses.

Finally, on August 25, 1974, Public Law 93-360 was put into effect; it amended the Taft-Hartley Act to provide economic security programs for those employed in nonprofit hospitals and brought health care facilities and their employees under the jurisdiction of the NLRB. Nonprofit hospitals were legally required to bargain with nurses for better wages, hours, staffing conditions, patient–nurse ratios, and a voice in hospital governance in general. To ensure that the public would be protected from strikes or work stoppage, several amendments were attached to the NLRA passed in 1974, such as longer notification periods and provisions mandating participation in mediation.

In 1994, a nursing home argued before the Supreme Court that the licensed practical nurses in its employ were supervisors because of their role in directing nursing assistants in patient care and, therefore, were not protected by the National Labor Relations Act. The Supreme Court in a 5 to 4 decision ruled in favor of the nursing home. Nursing organizations engaged in collective bargaining have expressed serious concern regarding the implications of this ruling for all nurses. Labor groups expect to lobby for legislation that would alter this interpretation of the NLRB ("Striking at Bargaining," 1994).

Understanding the Basic Language

Intelligent bargaining begins with an awareness of the process itself. As the word "bargaining" implies, collective bargaining consists of a set of procedures by which employee representatives and employer representatives negotiate to obtain a signed agreement (contract) that spells out wages, hours, and conditions of employment that are acceptable to both. A key word in this definition is *negotiate*.

BARGAINING AND NEGOTIATING

To negotiate means to bargain or confer with another party or parties to reach an agreement. *Bargaining* implies a discussion of the terms of the agreement and suggests that there will be give and take, that neither party will obtain all items asked for in the contract. Ideally, negotiations would proceed in a somewhat philosophical vein, moving toward reasonable compromises that could allow each side to achieve many of the conditions it is requesting, but this does not always occur.

Common interest bargaining refers to a process in which the employer and employee representatives begin by identifying those areas in which they agree and those goals or values held by both parties. Based on shared values and goals, the two parties then begin to work out their differences in regard to specific policies and conditions. Although relatively new as an approach to collective bargaining, common interest bargaining is gaining attention as a less adversarial process that may preserve effective working relationships and lessen feelings of alienation between supervisory personnel and employees involved in the union.

UNION AND COLLECTIVE ACTION

Collective bargaining allows employees working together as an organized unit to negotiate. A *union* is a legally authorized organized group of employees that negotiates and enforces labor agreements. Its major concern is the improvement of wages, hours, and working conditions of its members. Collective bargaining units tend to become organized when a group of persons in an institution identify common problems and concerns and become interested in forming a unit (Flanagan, 1992). When a branch or part of a professional association assumes this responsibility, as often occurs in nursing, the negotiating group may be known as a *collective action division*. The activity of the group may be referred to as *professional collectivism*, which supports the premise that the quality of patient care is directly tied to working conditions and that collective action is a professional responsibility. A professional organization must work under the same legal constraints as unions. It provides legal counsel and representatives to assist with negotiations, may lobby on behalf of issues, or may participate in other activities that would further the economic welfare of nurses. It oversees the development of the contract.

THE CONTRACT

The conclusion of the bargaining process should result in a signed contract that converts to writing the agreements that have been reached. A *contract* is "a legally binding agreement made between two or more persons to do or to refrain from doing certain actions" (Guido, 1988, p 167). In most instances a contract need not be in writing, but it is much easier to implement if it is written and signed by all involved. The contract remains in effect until breached or terminated. Most negotiated contracts define the period of time to be covered by the established conditions, usually 2 or 3 years.

Before being put into effect a contract must be *ratified*. This means that the terms of the contract must be accepted by the members of the bargaining group. This is usually done by a vote of the membership.

SOME RULES GOVERNING LABOR RELATIONS

When two parties agree to begin the negotiation process, it is understood that both will *bargain in good faith*. Bargaining in good faith is a poorly understood term, but generally it means that the parties will meet at regular times to discuss, with the intent to resolve, any differences over wages, hours, and other employment conditions. Failure to carry out these activities could fall into the category known as an *unfair labor practice*.

An *unfair labor practice* is any action that interferes with the rights of employees or employers as described in the amended NLRA. It is not possible to discuss all of these in detail; however, some examples follow. An employer must not interfere with the employee's right to form a union or other organized bargaining group, join the group, or participate in the group's activities. The employer may not attempt to control a group, once organized, or to discriminate against its members in regard to hiring or tenure. Most important, the employer must bargain collectively and in good faith with representatives of the employees.

Likewise, labor organizations have constraints placed on their activities. They, too, must bargain in good faith. They must not restrain or coerce employees in selecting a bargaining group to bargain collectively. They may not pressure an employer to discriminate against employees who do not belong to the labor organization.

One of the issues frequently brought up in negotiations that usually results in a dispute is that of *agency shop*. If an agency shop clause is in effect, all employees are required to pay the dues for membership. The obvious advantage of this requirement, from the workers' point of view, is encouraging membership in the union. The union is required to represent all employees, members or not. Negotiating a contract, monitoring compliance with its provisions, and facilitating the grievance process may be costly. The union, therefore, desires to have a greater percentage of paying members to support these activities. There are several variations in provisions related to agency shop. If, because of religious or philosophical beliefs, employees are unwilling to pay dues to the bargaining group, provisions may be made to pay the same sum to a nonprofit group such as a church or foundation. In some instances, those who are already members of the union are required to remain members for the life of the contract although no one is required to become a member. In some states laws referred to as "right to work laws" forbid the establishment of an agency shop.

Settling Labor Disputes

When labor disputes arise, several actions can be taken to help resolve the differences. Initially, of course, the parties continue to negotiate and may agree to extend the negotiation period if progress in settling differences is being made.

When the parties doing the negotiating cannot come to agreement on an issue, they are considered to be *at impasse* or the two groups are *deadlocked* on the issue.

MEDIATION AND ARBITRATION

Perhaps the most commonly used method of seeking agreement between parties is through *mediation* and *arbitration*. A *mediator* is a third person who may join the bargainers in early sessions to assist the parties to reconcile differences and arrive at a peaceful agreement. Mediation involves finding compromises, and the mediator is to assist with this. He or she must gain the respect of both parties and must remain neutral to the issues presented.

An *arbitrator* is technically defined as a person chosen by agreement of both parties to decide a dispute between them. The primary difference between a mediator and an arbitrator is that the mediator assists the parties in reaching their own decision, whereas the arbitrator has the authority to actu-

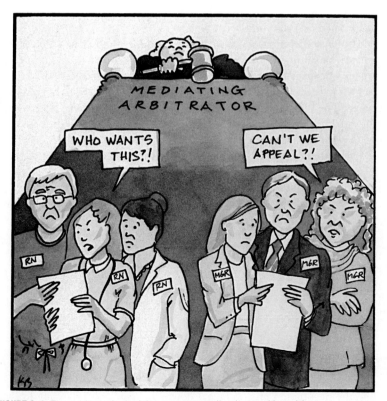

FIGURE 9–1 The arbitrator's decision may not really please either side.

ally make the decision for the parties if necessary. However, the terms *mediator* and *arbitrator* and *mediation* and *arbitration* often are used interchangeably, and, in fact, a mediator may also serve as an arbitrator.

Arbitration may take several forms. It may be mediation–arbitration, in which a third person joins the parties in the negotiation process before any serious disputes arise. This person's role is to act as a mediator who will attempt to keep the parties talking, suggest compromises, and help establish priorities. If an agreement is not reached by a specified date, or if it appears that neither party is willing to compromise on an issue (called a *deadlock*), the mediator then assumes the role of an arbitrator and gives a decision based on the information gained in the role of mediator.

Another form of arbitration is called *binding arbitration*. This means that both parties are obligated to abide by the decision of the arbitrator. Some people see this as the least desirable alternative in settling disputes because it may result in a decision that is not satisfactory to either side but one by which both must abide. It has been suggested, in instances in which binding arbitration is to be used, that the parties spell out exactly which of the issues are to be decided by the arbitrator. Binding arbitration has the advantage of resolving deadlocked issues without a strike being called. It also encourages both parties, knowing that the arbitrator's decision may not please either side, to reach a compromise on their own.

The *final offer* approach is a type of binding arbitration. Employer and employee bargaining representatives reach agreement on as many issues as possible. The deadlocked issues and a final position from each side are then presented to the arbitrator, who is obligated to select only the most reasonable package. The arbitrator may not develop a third alternative, which would "split the difference." The final offer approach encourages both sides to come up with a fairly realistic package and serves to close the gap on issues.

One criticism of any type of arbitration is the expense involved. Arbitrators must be paid for their services. It is also criticized because it undermines voluntary collective bargaining and allows parties to avoid unpleasant confrontation with their own difficulties by shifting that responsibility to a public authority. However, this is useful in preventing the disruption of services.

Arbitration may be requested from the American Arbitration Association or from available state public and private mediation and conciliation services. The American Arbitration Association is a nonprofit, nonpartisan organization that, for a nominal fee, will provide a list of qualified arbitrators. Most states also have available groups such as the Public Employees Relations Commission that also can provide a list of mediators and arbitrators.

STRIKES AND LOCKOUTS

When the negotiation process breaks down, lockouts and strikes are likely to occur. A *lockout* occurs when an employer closes a factory or other place of business to make employees agree to terms. One can readily see how undesirable this would be in the health care system, but it has occurred in some instances.

A *strike* occurs when workers refuse to work, thus imposing economic hardship and pressure on the employer. When the negotiation process breaks down, employees use the strike to emphasize their position. Workers may be striving to improve their own working conditions, salaries, and benefits. The most recent strikes by nurses, however, have been over issues related to patient care rather than those related to the economic status of the nurses. Striking places a serious economic hardship on employees and therefore is not undertaken lightly. Sometimes a strike is used to gain public attention to the labor dispute and to create public pressure for a settlement. This is only successful if the public agrees with the position of the striking workers.

REINSTATEMENT PRIVILEGE

A *reinstatement privilege* is a guarantee offered to striking employees that they will be rehired after the strike, provided that they have not engaged in any unfair labor practices during the strike and provided that the strike itself is lawful. The hospital may replace a striking nurse during the strike. If strikers agree unconditionally to return to work, the employer is not required to replace the striking nurse at that time. However, recall lists are developed, and if the nurse cannot find regular and equivalent employment, he or she is privileged to recall and preference on jobs before new employees may be given employment.

Nurses may lose their reinstatement privileges because of misconduct during a lawful strike. For example, strikers may not physically block other nurses and personnel from entering or leaving a struck hospital. Strikers may not threaten nonstriking employees and may not attack management representatives. These types of activities usually do not occur in strikes conducted by nurses but are not outside the realm of possibility.

OTHER METHODS OF INFLUENCING SETTLEMENT

One method of reaching solution is to employ an *authoritative mandate*, by which a peaceful settlement will be encouraged by a president, secretary of labor, or other high-ranking or influential person.

Another technique is *informational picketing*, which involves employees carrying informational signs outside of the institution. Informational picketing is not designed to stop work but rather to inform the public of the concerns under dispute. This tactic is designed to create public pressure on the behalf of the union and the employees.

In other instances, an *injunction* may be requested. This results in a court order that requires the party or parties involved to take a specific action or, more commonly, to refrain from taking a specific action. Employers may use this measure to forestall a strike. Unions may use this measure to stop a lock-out.

In still other instances the institution or company may be subjected to *government seizure and operation.* Government employees are then used to run the plant, firm, or industry in question. This is seldom seen in the health care industry for obvious reasons. However, this option was used in Montana in 1991 when state employees decided to strike. The National Guard was called in to replace striking state patrolmen.

What to Look for in a Contract

The negotiation process should ultimately conclude in the development of a written contract that is signed by both bargaining group and management representatives. The contract establishes guidelines for working conditions such as overtime, floating, work schedules, job security, and retention and recruitment of staff (Boisvert, 1991). It usually spells out certain other privileges to be provided to employees such as in-service education, leaves, health and safety provisions, committee participation, and tuition reimbursement (Flanagan, 1992). The contract may also provide guidelines for the grievance process.

A contract must meet certain specified criteria to be legally binding. It must result from mutually agreed-on items arrived at through a "meeting of minds." Something of value must be given for a reciprocal promise, that is, professional duties for an agreed-on sum. Contracts can be enforceable whether written or oral, but it is easier to work with those that are written (Rothman and Rothman, 1977).

Although each agreement will differ, most contracts have a fairly general format that will include:

- A preamble stating the objectives of each party
- A statement recognizing the official bargaining group
- A section dealing with financial remuneration, including wages and salaries, overtime rates, holiday pay, and shift differentials
- A section dealing with nonfinancial rewards, that is, fringe benefits such as retirement programs, types of insurance available, free parking, and other services provided by the employer
- A section dealing with seniority in respect to promotion, transfer, work schedules, and layoffs
- A section establishing guidelines for disciplinary problems

- A section describing how grievance procedures will be resolved
- A section that may explicitly state codes of conduct or professional standards

Several other areas that are negotiable are important and should be incorporated into the contract. These may be included in the section dealing with professional standards or nursing care. Cleland (1981) outlines the following items that should be considered in a contract that involves professional nurses. First, the contract should provide for shared governance, that is, that professional policy decisions should be developed by professional staff and administration who work jointly on the policy. This often takes the form of a nursing practice council or a professional performance committee. Second, the contract should provide for individual professional accountability. This would ensure peer evaluation of a practitioner's competence. Third, the contract should define the collective professional role. This spells out the responsibility of registered nurses as professional practitioners and describes their part in the planning of patient care. The purpose of this is to strengthen nurses' influence on the quality of care.

It is important that, as a new graduate, you know whether there is a contract in effect in the institution from which you seek employment or in the community in which you plan to work. You should also be knowledgeable about the terms of the existing contract so that you might best fulfill your obligations and recognize and benefit from the provisions to which you are entitled. The organization to which you are applying for employment can provide you a copy of the current contract. The state nurses' associations can be contacted for information regarding the organization that represents nurses in a particular hospital or facility. They can also provide a copy of any contracts that have been negotiated for which they represented the nurses.

The Grievance Process

Although the grievance process is a somewhat different subject than collective bargaining, it is usually one part of a negotiated contract and therefore deserves some mention here. Effective contracts will include, in addition to wages, hours, working conditions, and other items, a section that spells out the grievance procedure.

A *grievance* is a circumstance or action believed to be unjust and in violation of the contract. The *grievance process* represents an established and orderly method to be used in the adjustment of grievances between parties. In this sense, it represents a problem-solving mechanism. Grievances are usually related to interpretations of the contract. They generally occur as a result of a

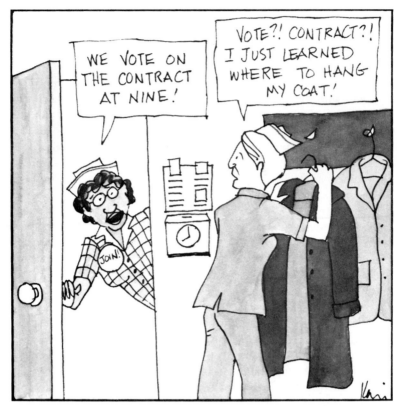

FIGURE 9–2 As a new graduate, you may find yourself poorly prepared to make decisions that are involved in bargaining issues.

misunderstanding or difference of opinion about the contract or its language or as direct violations of the contract. Although grievances can be filed by either the management or the employee, most cases are filed by the employee.

The grievance process spells out in writing in the contract a series of steps to be taken to resolve the area of dissension. Initially the employee and the immediate supervisor attempt to resolve the disagreement through informal talk. If no resolution occurs, the discussion moves into the steps of the grievance process. Typical steps are:

1. A written request for the next step is given to the immediate supervisor. Generally a time stipulation (eg, 10 days) is established for submitting the written request. A written response is required that also carries a time limit. From this point on in the deliberation, a representative from the bargaining unit may be present.

2. Assuming that the written response does not result in settling any problems, the grievance is submitted to a higher authority within the organization for appeal. Time lines are in effect and failure to comply with those time lines results in the discussion coming to a halt.

3. The employee, his or her representative, the appropriate representative from management (perhaps the Director of Nursing Service), and the grievance chairperson (who may be an officer in the bargaining unit) meet for discussion. The meeting may also include the personnel director, especially if the grievance relates to personnel policies. Once again, the contract usually specifies the number of days in which this must occur.

4. If no solution evolves following discussion, a neutral third party (arbitrator) is designated and is present at the deliberations. If no agreement is reached the arbitrator will rule on the situation. The decision of the arbitrator is usually binding.

It is important to discriminate between complaints and grievances. Employees may have complaints that are not violations of the contract. For example, Nurse No. 1 may object that she was required to float from the postpartum unit to the nursery. She had been oriented to the nursery but preferred to work in the postpartum unit. Nurse No. 2 was required to float from a medical unit to a surgical unit to which she had not been oriented. If the contract in this hospital stipulated that no one would be floated to a unit to which he or she had not been oriented, Nurse No. 1 had a complaint, whereas Nurse No. 2 had a grievance.

Hoover and colleagues (1990) point out that all organizations have problems. The absence of grievances may not be the best indicator of the health of the organization. It is entirely possible that problems are not being addressed. On the other hand, a high number of grievances is an indication of problems within the organization. These problems often relate to the language of the contract or the education of the employee to the conditions of the contract. Another barometer of the health of the organization is the level at which the grievances are resolved. It is most desirable to settle most grievances at the informal level and without the involvement of an arbitrator.

The grievance procedure may sound like many steps that may take a great deal of time, and indeed this is true. Although most grievances are settled short of arbitration, they are still time and energy consuming. Grievances can be best avoided if everyone has a good understanding of the terms of the contract and if sound personnel policies are developed and applied consistently and equitably. Open discussions between the employees and management to review mutual concerns and share information help reduce the number of grievances. Mutual respect is a critical element in any organization.

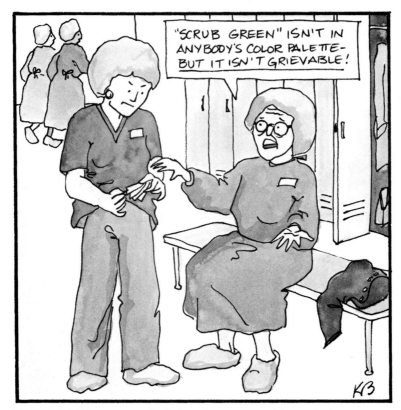

FIGURE 9–3 It is important to discriminate between complaints and grievances.

Issues Related to Collective Bargaining and Nursing

Three major issues of collective bargaining affect the nursing profession. The first of these relates to the fact that some nurses see collective bargaining as unprofessional. The second is the issue of which bargaining group will represent nursing if nurses do participate in collective bargaining. The final issue is an individual one and relates to the question of whether to join a union when one exists.

At one time the issue of whether nurses should participate in strike activities was of much concern. Many nurses found the withholding of services from patients to be unprofessional, and therefore, personally unacceptable. Others viewed the strike as the final method to bring attention to the needs of the nurse as a citizen. Fortunately, as bargaining groups representing nurses have become more knowledgeable and skilled in the process, strikes occur less frequently. Disagreements at the bargaining table are more commonly resolved through mediation and arbitration, much to the relief of many professionals.

These issues may take on greater or lesser importance depending on the area of country involved, the length of time the nurses in that area have been participating in collective bargaining, and the group chosen to represent the nurses at the bargaining table.

PROFESSIONALISM AND COLLECTIVE ACTION

Among the issues related to collective bargaining, the strain that exists between professionalism and collective action has probably received more space in recent nursing literature than has any other.

The argument against unionism has its roots in the history of nursing itself. Nursing was perceived by many, including nurses, as a selfless, all-serving, altruistic calling. The act of caring for others, even if that meant subordination of the individual to the goals of that care, was to be compensation enough for the services rendered. The strong religious influence that pervaded the early development of nursing added to this concept of the profession. Early leaders in nursing espoused this dedication to its arts. In 1893, Lavinia Dock stated:

> Absolute and unquestioning obedience must be the foundation of the nurse's work, and to this end complete subordination of the individual to the work as a whole is as necessary for her as for the soldier. (Cited in Bullough and Bullough, 1966, p 96)

Another factor that has hampered the strong development of unionization in nursing is the fact that nursing is primarily a women's profession. Although more men now enter nursing, only about 3% of the registered nurses in the United States are men.

Early social beliefs that woman's role should be submissive, supportive, and obedient were extremely compatible with pervading concepts of the expectations that our society placed on nurses. The paternalism that has existed in the health care delivery system has also made the process of collective bargaining for nurses a slow one (see Chapter 1). The combination of the role of women and the role of the nurse under earlier paternalistic practices had the nurse caring for the "hospital family," looking out for the needs of all, from patient to physician, and being responsible for keeping everyone happy (Ashley, 1976). The tendency to see the physician as the father figure in the health care system, the nurse as the corresponding mother figure, and the patients as the children has done little to promote the autonomy of nursing as a profession. A quote by Campbell (1980, p 1286) demonstrates the use of the family concept in health care: "If we are to keep unions out of the profession we, as nurses, must make every effort to build loyalty and a family feeling among our fellow nurses."

Despite the fact that nursing has a history of ambivalence toward union negotiations, today we see nurses involved in collective bargaining in greater numbers than ever before. Several factors are responsible for this change. Wilson and colleagues (1990) have identified these as the focus on the continued high cost of health care and the need to examine this rise, the scrutiny that has been placed on employee's salaries as part of this process, the fact that nurses comprise the largest number of employees in hospitals (nearly half), and changes in the NLRA allowing nurses to bargain collectively. Various sources differ with regard to whether unionization of hospital employees results in higher hospital costs.

In the early years of collective bargaining by nurses, there was some reticence to use the term "unionism." Much of the nursing literature surrounding the issue used appropriate and less emotionally charged synonyms. Today the term "unionism" is used with increasing frequency, reflecting a change in sentiment that supports the belief that nurses should be involved in collective bargaining. Unionism to some means gaining coercive powers and thus creating a public image of nurses and nursing that would have a detrimental effect on the profession. Some have feared that their white collars might turn "blue," recalling the traditional association of unionism with blue-collar workers. However, most of the literature of today has stopped quibbling over the word "unionism."

Many have come to believe that the collective action of nurses provides one of the best avenues for achieving professional goals and exercising control over nursing practice. As nurses are called on to assume greater and greater responsibility for complicated decisions, collective bargaining through a professional organization may provide the means to implement the concept of collective professional responsibility.

Certainly the way that collective bargaining will be perceived by the nurse and by the public that is served will be primarily determined by the manner in which the bargaining is conducted. Nurses as a group need to develop the skills necessary to communicate to the public the importance of their role in health care delivery. They must be able to handle conflicts and work toward resolution while maintaining integrity and dignity. Nurses need to become enlightened and informed, and they need more than a superficial understanding of the process of collective bargaining.

Nurses may benefit from broadening their perceptions. This applies to many areas of practice in addition to that of collective bargaining, particularly bioethical issues (see Chapter 7). Many nurses dichotomize issues into categories such as good/bad, right/wrong, best/worst. Nurses need to work toward understanding and accommodating differing points of view and acknowledging that areas of compromise can exist.

REPRESENTATION FOR NURSES

Of far greater controversy than whether nurses should unionize is the issue of which organization should represent nurses at the bargaining table. This is determined by elections that are supervised by the NLRB. To become the certified collective bargaining representative of a group of employees, the organization in question must receive 50% of the votes cast, plus one.

When nurses first began to organize, the ANA, through the state nurses' associations, was the bargaining representative. This group still represents more nurses than all the other organizations combined. In 1991, across the country state associations represented more the 139,000 registered nurses through more than 840 bargain units (Fuller-Jonap, 1994). However, there has been a strong movement on the part of other organizations to vie for the representative position. It has been estimated that more than 30 labor organizations represent health care workers (Miller, 1980). The ANA has been representing nurses since 1946. The National Union of Hospital and Health Care Employees (representing nurses since 1977) and the SEIU have voted to unite, creating something of a "super union" for health care workers. The Federation of Nurses and Health Professionals began organizing nurses in 1978. Other groups representing nurses in various parts of the country include the United Food and Commercial Workers, the Teamsters Union, and the American Federation of Teachers.

Nurses face a difficult decision when trying to decide which group can represent them best. In recent years, perhaps this decision has occupied more time and effort on the part of nurses than has the actual bargaining. Those who have strong allegiance to the ANA contend that only registered nurses should bargain for registered nurses. One of the reasons given for this position is that in collective bargaining, nurses face different issues than do other workers. In addition to concerns about salary, benefits, working conditions, and the like, nurses want also to negotiate questions pertaining to staffing, patient care concerns, and participation on joint hospital committees. Many believe that only nurses can effectively negotiate such items. These people contend that hospital administration, fearing the power of labor unions, will bargain more constructively and positively with nurses themselves. They also believe that the ANA will be a stronger, more united organization if it serves as both the professional association and the bargaining agent.

Others believe that nurses compromise their collective bargaining powers when the recognized union is a group other than the state nurses' association. They think that when nurses do not bargain for themselves, the "organization shrivels and their influence on health care weakens" (Mallison, 1985, p 943).

Some parts of the country are experiencing a trend toward having an organization other than the professional nurses' association represent nurses. Chief among the arguments for bargaining conducted by another group is the issue of supervisor membership in the professional association (discussed earlier in this chapter). Proponents of this position would also contend that it is not realistic for one group (ie, the ANA) to work with the professionalism aspect of nursing as well as with the issues of wages, benefits, and working conditions.

Some would argue for two organizations, one to represent issues related to professionalism and another to negotiate salaries. If nurses choose to have one group involved in professional concerns (eg, codes of ethics, standards of care, and updating skills required in the practice of the profession) and a second group representing them at the bargaining table, there are some obvious drawbacks. First and foremost is the matter of cost because both organizations would be collecting dues. Many perceive the cost of belonging to the ANA and the state associations as very high, with dues of approximately $350 per year. Additional membership dues in another organization, which are equally as expensive, might be prohibitive. Second, many believe that the union would become the dominant force between the two groups because money and working environment issues both speak strongly. There are no easy answers to this question, and it will certainly be one of the biggest issues facing nurses in the future.

TO JOIN OR NOT TO JOIN

Once the individual nurse has gained an understanding of collective bargaining and has developed a personal philosophy about the professional role, he or she will be ready to make a decision in regard to membership in the bargaining unit.

In working with students who are soon to embark on professional careers, we find that it is easier for them to decide whether to bargain collectively than it is to decide to part with the money that is required for membership. Many nurses want better working conditions and higher salaries but are all too willing to let someone else fund these endeavors and work to achieve them.

It is in response to these concerns that many "agency shop" clauses have been added to contracts. Those who are members and are active in the negotiation process believe it is inappropriate for some to benefit from the labors of the bargaining process without having contributed, at least financially, to the effort. The presence of agency shop clauses may serve as either an asset or a deterrent to recruitment, depending on the applicant's viewpoint.

Changing Trends With Regard to Collective Bargaining

At one time economic concerns and working conditions may have been the principal motivators for collective action. However, by the mid-1980s subtle, and at times not so subtle, changes were occurring throughout the United

States with regard to collective bargaining, unionism, and labor–management relations. Some working in the area of contract management would report a shift from the adversarial relationship that had historically existed between the employee and the employer, which focused on salaries, work hours, and the like, to one that placed greater emphasis on the quality of work life.

CONCESSION BARGAINING

Concession bargaining is a process by which there is an explicit exchange in labor costs for improvements in job security. This has been seen to occur with increasing frequency. An example would be a shift in emphasis from one that asks for increases in salary to one that focuses on eliminating the practice of calling nurses and telling them not to report for work because the census has dropped. On these days the nurses do not receive salary. These changes have been seen in industry more than in nursing, although the strike of 6000 Minnesota nurses was triggered by hospital practices related to the layoff of staff and the involuntary reduction of hours (6000 Minnesota RNs, 1984).

"UNION BUSTING"

A trend seen in health care institutions during the 1980s and persisting in some areas today is an effort toward "union busting." Although technically illegal when referring to methods used to get rid of an existing union, the term *union busting* has been expanded to include a wide range of legal activities that slow down collective bargaining. Pressured by rapidly escalating health care costs and influenced by the changing attitudes toward work, hospital administrators have hired consultants and law firms to assist and advise in discouraging and impeding organizational activities. This is also a counteraction to the courting by unions of the expanding groups of previously unorganized professional groups, such as physicians and nurses. Antiunion organizing campaigns are usually aimed at strategies that will delay and thus drag down the momentum of organizing efforts. This could include challenging union membership, attempting to decertify elections, and failing to bargain in good faith, thus drawing out the negotiating process (Ballman, 1985).

ISSUES OF DISCRIMINATION

As nurses have become more comfortable and knowledgeable about the bargaining process, their energies have been directed toward a variety of issues. This would include such concerns as pay equity, discrimination against female employees, comparable worth, and the right of the employee to know the hazards within the work environment (see Chapter 11). In some instances, discriminatory practices against male nurses have also been an issue.

CHANGES IN THE NUMBER OF BARGAINING UNITS

Within the organization of hospitals are many different positions and job titles ranging from the professional staff through office staff to those responsible for hospital maintenance. In nursing alone are groups of registered nurses, licensed practical nurses, and nursing assistants. As these various groups have been granted authority to organize into bargaining units, concern has been expressed about the number of various unions with which any hospital administration must bargain at any given time. Some fairly elaborate estimates have been made regarding the amount of time demanded by the collective bargaining process.

When the NLRA was first passed in 1974, the NLRB specified that seven employee bargaining units would exist within the health care industry (Wilson, Hamilton, and Murphy, 1990, p 37). Those seven groups were registered nurses, physicians, other professional employees, technical employees, business office and/or clerical employees, and skilled maintenance employees.

In 1984, the NLRB determined that bargaining units would be decided on a case-by-case basis. This resulted in the number of bargaining units being reduced to three: all professionals, all nonprofessionals, and guards.

In 1989, the NLRB once again proposed new rule changes that resulted in the establishment of eight collective bargaining units. At this time it was also determined that the rule would apply to all hospitals of all sizes. In response the American Hospital Association (AHA) sought and obtained a permanent injunction against the rule. Subsequently, "all-RN" units were legally approved. As might be expected the AHA and the ANA occupied opposite points of view with regard to this issue.

THE WORKPLACE ADVOCACY INITIATIVE

One of the most recent activities has been a move on the part of the ANA to improve their work environment and gain control over nursing practice. Ideally this would result in an assurance that patients would receive the best possible nursing care.

In moving toward this objective, in 1991 the ANA selected 16 states to receive grants to initiate or improve the workplace advocacy programs. Two grants focused on exploring new methods to ensure that nurses are involved in decisions that affect the quality of their work environments in states where the state nurses' association does not represent nurses at the bargaining table. The other grants were used to mount organizing campaigns that would result in strengthening the bargaining programs of the state association.

Other aspects of the ANA Workplace Advocacy Initiative included providing data about salaries and related economic and employment issues; providing information related to health, safety, and other workplace concerns; developing systems of analysis of compensation packages; consultation; and supporting networks for sharing information and providing mutual support.

The Impact of Shared Governance on Collective Bargaining

Few areas have felt the impact of technology as much as has health care. Ranging from new systems of information and communication to different administrative structures, to changing approaches to systems of evaluation, the health care delivery system has seen a radical acceleration in all forms of technology. In the realm of administrative structure, one of the more important of these has been the recent move to a pattern of shared governance within health care agencies.

In a shared governance model, nursing staff are provided with more autonomy. This structure allows nursing staff to make major decisions within the organization, attempting to get the decision-making process as close to where the action is occurring as is possible. Often this pattern of organization is paired with concepts of total quality improvement (TQI), which has as it hallmark, emphasis on the customer. Alexander, Bourgeois, and Goodman (1994, p 283) state "TQI and shared governance (1) empower all employees, (2) encourage decision making at the appropriate level within the organization, (3) promote teamwork with consensus and shared responsibility, (4) encourage and recognize employee contributions, and (5) provide opportunities for personal growth."

In this environment, much of the direction for the organization is developed through committees or councils resulting in staff actively participating in management. Often councils will report to a nursing executive board that serves as a coordinating and approval body. Within this framework, the nurse is held to greater accountability within the context of peer-defined and peer-operated parameters (Porter-O'Grady, 1990). The traditional role of the supervisor as one who hires, evaluates, promotes, and fires has become a thing of the past. Peer evaluations may have taken its place.

The greater involvement of staff nurses in health care agency decision-making may have a significant impact the collective bargaining process. Many of the issues that historically were resolved at the bargaining table, such as the use of agency nurses, work load, and policies regarding floating from one unit to another, are now developed at the committee or council level. Each nurse has greater accountability for participation in decision-making outside of the bargaining process and for implementing decisions that have been made.

With mechanisms for change built in to the operational pattern of the health care agency, nurses may find less to negotiate at the bargaining table and, in reality, the processes may provide some duplication of one another.

Key Concepts

▷ Since 1974, it has been possible for nurses to bargain collectively for salaries, working conditions, and fringe benefits. This process also allows for their participation in committees focusing on improved patient care and patient care standards.

▷ The collective bargaining process culminates in a contract that places in writing the decisions reached at the bargaining table. As a new graduate you should know whether the health care agency at which you are seeking employment has a contract in effect.

▷ A contract usually includes a section that spells out the process to be used in a grievance. It is important, should a grievance arise, that all steps be followed as outlined in this document.

▷ One of the issues surrounding nurses and collective bargaining is related to which group should do the bargaining for nurses. Many believe this process is best conducted by the professional organization; others believe they will be best served by an organization that has collective bargaining as its major focus.

▷ Trends with regard to the collective bargaining process include concession bargaining, "union busting," issues of discrimination, and changes in the number of bargaining units.

▷ The advent of shared governance in hospitals has caused nursing to move away from the traditional hierarchy. As more and more facilities adopt shared governance structures, the collective bargaining process will change.

CRITICAL THINKING ACTIVITIES

1. Do you support the concept of nurses becoming members of a union? If so, should all employees of an organization be required to pay membership fees? Give the rationale to support your views.

2. Outline the major disadvantages of unions in nursing and give examples to demonstrate the disadvantages you perceive.

3. If the collective bargaining agent in the hospital in which you worked was other than the state nurses' association, would you belong to both organizations? What factors would you use to support your decision?

4. What are the reasons that grievance processes need to be spelled out in the contract?

5. In what way do you think shared governance will have an impact on collective bargaining? Support your ideas with examples from the literature.

References

Alexander MK, Bourgeois A, Goodman LR. Total quality improvement: Bridging the gap between education and service. *In* Strickland OL, Fishman DJ. Nursing Issues in the 1990s. Albany, NY: Delmar Publishers, 1994:280–289

Ashley JA. Hospitals, Paternalism and the Role of the Nurse. New York: Teachers' College Press, 1976

Ballman CS. Union busters. Am J Nurs 85(9):963–966, 1985

Boisvert SC. Collective bargaining: Another view. Maine Nurse 78(4):5, 1991

Campbell GJ. *In* Opinions: Is bargaining unprofessional for nurses? AORN J 31(6):1289, 1980

Cleland V. Taft-Hartley amended: Implications for nursing—the professional model. J Nurs Admin 11(7):18–22, 1981

Dock LL. Nurses should be obedient. *In* Bullough V, Bullough B: Issues in Nursing: Readings Selected From Books and Periodicals to Form a Basis for Discussion of Problems in Nursing Today. New York: Springer-Verlag, 1966:96

Flanagan, L. How collective bargaining benefits nurses. Directions: American Nurse Supplement. October:8–9, 22, 1992

Fuller-Jonap F. Collective bargaining in nursing: Benefits, issues, and problems. *In* Strickland OL, Fishman DJ. Nursing Issues in the 1990s. Albany, NY: Delmar Publishers, 1994:33–45

Guido GW. Legal Issues in Nursing: A Source Book for Practice. Norwalk, CT: Appleton & Lange, 1988

Hoover K, Sanders EM, Colin JM. What's right about grievances? Am J Nurs 90(11):45–46, 1990

Mallison MB. Weathering the economic climate. Am J Nurs 85(9):943, 1985

Miller RU. Collective bargaining: A nursing dilemma. AORN J 31(6):1197, 1980

Muff J. Altruism, socialism and nightingalism: The compassion traps. *In* Muff J: Women's Issues in Nursing: Socialization, Sexism, and Stereotyping. Prospect Heights, IL: Waveland Press, 1988:234–247

Porter-O'Grady T. Nursing governance in a transitional era. *In* Chaska NL: The Nursing Profession: Turning Points. St. Louis: CV Mosby, 1990:432–439

Rothman DA, Rothman NL. The Professional Nurse and the Law. Boston: Little, Brown, 1977

6,000 Minnesota RNs strike back at layoff trend. Am J Nurs 84(7):941, 948, 1984

Striking at bargaining rights, court says RNs are supervisors. Am J Nurs 94(7):67, 70–71, 1994

Supreme Court okays all-RN unit. Am Nurse June:1, 1991

Wilson CN, Hamilton CL, Murphy E. Union dynamics in nursing. J Nurs Admin 20(2):35–39, 1990

Further Readings

Beletz E, Meng MT. The grievance process. Am J Nurs 77(2):256–260, 1977

Browne MN, et al. Litigation and collective bargaining: Two pay equity strategies. A D Nurse 3(6):18–20, 1988

Castrey BG, Castrey RT. Mediation: What it is, what it does. J Nurs Admin 10(9):18–21, 1980

Eldridge I, Levi J. Collective bargaining as a power resource for professional goals. Nurs Admin Q Winter:29–40, 1982

Flanagan L. All-RN rule to have major impact. Am Nurse March:26, 1982

Gross JA. Conflicting statutory purposes: Another look at fifty years of NLRB law making. Indust Labor Rel Rev 39(10):7–18, 1985

Hudacek SS. Collective bargaining—not a dinosaur of the past. Adv Clin Care 5(1):27–28, 1990

Ketter J. Staff nurses celebrate 20 years of NLRB protection. Am Nurse 26(6):3, 9, 1994

McCarty P. ANA launches workplace initiative—SNAs get grants for RN advocacy, new organizing. Am Nurse April:1, 7, 1991

Pettengill MM. Collective bargaining: Impact on nursing. *In* Chaska NL: The Nursing Profession: Turning Points. St. Louis: CV Mosby, 1990:454–463

Pettengill MM. Multilateral collective bargaining and the health care industry: Implications for nursing. J Prof Nurs 1(5):275–282, 1985

Scott K. SNA representation means increased job satisfaction. Am Nurse, January:24, 1993

Smith GR. Unionization for nurses: An issue for the 1980s. J Prof Nurs 1(4):192–201, 1985

Stickler KB. Union organizing will be divisive and costly. Hospitals 64(13):68–70, 1990

Targeting charge nurses, hospitals move to prove RN "supervisors." Am Jrnl Nurse 94(9):75, 1994

10

The Political Process and Health Care

Objectives

After completing this chapter, you should be able to

1. Explain the relevance of the political process to nursing.
2. Discuss seven ways you might influence the political process.
3. Outline the current U.S. federal governmental role in health care.
4. Discuss the various proposals related to a national health care system.
5. Explain common state legislative concerns.
6. Discuss common local political concerns.
7. Identify how politics is relevant to your participation in organizations.

Ellis JR, Hartley CL: NURSING IN TODAY'S WORLD:
CHALLENGES, ISSUES, AND TRENDS, 5th ed.
© 1995 J.B. Lippincott Company

Politics is the way in which people in a democratic society try to influence decision-making and the allocation of resources. Because resources (money, time, or personnel) are limited, choices must always be made as to their use. There is no perfect process for making optimum choices because in every instance in which one valuable option is chosen, some other option must be left out. Politics is a part of every organization as well as part of government at every level. In this chapter we hope to help you to understand the political process as we discuss some of the current issues in regard to political decisions and describe ways you can play a role in the political arena.

Relevance of the Political Process for Nurses

Nurses have always been involved in politics. Florence Nightingale used her contacts with powerful men in the government to obtain supplies and the personnel she needed to care for wounded soldiers in the Crimea (Woodham-Smith, 1983). Hannah Ropes was able to fight incompetence and obtain decent care for wounded Civil War soldiers because she understood who were the influential people in Washington and who would be receptive to her efforts on the soldiers' behalf (Donahue, 1985).

Modern times are no different. With all the many different voices competing to be heard in the decision-making circles of any nation, the person who understands power and how the system works is better prepared to achieve desired ends.

Health care is costly, and public dollars can be and are spent in many ways to provide health care. What part of the federal budget should be allocated to health care? What part of the state budget? The local governmental budget? Of the money allocated, what part should be used for preventive health programs? What part for research? What part for care and treatment? What part for education? These questions are answered by legislation and by administrative decisions made by governmental agencies.

If you have opinions regarding an appropriate government role in health care, then politics is for you. If you disagree with the priorities as they are set currently, then politics is for you. If you have ever been blocked in your attempt to provide health care to a client and family because funds or programs were not available, then the political process is relevant to you.

Your practice as a nurse is controlled by a wide variety of governmental decisions. One of the most basic is the Nurse Practice Act of your state. In that document, nursing is defined legally and the scope of nursing practice is outlined. This document affects what you do each day that you practice. All of the philosophical discussions about the role of the nurse must return to the reality of the nurse's role as legally defined in the state's practice act. Do you care what that role is now or what changes are made in it? Does it make any difference to you what education is required in that law or if that law requires continuing education? Answering "yes" to any of these questions underlines the relevance of the political process for you.

Many decisions are made within the various nurses' organizations (see Chapter 13). These organizations speak for nurses in a variety of settings. Are you happy with the way they are spending funds paid in dues? Do you agree with all of the public statements they make? Do you support their mechanisms for decision-making? Are you happy with the image of nurses and nursing the public receives from these organizations? Do you care what these organizations do with their resources? The political process is an important part of their functioning, too.

Influencing the Political Process

Once you have decided that the political process affects you and your practice as a nurse in many crucial ways, your next concern is how to influence the process by which those decisions are made. Can you as an individual have an effect on such things as what legislation is submitted, what is passed, and the content of that legislation? The answer is yes you can, but not without effort and concern on your part. Each person must determine his or her own level of personal involvement, but there is, in the broad realm of the political process, a place for everyone to function in a way that is comfortable. Some of the ways are outlined here.

BEING INFORMED

To be informed about legislation and health care, it is necessary to become familiar with the sources of information. Your daily newspaper can be an excellent source regarding significant legislation being proposed. This source is not complete, however, and you often learn of legislation after it has already been passed.

Television and radio news reports are valuable but may give only an overview of a particular piece of legislation being introduced. This overview may be helpful in alerting you to something that you want to study more intensively. Some television programs do discuss issues in depth. In an attempt to meet the Federal Communications Commission rules regarding equal time, these programs usually make an attempt to present both sides of any issue.

Professional journals usually devote some space to current legislative issues. This is done routinely in the *American Journal of Nursing* and in the *American Nurse*. When major issues are being discussed, other nursing periodicals frequently contain articles of interest.

Nursing organizations or other health-related organizations may hold open meetings to present and discuss legislative issues. Often knowledgeable speakers are present who can help you to understand what is being proposed and the various potential effects. Nursing organizations may present the best opportunity for you to be current and informed because they often are in touch with lobbyists or congressional staff persons who follow issues critical to nursing.

Newsletters or journals of organizations that have a political focus provide information on what they see as current issues. These include consumer groups such as Common Cause, political groups such as Young Democrats and Young Republicans, and nonpartisan groups such as the League of Women Voters.

Copies of legislation are usually available through your congressional representatives (for federal matters) or your state representatives (for state matters). Along with copies of the legislation you may receive other informational material from a legislator. Government agencies affected by proposed legislation may also provide information about its potential effect.

Each source of information is valuable to you but should be weighed in terms of its known biases. Even the most objective-sounding report may be as greatly shaded with meaning by what is not reported as by what is reported. Identifying the groups that support and the groups that oppose a particular viewpoint may help in recognizing bias. Speculate whether the group and its members would tend to gain or lose personally by the passage of proposed legislation. Are special interest groups voicing an opinion? When biases are evident, it is advisable to obtain information from those with divergent viewpoints. Decisions need to be based on firm factual data.

Once you are informed about the current issues in legislation, you are better prepared to form a personal opinion about them and to try to influence the outcome of the political process. There are many ways you can affect that process.

VOTING

Your individual vote on a ballot issue is significant. One of the unfortunate statistics in the United States is the low percentage of those eligible who are registered and voters. Nurses, as a group, have a high percentage who are voters. When legislators hear statistics such as "1 in 17 women voters is a nurse," or "1 in every 44 voters is a nurse," they pay attention to the opinions of nurses. Although you cannot vote directly on most legislative issues, you can vote for candidates whose positions you support and who share your values. Absentee ballots are always available for those who cannot be present at their polling place on the day of the election. These must be requested well in advance of the election, however.

It is a common practice to belittle the importance of the individual vote in any election. Recent major elections in this country have demonstrated again how important those votes can be. Recounts were necessary in several elections because the margin between the two candidates was only a few hundred votes out of the thousands cast. Even one-sided votes with overwhelming support for or against one candidate or issue may strongly emphasize the position of the voting public, and thus influence subsequent legislative and governmental decisions.

SHAPING PUBLIC OPINION

Public opinion does influence the actions of legislators and regulatory bodies. You may help to shape that public opinion. As a registered nurse, your opinion about matters that affect health care may help others make their own decisions. Share the knowledge you have gained through your personal experience and research. Do not be afraid to state your own opinion, although you must be prepared with evidence to support that opinion to be accepted as a thoughtful health care professional. This does not mean that you must become an orator on every social occasion, but that you should use opportunities that arise to present your concerns to others.

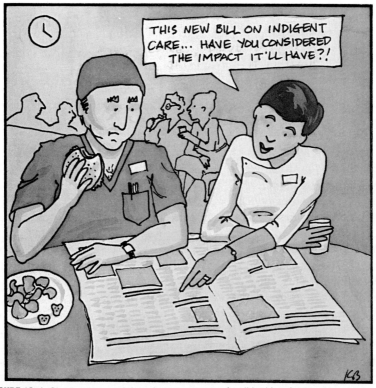

FIGURE 10–1 Sharing your opinions is one avenue of political involvement.

COMMUNICATING WITH LEGISLATORS AND OFFICIALS

Legislators are affected by the views of their constituents. Letters received usually are reviewed by the legislator's staff; views are tabulated, and letters with significant opinions or information are directed to the legislator for individual consideration. Form letters and postcards receive the least attention from a legislator. A carefully written personal letter that reflects thoughtful and informed opinions on an issue that person is competent to evaluate receives the most attention.

As a registered nurse you have expertise in an aspect of health care that can provide a valuable viewpoint. Identify yourself as a registered nurse in your letter and outline why you are concerned about the issue in question. Legislators often appreciate personal anecdotes from your practice (with identities concealed, of course) that underscore your point.

Concern regarding rules and regulations of a specific department of government can be addressed to officials of that department. It is possible for officials to become insulated from the effects of their decision-making. Communication from concerned citizens is important to them as well as to legislators. Letters to officials should reflect the same careful professional view as letters to legislators do to be most effective in influencing regulations.

Telephone calls cannot usually be made directly to a legislator but can be made to the legislator's office. Staff keep a record of all calls and the positions of callers. In some states a toll-free number is maintained for calls to state legislators during the legislative session.

For those with access to E-mail, many governmental agencies now have E-mail addresses that allow you to send a message electronically. As the "information highway" becomes more widely accessible, this avenue of communication will become easier to use.

Telegrams are delivered by telephone within 5 hours of being sent. A mailgram is a less expensive type of telegram that is delivered in the regular mail on the next business day after you send it. These are especially useful right before an important vote or committee deliberation.

Visits to congressional or state representatives may also be an effective means of expressing your concerns. One of the best ways to arrange to speak to congressional representatives and senators is to contact their local offices. Through these offices you may receive assistance in arranging your visit. They may also help you to arrange other interesting and valuable experiences such as attending committee hearings, taking tours, and visiting Congress in session. Appointments should always be made well in advance, or the person may not have time to speak with you. If your time is circumscribed (such as a limited visit to Washington, DC), you may have to modify your expectations and meet with a staff member who will relay your concerns. Plan carefully for your visit. It is often helpful to write out concerns and questions. Be sure to leave time for

HOW TO WRITE YOUR CONGRESSMAN

How to learn their names . . .

Call your public library, local newspaper, or chapter of the League of Women Voters to learn the names and addresses of your U. S. senators, your representative to congress, and your state senator(s), and your state representative(s), (called assemblyman in California, New Jersey, New York, and Wisconsin; delegate in Virginia and West Virginia).

How to obtain a copy of a bill

For a Senate bill, write or visit (no telephone requests filled) the Senate Documents Office, Washington, DC 20510; for a House bill, write or visit the Doorkeeper of the House, U. S. Capitol, Washington, DC 20515.

Ask for the bill by number and enclose a self-addressed and gummed label for fastest service. There is no charge.

Requests are normally filled the day received, unless the bill is out of print, and sent via first class mail. There is a limit of six items per day per person, and of three copies of one bill per person (or of one copy per bill if the bill is 60 pages or longer).

Request a copy of a state bill from the appropriate state legislator.

Copies of hearing record can be requested from the committee conducting the hearing, although they usually are not ready for distribution until several weeks after the hearing.

An alternate to the above procedures, for federal bills and hearing records, is to request a copy from your appropriate senator or representative.

(Reprinted by permission of the N.A.A.C.O.G.)

Fundamentals:

1. Address your letter properly: "Hon. _____, House Office Building, Washington, DC 20515", or "Senator _____, Senate Office Building, Washington, DC 20510".
2. Identify the bill or issue. Try to give the bill number or describe it by popular title.
3. Watch your timing. Inform your congressman while there is still time to take effective action.

Write to the right persons:

Concentrate on your own delegation. The representative of your district and the senators of your state cast your votes in the Congress and want to know your views.

Be brief:

Be reasonably brief. Your views and arguments stand a better chance of being read if they are stated as concisely as the subject matter will permit. It is not necessary that letters be typed — only that they be legible — and the form, phraseology, and grammar are not important.

Do:

1. Write your own views — not someone else's. A personal letter is far better than a form letter or signature on a petition. Form letters often receive form replies.
2. Give your reasons for taking a stand. The effects of a bill on a certain constituency will be far more helpful.
3. Be constructive. If a bill deals with a problem, but you believe the bill is the wrong approach, outline the correct approach. If you have expert knowledge, share it with your congressman.
4. Say 'well done' when it is deserved. Congressmen appreciate this from people who believe they have done the right thing.

Do not:

1. Don't make threats or promises.
2. Don't berate your congressman. If you disagree with him, give reasons for your disagreement.
3. Don't become a 'pen pal'. Quality is more important than quantity.
4. Don't demand a commitment before the facts are in. A bill rarely becomes law in the same form as introduced, it is possible for a writer to change his or her position once a bill reaches a floor.

The above material, excerpted from *Congressional Record, Nov. 2, 1977,* by Morris K. Udall, was prepared by the Washington office of The American College of Obstetricians and Gynecologists.

FIGURE 10–2 How to write your congressman.

answers to the questions that you pose. Even when you disagree with the position taken by your legislator, be polite and present your concerns calmly. Rudeness will result in an unwillingness to listen to what you have to say.

(*text continues on page 350*)

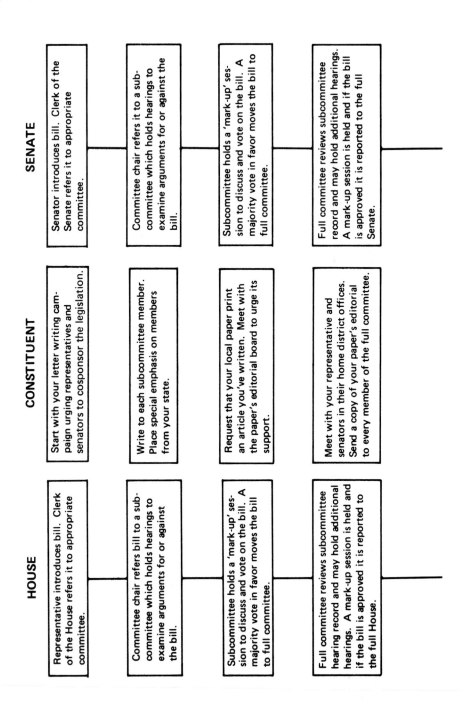

HOUSE

Representative introduces bill. Clerk of the House refers it to appropriate committee.

Committee chair refers bill to a sub-committee which holds hearings to examine arguments for or against the bill.

Subcommittee holds a 'mark-up' session to discuss and vote on the bill. A majority vote in favor moves the bill to full committee.

Full committee reviews subcommittee hearing record and may hold additional hearings. A mark-up session is held and if the bill is approved it is reported to the full House.

CONSTITUENT

Start with your letter writing campaign urging representatives and senators to cosponsor the legislation.

Write to each subcommittee member. Place special emphasis on members from your state.

Request that your local paper print an article you've written. Meet with the paper's editorial board to urge its support.

Meet with your representative and senators in their home district offices. Send a copy of your paper's editorial to every member of the full committee.

SENATE

Senator introduces bill. Clerk of the Senate refers it to appropriate committee.

Committee chair refers it to a sub-committee which holds hearings to examine arguments for or against the bill.

Subcommittee holds a 'mark-up' session to discuss and vote on the bill. A majority vote in favor moves the bill to full committee.

Full committee reviews subcommittee record and may hold additional hearings. A mark-up session is held and if the bill is approved it is reported to the full Senate.

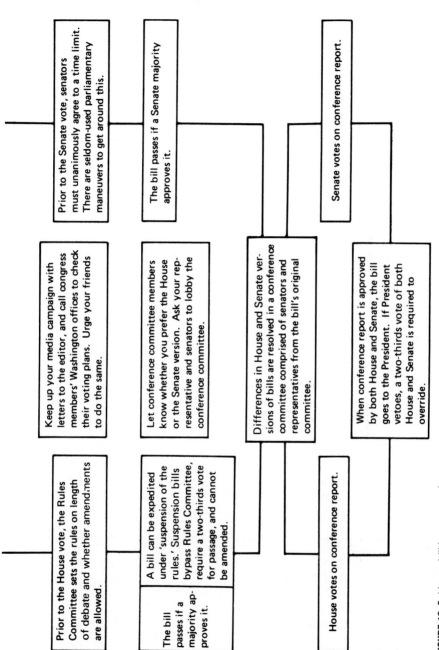

FIGURE 10-3 How a bill becomes a law.

Prior to the Senate vote, senators must unanimously agree to a time limit. There are seldom-used parliamentary maneuvers to get around this.

The bill passes if a Senate majority approves it.

Senate votes on conference report.

Keep up your media campaign with letters to the editor, and call congress members' Washington offices to check their voting plans. Urge your friends to do the same.

Let conference committee members know whether you prefer the House or the Senate version. Ask your representative and senators to lobby the conference committee.

Differences in House and Senate versions of bills are resolved in a conference committee comprised of senators and representatives from the bill's original committee.

When conference report is approved by both House and Senate, the bill goes to the President. If President vetoes, a two-thirds vote of both House and Senate is required to override.

Prior to the House vote, the Rules Committee sets the rules on length of debate and whether amendments are allowed.

A bill can be expedited under 'suspension of the rules.' Suspension bills bypass Rules Committee, require a two-thirds vote for passage, and cannot be amended.

The bill passes if a majority approves it.

House votes on conference report.

GROUP ACTION

The political process within the nursing profession takes many forms. On one level it is the involvement of nurses in legislative and ballot issues. Nurses can be involved as individuals, but they are far more effective when they work in groups. As the largest single health care occupation, nurses have many votes. This makes legislators pay attention to positions that are held by a group of nurses. In addition, although nurses do not have high incomes, when gathered together their financial contributions can be significant to a candidate or issue.

Nonlobbying Nursing Organizational Effort

Most traditional nursing organizations are nonprofit groups and therefore are limited in their political activity. The major role of these groups in politics is testifying as to facts and concerns within the health care area. The American Nurses Association (ANA) has an office in Washington, DC, and tries to keep the nursing profession informed about legislative matters of importance to health care. The ANA also provides experts in the nursing profession to testify about proposed legislation. The ANA recently organized the Nurses Strategic Action Team (N-STAT) to provide nurses with a means to mobilize quickly to influence legislative policy. This is aimed at grassroots involvement in legislative issues and includes meeting with members of Congress, writing letters, and making phone calls. It involves some 8000 nurses.

Other nursing organizations such as the National League for Nursing (NLN) and the Association of Colleges of Nursing also testify on pertinent issues before the federal government. The Tri-Council is a coalition of the ANA, the NLN, the American Association of Colleges of Nursing, and the National Organization of Nurse Executives that functions at the national level. This organization provides expert testimony for committees and commissions that are considering health-related legislation. By coordinating efforts, the member organizations are able to present a more united front and a stronger voice for nursing.

Most state and district nurses' associations have legislative committees that monitor legislative and regulatory actions in their area. They may provide educational events for nurses in regard to current issues and testify at hearings regarding health-related issues.

Political Action Committees

To take a more active role in seeking passage of desired legislation, defeat of undesired measures, and election of candidates, groups form organizations called political action committees, often referred to as PACs. These organizations are registered as political action groups and are free to try to affect the political process. However, they are not considered nonprofit organizations and donations to them are not tax deductible because they are used for political purposes.

The ANA Political Action Committee (ANA-PAC) is a political action organization formed by the ANA. ANA-PAC actually lobbies for the passage or defeat of bills and supports candidates for public office. Since the 1976 federal elections, ANA-PAC has raised funds to support candidates for the Senate and the House of Representatives based on their expressed and demonstrated stands on key health issues, such as health care reform proposals, funding for nursing and biomedical research, extension and funding of nursing education, and third-party reimbursement for nurses. Not all endorsed candidates were supported financially because of the limitations of the funds available. Candidates' successes are attributable to many factors, but the effect of nursing support has been demonstrated. Many state nursing associations also have political action organizations. These groups serve the same function on the state level as the ANA-PAC does on the national level. Many candidates actively seek the endorsement of nursing organizations because they perceive them as influential with voters.

The Nurses' Coalition for Legislative Action is an organization of 28 specialty nursing organizations that works to support the positions of its member organizations at the federal level. Nurses in specialty organizations have supported this organization as a way to bring a larger voice in support of issues that affect nursing specialty practice.

Although growth in size of these nursing political action groups has not been rapid, it has been steady. In addition, nurses are gaining more sophistication in the political process. Both of these factors result in nurses gaining increased power. There is still a long way to go before nurses have the same kind of power as that wielded by such groups as labor, education, and medicine, but change is occurring.

Other Politically Important Groups

In addition to these specific nursing-related groups, other organizations are concerned about health and social issues. Some are official lobbying groups and others provide information resources. These groups such as Common Cause (a consumer lobbying group), the League of Women Voters, and even church organizations often act to affect the political process. You may support these groups by simply donating money for their needs or by being actively involved in their work.

TESTIFYING FOR DECISION-MAKING BODIES

Many decisions relative to health care in general and to nursing are made by committees and commissions of the various levels of government. They

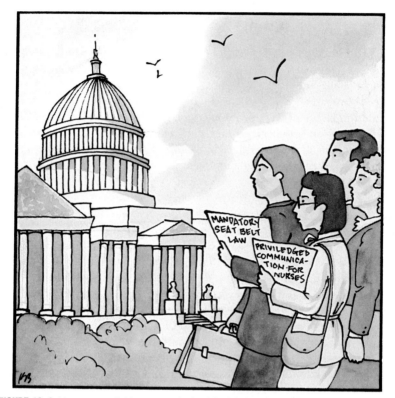

FIGURE 10–4 Nurses may lobby to get desired legislation passed by visiting legislators, by presenting information and arguments about the bill, and by writing letters.

frequently have hearings to gather information before decisions are made. As a nurse your testimony may have particular value when certain areas of health care are being considered. A nurse may testify as either an official representative of an organization or an independent individual.

You may learn of opportunities to testify through announcements in the newspaper or through professional publications. In general, you must register in advance to testify. In some instances, this may occur at the door before the meeting begins, but for more formal situations, you may have to notify the committee in advance that you wish to testify.

If you have an opportunity to testify, be sure to make your position clear so the decision-makers know whether you speak for yourself or for a larger group. Prepare your testimony ahead of time, but try not to just read a statement. A less formal presentation is usually more interesting for the listener. Be prepared with sources for any facts and figures you present and explain any technical terms you use. There may be a time limit for each testimony. Check on this before you begin and make sure that you present your most important arguments and facts first. Most committees will accept written testimony if you cannot be there in person, but the personal presentation is usually more effective.

INDIVIDUAL SUPPORT FOR LEGISLATION AND CANDIDATES

As an individual you may choose to support a specific piece of legislation by contributing money for publicity and campaigning or by personally working on a committee that is striving for passage of the proposal. Funds are needed for printing and distributing literature, newspaper ads, and television and radio announcements. Workers may be needed for secretarial tasks, to contact people in a door-to-door campaign, and to speak on behalf of the issue.

Supporting a candidate for public office is done in the same way. In our political system the reality is that those who have actively supported a candidate during an election campaign are listened to more closely when decisions are made. Working for a candidate is one way to make your view known. It is also an excellent way to gain first-hand knowledge of the political process.

HOLDING OFFICE

Whether you are involved with your local nursing organization or the U.S. Congress, those who have been elected or appointed to office have considerable power to affect outcomes. Leaders in nursing organizations help to shape the direction and efforts of those organizations. As members of the state legislature, nurses have been effective in shaping health policy in their respective states. Eddie Bernice Johnson, elected as a Congresswoman from Texas in 1994, was the first nurse to hold an elective federal office. Nurses have been appointed to major administrative positions in state and federal health agencies and the staffs of several senators and representatives. Nurses have a promising future in the health policy arena.

LIMITATIONS ON YOUR POLITICAL ACTIVITY

If you are an employee of any governmental agency, such as a public health department or the Veterans Administration, there are restrictions on your political activity that do not apply to the general public. For the federal government, these restrictions are defined in the Hatch Act. The main focus of prohibited activities are those that have to do with supporting a particular political party by being an officer or party spokesperson. The Hatch Act also prohibits any activities on behalf of a party or in support of legislation that could be construed as providing support from the agency that employs you.

This act does not interfere with your rights as a private citizen to support parties and candidates financially, to join political parties, to work for or against measures that will appear on a ballot, or to participate in nonpartisan (ie, not connected with a political party) elections as a candidate. Each state has its own version of the Hatch Act. If you are employed by a governmental agency of any kind, you should investigate the limitations that it may place on your political activity.

The Federal Government's Role in Health Care

Federal legislation has critically affected nursing and health care. If you understand key concepts regarding the way in which the federal government is already involved in health care and how federal legislation has affected health care delivery, you will be more effective in the political arena.

FEDERAL AGENCIES RELATED TO HEALTH CARE

The federal government operates in the health care field in complex ways, as mentioned in Chapter 8. Literally dozens of federal agencies relate to health in some way. The following overview may help you to place some agencies in context.

The Department of Health and Human Services (DHHS) is a cabinet-level administrative unit of the federal government. It was originally created in 1953 as the Department of Health, Education, and Welfare. The date of its origin points out how recent has been the view that the federal government should have a major responsibility toward health care or that health should have status equal to defense at the federal executive level. In 1980, a separate department was created for education and the remaining functions were retitled the Department of Health and Human Services. There are four major service divisions of DHHS (Table 10–1).

The Office of Human Development Services is responsible for four sections. The activities of these sections are primarily in the health prevention and welfare field.

The Public Health Service (which contains the Centers for Disease Control and Prevention and the National Institutes of Health [NIH]), the Food and Drug Administration, the Health Resources Administration, and the Health Care Financing Administration (which administers Social Security, Medicare, and Medicaid) are all part of the DHHS. The Public Health Service has also historically operated hospitals for merchant seamen and the Coast Guard. These facilities are also available to veterans and certain government employees. Many of these public health hospitals have been closed in recent years and care transferred to community resources.

Within the Department of the Interior, the Bureau of Indian Affairs has operated hospitals and clinics on Indian reservations. Within the Defense De-

TABLE 10–1 Major Service Divisions of the Department of Health and Human Services

Office of Human Development Services	Social Security Administration
Administration on Aging	Systems
Administration for Child, Youth, and Families	Governmental Affairs
	Family Assistance
Administration for Native Americans	Hearings and Appeals
Administration for Public Service	Operational Policy and Procedure Assessment

Public Health Service	Health Care Financing
Centers for Disease Control and Prevention	Health Standards and Quality Bureau
Food and Drug Administration	Bureau of Quality Control
Health Resources Administration	Bureau of Program Operations
Health Services Administration	Bureau of Program Policy
National Institutes of Health	Bureau of Support Services
Alcohol, Drug Abuse, and Mental Health Administration	Office of Child Support Enforcement

partment, the military branches operate hospitals and clinics for service members and their families and also has an extensive program for financing health care by civilian health providers through a program known as CHAMPUS. The Department of Veteran's Affairs operates many hospitals and nursing homes for veterans.

When all of these programs and agencies are considered together, it is clear that the federal government is a major force in health care. Some individuals express concern about changes in our health care system that they see as indicating governmental involvement. For good or ill, the federal government already controls many aspects of health care.

THE FEDERAL BUDGET PROCESS

Because funding is a driving force in all decision-making, you will find it useful to understand something of the federal budget process. The money actually available from the government for each federal program depends on two separate legislative actions. The first action is the authorization act. This is a bill, passed by both the House of Representatives (where any revenue bill must originate) and the Senate, that describes the program and outlines the rules under which funds can be expended. It also sets a ceiling on the amount of money that can be provided. It is under these acts (often referred to by the "title" of the section of the authorizing act) that funds are dispensed for all the health-related activities described in this chapter.

The second necessary legislative action is the appropriations act. In the appropriations process the federal budget is established and specific amounts of money are appropriated for actual spending for each program previously authorized. Both the House and the Senate pass a budget appropriations act. Then a joint House and Senate committee meets to achieve a compromise that both will accept. The final result is entitled the "Omnibus Budget Reconciliation Act" (OBRA), which includes the compromises the budget committee has worked out between the House and Senate versions of the budget. The amount appropriated for any program cannot be more than the amount originally authorized, but it can be, and frequently is, less. Sometimes this is confusing because two monetary amounts may be reported in regard to the same act, the authorized amount and the budgeted (or appropriated) amount.

The budget act may also contain requirements or controls on those people and organizations who receive federal support. It is under this authority that the federal government sets standards for nursing homes that receive reimbursement through Medicaid and Medicare. The rules and regulations for nursing homes included in OBRA '87, the budget reconciliation act for 1987, were very extensive. These rules and regulations took effect on October 1, 1990. This allowed the affected organizations to begin the process of change to meet the new requirements.

Historically, a third factor has affected the amount of money available for a specific federal program. The executive branch makes decisions about how and when available funds will be spent. If money that has been authorized and appropriated has not been spent by the end of the budget period, it is lost. The funds must then be reauthorized and reappropriated. The executive branch has used this mechanism to withdraw support for programs it opposed.

FEDERAL SUPPORT FOR NURSING EDUCATION

The Nurse Training Act of 1964 (Title VII of the Public Health Service Act) was a significant factor in the growth of nursing education. It provided for financial assistance to schools of nursing and to students in those schools for 2 years and was renewed in 1966 for 2 additional years. In 1968, financial assistance to schools and students was continued under Title II of the Health Manpower Act. In 1971, federal aid to nursing education was again expanded. Monies for constructing schools of nursing and for aiding the educational program were provided. Many of you have been educated in buildings or practice laboratories whose construction was funded under this act. Individual financial aid to students was also provided. A large number of your instructors may have had their graduate education made possible by this funding.

Although nurses think that the funds were well used in a responsible manner, continued funding was not automatic. In 1973 and 1974, the Nixon administration made a concerted effort to curtail money spent on nursing education as well as on other health-related endeavors. Later both the Ford and the Carter administrations proposed drastic cuts in money allocated to nursing education. Nursing organizations fought long and hard through testimony and through providing public information to achieve passage of new Nurse Training Act legislation. This was finally accomplished, although there were many compromises over what nurses had originally wanted to see passed.

A different version of the Nurse Training Act was passed in 1979 as Public Law 96-97 and was referred to as the Nurse Education Act. In addition to support for nursing students, nursing schools, and nursing research, this bill provided for an independent study of nursing personnel needs. However, the total amount of money appropriated was less than previous acts had provided.

Funds currently appropriated through the Nurse Education Act are limited. They primarily support education for advanced nursing practice and graduate degrees. Every 2 years at the time the biennial budget is passed, nurses have supported legislation to reinstitute the Nurse Education Act. Although there has been consistent support from some legislators, funds available have been limited.

The budget proposed by President Clinton for Fiscal Year (FY) 1995 consolidates approximately 30 programs related to the health care workforce and are scheduled to be introduced in legislative form. This change would also result in categorizing health professions programs into five grant programs: primary care, minority and disadvantaged assistance, consolidated loans, priority nursing, and health professions research and data. Priority nursing would set aside $38 million for nurse anesthetists, nurse special projects, professional nurse traineeships, and advanced nurse education. The nursing community is supporting the expansion of graduate nursing education, advanced nursing practitioner education, nurse anesthetist education, nursing student loans, and special programs to forgive loans for those working in underserved areas.

MEDICARE AND MEDICAID

In 1965, after years of effort and testimony by many health-related groups, (including the ANA) and with widespread public support, an amendment of the Social Security Act was passed. Title XVIII of the act, which was termed *Medicare*, provided payment for hospitalization and insurance that could be purchased for meeting physicians' fees for people over age 65. Title IX of the act, which was termed *Medicaid*, provided funds for health care for the dependent population. Medicaid is administered by the states, which determine eligibility and level of coverage.

Medicare and Medicaid have supplied an important health care resource but have not been without problems. Costs have been much larger and have risen faster than anticipated. There has been a great deal of publicity over instances of abuse and even fraud that have occurred in connection with these two programs. The goals of providing cost-effective, adequate health care for elders and the indigent through these programs has yet to be achieved.

In 1982, Medicare was revised by the 97th Congress to address the problem of rapidly escalating costs. The premium for Part B of Medicare (the optional portion that provides for out-of-hospital and physician care) and the deductible that the individual had to pay for covered service were increased. The system of payment was changed to prospective payment based on diagnosis-related groups. Many items that were previously funded separately were now included in the one prospective rate. A mechanism for reimbursing hospice care was included.

There was still separate support for medical education and nursing education programs that were under the control of the hospital in which they occurred. This was meant to compensate for additional costs related to the teaching responsibilities of and the services rendered by those in such programs. Although the largest share of this fund was for residency programs for physicians, significant support was available for hospital-based nursing programs. This funding source for nursing education programs in hospitals is now in jeopardy as increased efforts are being made to cut Medicare costs even further.

EVALUATION OF HEALTH SERVICES: PEER REVIEW AND QUALITY ASSURANCE

The first provision for the systematic evaluation of health care services provided to the consumer was established through the Professional Standards Review Organization and utilization review set up by Medicare and Medicaid. As part of the 1982 revisions of Medicare, the evaluation process was altered to require that hospitals contract with an external medical review organization, called a Utilization and Quality Control Peer Review Organization (abbreviated PRO). These organizations have been established through contracts awarded by the Secretary of Health and Human Services through competitive bidding. Most of the PROs are statewide in scope and are required to have a substantial number of physicians represented in the organization to effectively set standards and review care.

Evaluation may include preadmission, preprocedure, concurrent, or retrospective reviews. The purpose of the reviews is to determine whether the care given was necessary and whether it was given in the appropriate manner. For example, the reviews have resulted in an increase in the number of

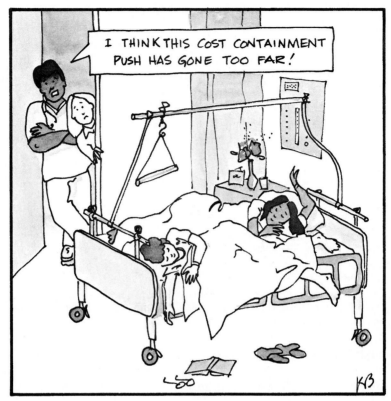

FIGURE 10–5 Federal legislation is encouraging hospitals to stop the rapid rise of health care costs.

surgeries performed as day procedures on outpatients rather than as inpatient surgeries. This results in a significant economic saving. The PRO is also required to evaluate outcomes of care to ensure that the changes made do not jeopardize clients.

OCCUPATIONAL SAFETY AND HEALTH

There has been a great deal of controversy over the provisions of Occupational Safety and Health Act (OSHA), which is designed to improve the safety of the working environment. The act provides a mechanism for establishing safety standards for all occupational settings. OSHA regulations have been used to mandate that hospitals place "sharps" containers to safeguard employees from inadvertent needle sticks in all areas where needles are used, that hepatitis B immunization be provided to those who are at risk based on the work setting, and that supplies necessary to protect oneself from blood-borne pathogens be readily available.

Many people think that the rules and regulations created by this act are too extensive and cumbersome. For example, the rules regarding ladder safety are extremely detailed and cover several pages. When one considers the enormous number of different pieces of equipment and envisions the quantity of regulations that exist to cover all these items, it is apparent that it would be almost impossible for any one person to know all the applicable regulations.

Nevertheless, the concern for the safety of the working person is of real importance to nurses. Occupational injuries are a major health problem in the adult population. They are costly not only in terms of health and personal loss but also in terms of lost productivity. Nurses are affected by the provisions of this act in their work environments. They, too, are subject to injury and accident on the job. Concerns related to safety for nurses in the workplace are discussed in Chapter 11.

Nurses in occupational health nursing are involved in another way. They may be part of the program for educating workers about job safety. In some situations safety precautions are time consuming and uncomfortable, and workers may be tempted to ignore them. Nurses may be able to help workers understand the importance of following health and safety regulations. Occupational health nurses also work with management in planning to make the environment safe and in establishing appropriate procedures in caring for injuries.

NURSING HOME REGULATIONS

OBRA '87 was briefly mentioned in the discussion of the federal budget process. This legislation contained regulations that for the first time mandated a national standard for quality of care in long-term care facilities.

Included in this legislation was the mandate for an admission assessment for every individual admitted to long-term care. As part of this admission assessment, the collection of a minimum data set (MDS) to facilitate research in long-term care was required. Based on critical data, resident assessment protocols (RAPs) and plans of care must be established. There were also regulations to limit the use of both chemical and physical restraints and to require programs to maintain individuals at their highest level of functioning. Training for nursing assistants was mandated, and the requirements for supervision by licensed nurses were increased. Although the provisions of this act were set to take effect in October 1990, there was delay based on legal challenges to the requirements and the time needed to establish monitoring mechanisms. Therefore, some of the provisions of OBRA '87 took effect as late as 1994.

FAMILY HEALTH CONCERNS

The Maternal-Child Health Act, Title V, was planned to improve health in the nation through benefits such as nutritional support, health supervision and well child care to mothers and children. Part of the money appropriated was earmarked for nursing research projects and nursing research training. Nurses who provide care are directly affected in their practice because the provisions of the act outline what care is funded and to whom that care can be provided. Since its inception, the Maternal-Child Health Act has never been fully funded. This means that even those who are eligible for services under the provisions of the act may not receive them because of budget limitations.

The Americans with Disabilities Act of 1990 brought to fruition an effort that had begun 20 years earlier to guarantee that those with disabilities were ensured of equal access and opportunity. A disability is defined in the act as "a physical or mental impairment that substantially limits activities of daily living" (Watson, 1990, p 325). In 1973 the Rehabilitation Act began the effort by providing the disabled with physical and vocational access to organizations and institutions that received federal funds. The Americans with Disabilities Act moves beyond that basic support and provides the same rights to those with physical disabilities as had been provided to women and minorities under the 1964 Civil Rights legislation. The law requires accessible workplaces, nondiscriminatory practices, and access to public services, such as transportation and telephone, and provides legal avenues for redress when these provisions are not carried out. Nurses are key individuals in educating the disabled about their rights under the law and acting as advocates in the community (Watson, 1990).

The Women's Health Equity Act, which was first introduced in 1990, addressed the unmet health needs of the women of the United States. Although women make up 52% of the population, only 13% of the research dollars of the NIH are directed toward women's health issues (Sharp, 1990). For example, although heart disease is the major cause of death in women, no women were included in any of the major heart disease studies. This bill brought together concerns for adequate research into breast cancer, women's infertility and contraceptive needs, and the inclusion of women as subjects in other research studies (Sharp, 1990). Although the bill did not pass in 1990, the stage was set for changes in health care funding and research priorities that have occurred since that time. Nursing groups, particularly ANA, continue to ask Congress to remedy injustices related to disproportionate health care for women including lack of comprehensive benefits, limited access to health insurance, barriers to health care services, limitations on health care providers, gaps in knowledge in women's health research, and an overall male bias in treatment from the health care system (ANA testifies, March 16, 1994).

The Family and Medical Leave Act of 1993 provided a mandate for unpaid leave for those who wish to take time off without pay to care for an ill family member (Wimberly, 1993). There was opposition from those who believe that this will place an unfair burden on businesses. However, family leave is well established in European countries. There, leave with pay is available in some instances.

State-Level Legislative Concerns

Many issues that vitally affect the health care area are decided at the state level. Because issues in each state differ, only some general areas of concern are outlined here.

STATE AGENCIES AND HEALTH CARE

Types of state institutions range from those for the care of the mentally retarded and the mentally ill to penal systems and institutions of higher education. Health care is often a consideration in all of these settings. When budgets are planned, such diverse concerns as immunization and contraception may be part of the debate. Nurses often can advocate for those who are unable to speak for themselves in regard to their own health care needs. Sometimes nurses who work in these settings are unable to deliver quality care because of severe budgetary deficiencies. All nurses can support efforts to provide quality health care in such settings.

NURSE PRACTICE ACTS

Nurse practice acts are being discussed and revised in many states. The process is long and difficult and requires intense effort on the part of nurses. Once a bill that has been carefully developed has been submitted to the legislative body, nurses must remain alert to changes and amendments that may substantially alter the intent of the original proposal. The bill must be followed through the legislative process until its passage. One current concern related to opening nurse practice acts is the pressure to lessen the standards or allow unlicensed assistive personnel to perform more nursing tasks.

Local Political Concerns

The budgetary process always seems to be at the base of any political or legislative concern. Because only a limited amount of money is available, budgets are always developed with a series of compromises. To gain one objective it is sometimes necessary to recognize that there will be no funds for another. In most communities budgets for public health departments, school nurses, and so forth are developed over a period of several months. Hearings are often held, at which members of the public may ask questions and address the issues. Nurses have often found that involvement at this planning stage is most rewarding. Determining priorities for health is essential, and nurses often can speak with authority on these matters. Nurses actually employed in the department under consideration may be much more limited in making their views known because of regulations governing their action in the political sphere. For this reason it is significant that other nurses recognize the importance of community health. It is not only the practice of the public health nurse that is affected by the priorities of the agency. For example, the nurse who is employed in the hospital may wish to refer a discharged patient to a public health nurse for follow-up, only to find that, owing to changes in the ordering of priorities, home visits for the identified purpose are no longer being made.

In many communities decisions about the allocation of federal money are made at the local level. Support for alternative health care centers, blood pressure screening, and senior citizen centers may depend on whether those who are knowledgeable about the benefits of these services are willing to voice their advocacy.

Health Care Reform

The United States is the only major industrialized country other than South Africa that does not provide some type of government-sponsored health care for all citizens. Through Medicare, Medicaid, and the widespread effects of the military, public health, and Indian health systems, the federal government is already deeply involved in the provision of health care. How much greater that involvement should be is the subject of serious debate.

Some questions being raised are:

- Is there a right to health care?
- If there is a right, what level of health care does this cover—routine preventive services, surgery and hospitalization for all conditions or only for serious life-threatening conditions?
- Should catastrophic illnesses, transplantation, and experimental treatments be included?
- What about fertility-enhancing services? Should abortion services be available?
- How can health care in the United States be transformed into an effective, coordinated system?
- How would a changed health care system be financed?

These are difficult philosophical and ethical questions, and there are no simple answers.

FACTORS CREATING SUPPORT
FOR HEALTH CARE REFORM

Public opinion appears to be moving toward support of some type of nationwide health care reform. People are looking at health care as a right rather than as a privilege available only to those who can afford it. Costs of hospital and medical care have risen much more rapidly than the general rate of inflation. Part of this rise is caused by advances in treatment that require expensive equipment, laboratory work, and intensive care. However, criticism has been leveled at the profits being made in health-related corporations. Another area of criticism is the demand of individuals for unnecessary procedures and care.

One factor that is creating more support for some type of statewide or national health plan is the increasing amount of uncompensated care being provided by some of the nation's health care facilities. When people are unemployed or underemployed, they often do not have health insurance. These same people are often not eligible for public assistance for health care. They then do not receive preventive health care or prompt attention to health problems when they arise. When they have major health care needs they seek care in emergency rooms, one of the most costly areas supplying health care. Regulations require that emergency rooms provide care to those with critical problems; therefore, individuals are treated and may be admitted for surgery and major care. Costs may mount and bills simply remain unpaid. Hospitals historically have absorbed these costs through spreading them out to those who do pay their bills. As insurance companies and the government become more stringent about reimbursement, this is becoming increasingly difficult and some hospitals will be in serious financial trouble if some method of assisting with this problem is not found soon.

Another factor creating pressure is the number of working individuals whose employers do not provide health insurance coverage. In the past many of these individuals purchased private health insurance. This is becoming prohibitively expensive, leaving many people without coverage. Many express concern that they are gambling with their families' future, but do not see that they have a choice.

The number of people with chronic illnesses continues to grow as the population ages and those with chronic illness live longer lives. Many of these individuals find themselves completely excluded from health insurance coverage because of their "preexisting condition." These people are speaking out for the need for a system that will include them. Even those with chronic illness who now have coverage know they can never change their jobs because their coverage is only possible based on having had insurance before the condition manifested itself.

Businesses have noted the growing costs of health care that have escalated their health insurance premiums for employees. In an effort to curb
costs, businesses have instituted a variety of programs. However, many are becoming concerned that without changes in the system they will be unable to
keep up with these costs.

NURSING'S AGENDA FOR HEALTH CARE REFORM

The ANA, the NLN, and almost 60 other nursing organizations are cooperat-
ing in presenting Nursing's Agenda for Health Care Reform (American
Nurses Association, 1991) to legislators, health care agencies, and the public.
The decision was made to present a framework for health care reform when
research revealed that nurses hold a unique position of trust in the minds of
the public. In the Hart survey conducted for the NLN, 77% of those polled
believed that nurses took a constructive role in health care and were not
solely concerned with their own self-interest. This contrasted to 42% who believed that doctors had a constructive role, 19% who believed the federal government had a constructive role, and 11% who thought insurance companies
took a constructive role (National League for Nursing, 1991).

Nursing's agenda is based on a belief that any system must include quality health care, must have access for all citizens, and must be cost effective.
One aspect of this is a federally defined standard package of essential health
care benefits. This would include primary care and prevention and would be financed by a mix of public and private sources. Access has to do with geographical, economic, and cultural factors. Nursing suggests improving access
to health care by delivering it in schools, workplaces, and the home; controlling costs through managed care; and implementing the plan in steps.

One key concern of nurses is that nursing care needs to be directly reimbursed. This has been of special concern to primary health care nurses. The
availability of funding for the care to be provided by nurses will, to a great extent, determine whether the public is able to use such services. Physicians
(through the American Medical Association) have consistently supported
provisions that would result in direct payment only to physicians or for care
ordered by physicians. Other organizations of direct care providers, social
workers, nurses, psychologists, and so forth are seeking greater breadth in reimbursement. Third-party payment funds a large percentage of the health care
in the United States; if this avenue of funding is closed to nurses and other direct care providers, then their ability to provide services is severely curtailed.
Physicians believe that controlling access to third-party payment will control
costs of health care. This limitation also preserves for the physician a unique
position of power in the health care setting.

MAJOR FEDERAL HEALTH CARE REFORM PROPOSALS

Several health care reform proposals are before Congress at this time. Each of these has somewhat different characteristics. Any legislation passed is likely to be a compromise among all of the powerful players in the health care reform drama. Here we will present some of the major areas that you should examine and compare as each proposal is developed and promoted.

Determining Who Is Covered

Some plans are based on universal coverage for everyone in one system. Other systems would retain separate plans for Social Security, Medicaid, and those who chose independent coverage. Nursing has supported plans that would eventually cover all individuals although there is recognition that a gradual process of including people in the system may be essential to economic stability.

Benefits Included

What benefits will be included in any health care package will require considerable compromise. Some items, such as well child care and maternal-infant care are so well supported with research as to their cost effectiveness and so appealing to the public that they are included in everyone's planning. Services such as treatment for infertility and abortion are much more controversial and problematic. There are differences regarding the inclusion of high-cost services such as bone marrow and organ transplantation. You will want to compare any plans on the basis of the standard benefits included.

Sources of Financing

Whether the source of funds for those not currently covered in any plan should be general tax revenues, special taxes on such things as cigarettes and alcohol, changes in Social Security rules, or other governmental sources is a major area of controversy. Some proposals would mandate that all employers provide insurance to decrease the numbers of uninsured that would need to be covered by any governmental plan. One proposal has been to cover those without health care insurance by increasing the premiums or costs to all others to cover these costs. Savings from changes in the system are targeted as one source of funding. Comparing the proposals for sources of funding is important in understanding the individual plan. Another consideration is whether the proposed funding mechanism will actually generate enough funds to support the benefits included.

Mechanism for Managing Financing

The most universal and easy to understand proposal would mandate a single-payer system managed by the federal government. In such a system insurance companies would no longer operate as we know them now. A complex pattern of managed competition is found in some proposals. In this plan, insurers and health care providers would form large associations termed health care alliances that would bid to provide the mandated benefits for individuals. The competition of these alliances is expected to provide for cost reductions. In some of the plans, the financing system would basically remain the same with those not currently covered being insured through special pools with premiums paid by the government. Others suggest that each state be free to determine the system they would like for managing finances.

The Role of the States in National Health Reform

The role of the states in any national health care reform is another area of difference. Most of the plans place responsibility on the states for some aspects of managing the system. This may focus on evaluating services and the actions of care providers or may include extensive determination of benefits and providers.

MALPRACTICE REFORM

All of the plans address concerns regarding malpractice suits and the cost to the system of litigation. Most include some type of dispute mechanism other than a court proceeding. Plans differ on the presence of caps on awards, limits on attorney's fees, the approach to punitive damages, and the statute of limitations.

STATE INITIATIVES IN HEALTH CARE REFORM

Because the federal government has not acted at the time of this writing, many states are studying the problem from a state perspective. Each state that has approached the problem has found a somewhat different solution.

Hawaii has the oldest universal health care plan in the United States. Perhaps because it is less populated and is geographically small, its citizens were able to build a consensus regarding a coordinated health system for the state. Some individuals are covered through employers. For those without this coverage, health care coverage is available through a state system. One of the difficulties Hawaii has experienced is in distribution of health providers to smaller communities throughout the islands.

Oregon has drawn attention for its attempt to differentiate those services that should be included in a governmentally financed plan from those that will not be publicly supported. Based on hearings held throughout the state, the Oregon Commission developed a prioritized list of services. When the funding was identified, starting at the top of the list, items were designated to be included. When the funds would be exhausted, then items below that level were omitted from coverage. Prioritization was based on the importance of the service to saving life, the number of people served, and whether treatment would significantly alter health outcomes. This rationing of services is defended based on the rationale that without it, some individuals would have every possible service, whereas others would have no services at all. Oregon requested and received a waiver from Medicaid that has allowed them to include in the state plan any individual who does not have private insurance available. Previously, those not eligible for public assistance could not be provided any coverage through federal sources. Thus all Oregonians will have the basic benefit package. Those with private health care plans may still purchase and receive greater benefits. A unique and compelling feature of the Oregon plan has been the consumer involvement in its development.

Washington State passed a health care reform measure. This measure provided for a state-managed plan for the uninsured and mandated employer coverage for employers larger than a specific size. Unfortunately some high-risk groups such as migrant farm workers were originally excluded from the plan. The state plan requires that individuals in the state plan be part of managed care systems where a primary care provider takes responsibility for providing preventive health care services as well as treatment for illness and injury.

Other states are in the process of developing health care reform plans at this time. Many state legislators have decided that it is better for states to move ahead independently than it is to wait to find out what the Congress will do.

The Political Process Within the Nursing Profession

Any large group of people organized into a body has a political process. All of the earlier discussion about the traditional political process is equally applicable to the politics of the profession.

On an individual level, one is seldom able to influence such an organization meaningfully unless one is a member. This may create some conflict within the individual. If you do not agree with all that an organization is doing, the usual course of action is to withhold or withdraw your membership. When you are member of a profession, you may find that this course of action presents more difficulties. The organization may continue to speak for the profession. If you are outside of the organization, you may find yourself without a voice on significant issues affecting your professional life. By joining a professional organization and actively involving yourself in it, you may be able to make your concerns and viewpoints heard.

If you decide to join a professional organization, you have an obligation to be an informed and concerned member. Your vote on candidates for local, state, and national office is important. Your activity on a committee or as an officer is necessary for the organization to function effectively. You have an obligation to be informed on issues that are before the organization and make your viewpoint known. The concerned involvement of many individual members will make an organization an effective voice for a profession. Chapter 12 describes many organizations related to nursing.

Key Concepts

⇨ Because scarce resources are allocated through the political process, nurses will find understanding this process essential to influence the health care system.

⇨ Every individual has many opportunities to affect the political process. This may be done simply through keeping informed, through voting, or trying to shape public opinion. Communicating with legislators and officials can be done as an individual or as part of a group. Testifying presents issues of importance and individual support may be given to those running for office. You may even decide to run for public office.

⇨ The federal government is active in health care through many existing agencies, both those within the Department of Health and Human Services and through other branches of government as well. The federal budget process affects the services that are available through the many legislative acts affecting health care.

⇨ Many factors are coming together in support of health care reform. Nursing organizations are supporting efforts to reform health care that provide for access, quality, and cost control. Within the major reform proposals are different approaches to funding, managing reimbursement, determining who is covered, what benefits should include, malpractice reform, and the role of the states.

⇨ The political process is part of any large organization and nursing organizations are no exception. Understanding the political process will help you to be a more effective participant in a large organization.

CRITICAL THINKING ACTIVITIES

1. Identify a political issue about which you feel strongly. Write a letter to a governmental official that provides sound rationale in support of your position.
2. Identify an aspect of health care reform that concerns you. Analyze the various proposals currently before Congress in regard to that specific aspect. Rank the proposals in order of your preference, providing rationale for your decision-making.
3. In a small group, divide the various proposals for health care reform among all the participants. Hold a discussion in which you analyze the proposals.
4. Identify a current health care issue in your state or province. Investigate that issue and form a position supported with data.
5. Contact your state nurses' association and find out if your state has a political action organization. If it does, contact that organization and ask what the current issues are in the state. Investigate those issues.

References

American Nurses Association. Nursing's Agenda for Health Care Reform. Washington, DC: American Nurses Publishing Co., 1991

ANA testifies on women's health issues. Capital Update 12(5):5, March 16, 1994

Donahue MP. Nursing: The Finest Art. St. Louis, CV Mosby, 1985

Division of Nursing, Funding and Application Data for Grant Programs Administered by the Division of Nursing. 1964–1990

FY '85 health appropriations. Testimony of the American Nurses Association to the Labor, Health, and Human Services Subcommittee of the House Appropriations Committee. Publication No. 34-323. Washington, DC: U.S. Government Printing Office, 1985

Kalisch BJ, Kalisch PA. The Politics of Nursing. Philadelphia: JB Lippincott, 1982

National League for Nursing: Nursing introduces its national health strategy to the public. Public Policy Bulletin, March 1991. New York: National League for Nursing, 1991

Nurses' Coalition for Legislative Action. Correspondence. 1985

Sharp N. Women's Health Equity Act of 1990. Nurs Manage 21(12):21–22, 1990

Solomon S. Update: Nursing education funds, NIN, DRGs and education. Nurs Health Care 5(6): 302–303, 1984

Watson PG. The Americans with Disabilities Act: More rights for people with disabilities. Rehabil Nurs 15(6):325–328, 1990

Wimberly JW Jr. The family medical leave act of 1993. AAOHN J 41(11):551–557, 1993

Woodham-Smith C. Florence Nightingale. New York: Atheneum, 1983 (reprint of 1951 edition)

Further Readings

The American Nurse. Kansas City, MO: American Nurses' Association, monthly newspaper

ANA, AORN testify at OSHA hearing on employee regs. OR Manager 5(11):1, 4, 1990

Capitol Commentary. A monthly publication regarding federal health actions and activities published by the ANA.

Cassetta RA. ANA governmental affairs: Working for you in Washington. Am Nurse 26(4):16, 1994

Cassetta RA. RNs fight for recognition of women's health issues. Am Nurse 26(2):1, 16, 1994

Chinn P. Looking into the crystal ball: Positioning ourselves for the year 2000. Nurs Outlook 39: 251–256, 1991

deVries C, Vanderbilt M. The Grassroots Lobbying Handbook: Empowering Nurses Through Legislative and Political Action. Washington, DC: American Nurses Publishing Co., 1991

deVries C, Vanderbilt M. Key players on bill hear ANA input on reform. Am Nurse 26(4):1, 20, 1994

Elon R, Pawlson LG. The impact of OBRA on medical practice within nursing facilities. J Am Geriatr Soc 40(9):958–968, 1992

Fedor MA. AIDS: Advocacy and activism. Nurs Health Care 12(3):119, 1991

Fry ST. Ethical implications of health care reform. Am Nurse 26(3):5, 1994

Griffith HM. Needed–A strong nursing position on preventive service. Image 25(4):272–284, 1993

Headline News. American Journal of Nursing, 94(1):83, 88, 1994

Health care reform proposals compared. Nurs Health Care 14(9): 455–457, 1993

Ketter J. ANA, Dept of Labor discuss workplace issues. Am Nurse 26(6):1, 3, 1994

Nornhold P. 90 predictions for the 90s. Nursing 20(1):34–41, 1990

Scott K. RN career security is ANA goal for reform. Am Nurse 25(9):1, 6, 1993

Sharp N, Biggs S, Wakefield M. Public policy: New opportunities for nurses. Nurs Health Care 12(1):16–23, 1991

Simpson M, Hanley B. Nurse policy analyst: Advanced practice role. Nurs Health Care 12(1): 10–15, 1991

Stark PL. Health care under siege: Challenge for change. Nurs Health Care 12(1):26–31, 1991

Watts RJ. Democratization of health care: Challenge for nursing. Adv Nurs Sci 12(2):37–46, 1990

See also the official publication of your state nurses' association.

IV | Career Opportunities and Professional Growth

In this unit we present basic information about the employment world you will find in nursing. This will help you as you move from the student role to the role of the registered nurse employed within the health care delivery system. Chapter 11 looks at your personal relationship with this new role; Chapter 12 is designed to help you understand the organization itself. In Chapter 13, we present the variety of nursing organizations that may help you in your personal growth in nursing. These organizations will also provide you with opportunities to affect the nursing profession and make a personal contribution to nursing.

11

Beginning Your Career as a Nurse

Objectives

After completing this chapter, you should be able to

1. Discuss the historical development of employment roles for nurses.
2. Describe a variety of employment opportunities available to nurses today.
3. Explain the common competencies needed by the new graduate as outlined by the job analysis study.
4. Analyze the eight common expectations employers have of new graduates and relate them to your own background and education.
5. Develop a list of your personal short- and long-term career goals.
6. Describe how you plan to maintain your competence in nursing.
7. Create a personal resumé; sample letters of application, follow-up, and resignation; and a plan for your personal responses in an employment interview that can be used when you seek employment.
8. Explore strategies that you might personally use to prevent or alleviate reality shock.
9. Analyze your own values and life situation in relationship to your personal potential for burnout.
10. Discuss two areas of concern relative to sex discrimination in nursing.
11. Identify ways that you can act to protect the health of both yourself and others in the nursing workplace.

After completing an educational program, you, as a new graduate, will want to get out into the real world and practice your nursing skills. In the past such a goal was rather simple and straightforward, but a nursing career is now much more complex.

Historical Employment Opportunities in Nursing

Early in the 20th century almost all graduate nurses performed private-duty nursing. The nurse was hired by a patient or family to provide care during a particular episode of illness or disability. Some nurses specialized in maternity cases, in which they cared for new mothers and infants; others specialized in caring for persons with long-term illnesses, such as strokes. The nurse was expected to live at the patient's residence and assume 24-hour responsibility for the patient's care. This might even include preparing special foods for the convalescing patient and the family. Nurses hired as graduate nurses in hospitals usually were head nurses, supervisors, or directors. Patient care was usually provided by students (see Chapter 2).

By the 1930s the employment situation began to change. More graduate nurses were hired to provide patient care. Employment practices became modernized, and nurses were no longer expected to be on duty 24 hours a day when engaged in private-duty nursing. Most nurses were employed in a hospital or an institution. Regular work schedules were established in hospitals. Nurses still worked split shifts—morning and evening of the same day with several hours "off duty" in the afternoon. There were few employee benefits (paid holidays, vacations, insurance, and retirement plans), but the beginnings of change were there.

World War II had a major impact on nursing. Because women were essential to the war effort, it became acceptable for married women to continue working. Women nurses were valued members of the armed forces and attained elevated status by becoming officers in the military. These nurses had to learn to be assertive in managing their responsibilities, and many brought this quality back to the hospital. Wanting to be of service to a country at war, women who might never have considered nursing because of its previous status now entered the profession.

The expansion of the hospital or institutional job market for nurses was also influenced by population growth. Advances in medicine, which included more surgery being performed, resulted in special care that was available only in a hospital. The number of hospitals increased dramatically.

The noninstitutional job market also grew. Since the early 1900s, when Lillian Wald established a visiting nurse service, community health nursing has continued to develop. Nurses were pioneers in bringing health care to people's homes and in focusing on prevention of illness through consumer education.

Other areas of nursing in the community began to widen as well. More nurses were working in industry. Conditions for workers improved, and action regarding their health became part of law, custom, or contract. Nurses also worked in school districts, and the school nursing specialty started to expand.

Nurses began to provide primary health care. Primary care is that segment of health care that furnishes both the initial contact with the health care system and the longitudinal supervision of health care needs. Perhaps the first primary health care by nurses was provided by the midwives of the Frontier Nursing Service in Kentucky in the 1920s. These midwives assumed overall responsibility for the care of child-bearing women during pregnancy, delivery, and the postpartum period.

Another early group that expanded practice were the nurse anesthetists who organized the Association of Registered Nurse Anesthetists in 1931 and assumed responsibility for accrediting programs to prepare nurses in this specialty field. At this time nurses employed outside of institutions were a minority.

After World War II, nursing grew geometrically, extending to many areas at once, and the nation experienced a shortage of nurses. Because of this shortage, many other categories of health care workers were created, but roles and relationships were not carefully planned. The majority of nurses continued to be employed in hospitals. As the supply of nurses grew, new patterns of care delivery that capitalized on the skills of the registered nurse developed and primary nursing became widespread.

Employment Opportunities Today

The health care environment today is affected by all that has gone before. In some settings, there are remnants of the paternalistic attitudes that were prevalent in the years when women were expected to accept the hospital as the family surrogate during training and employment. This attitude may coexist with one that expects today's nurse to be an independent decision-maker. Emphasis is placed on the nurse's need for breadth and depth of theory to cope with the complexities of caring for the acutely ill. At the same time, pangs of nostalgia may be expressed for the days when nurses "really knew how to work" and did not worry much about "book learning."

Unlike graduates of the hospital programs of the past, you will have had fewer hours working in an employment-type situation. Your contact with employment settings may have been brief and you may not have experienced all of the many settings in which registered nurses are employed. You may have questions regarding employer expectations and your own role as a registered nurse employee.

As more and more care is delivered outside of acute care hospitals, the percentage of nurses working outside the hospital has increased. Home health, hospice care, community mental health centers, women's health care delivery systems, maternal-infant care programs, outpatient and primary care, and long-term care facilities are hiring increasing numbers of registered nurses as they care for clients with more complex needs.

The growth of autonomy for the registered nurse has been even more marked outside the hospital setting than in it. Community health nurses have always operated much more independently than hospital nurses. The focus on health care is shifting from illness to health. Because many of these positions require a baccalaureate degree, experience, or specialized educational programs, the new graduate is most often employed in the hospital or long-term care institution.

The number of positions for registered nurses in many settings other than those that provide patient care has also grown. Health care-oriented businesses such as insurance companies and medical equipment supply companies have found that it is easier to teach nurses about business than to teach business people about health care. As a result, nurses are being employed in what some individuals see as non-nursing positions. Others argue that these, too, should be considered nursing positions because the expertise that makes the individual successful is nursing expertise.

The number of men in nursing, which remained relatively small for many years, is beginning to increase as society reassesses its attitude toward labeling jobs as woman's or man's work. Men have been attracted by the opportunities and improving economic picture of nursing and in turn have not been reluctant to advance it still further.

The economic position of the nurse has improved for a variety of reasons. One reason is the extension of laws governing fair labor practices to nonprofit institutions and the advent of collective bargaining (see Chapter 9). Another major factor affecting the economic position of nurses was the nursing shortage of the 1980s. The demand for nurses rose faster than the supply; employers began increasing salaries and benefits to attract nurses. This was especially notable in urban communities.

Then in the 1990s the pressures of a changing health care system and cost containment created still more changes for nursing. Hospital stays shortened so dramatically that hospital censuses decreased across the country. The nursing shortage appeared to end abruptly as hospitals began reassessing their needs.

All of these factors bring you, as a new graduate, into a world of uncertainty but one also filled with opportunity and promise. Now you must determine your place in this world.

Competencies of the New Graduate

Recently you have heard the term *competency* used a great deal, especially as it applies to the new graduate. Competency, as used here, refers to the ability of the graduate to effectively and efficiently perform specified nursing skills including the application of critical thinking skills.

The most definitive statement on the competencies needed by the newly registered nurse has been developed by the National Council of State Boards of Nursing (NCSBN) based on its job analysis study that serves as the basis for the NCLEX-RN licensing examination (Chornick, Yocom, and Jacobson, 1993).

This study was based on responses by a stratified random sample of newly licensed, entry-level registered nurses most of whom were employed in acute care hospitals. Both the frequency of 270 nursing activities and their *criticality* was studied. Criticality refers to activities that cannot be delayed or omitted without a "substantial risk of unnecessary complications, impairment of function, or serious distress to clients" (Chornick et al., 1993, p 11).

Activities expected of newly licensed nurses that led the list for criticality were:

- Use universal precautions
- Report significant changes in the client's condition
- Perform cardiopulmonary resuscitation
- Perform Heimlich maneuver/abdominal thrust
- Provide emergency care for a wound disruption
- Recognize the occurrence of hemorrhage
- Manage a medical emergency until a physician arrives
- Implement measures to prevent circulatory complications (such as embolus, shock, hemorrhage, etc.)
- Respond to symptoms of fetal distress

Activities were further studied in terms of the frequency with which they were expected of newly licensed registered nurses. In all settings nurses were expected to:

- Coordinate care through working with others on the health care team and supervising delivery of care by assistive personnel
- Preserve the quality of care through such activities as acting as an advocate for needed changes in care, documenting errors or problems, intervening in situations involving unsafe or inadequate care
- Maintain the safety of the client as exemplified by verifying, identifying, reporting unsafe equipment, and following infection control guidelines

- Prepare clients and families for care that is to be done including proce-dures and treatments; and help them to understand expected outcomes
- Carry out procedures in a safe, effective manner

Physiologic integrity and psychosocial integrity were supported by a wide variety of individual actions. Some, such as assessing vital signs, seemed al-most universal. Others, such as monitoring for side effects of radiation ther-apy, were needed in a small minority of settings. Allowing clients to talk about their concerns and assisting them to communicate effectively were again al-most universal activities.

Activities that represent carrying out the nursing process in terms of as-sessment, analysis, planning, implementation, and evaluation applied to al-most all settings.

In addition to this study, statements regarding competencies of new grad-uates have been developed by the various educational councils of the Na-tional League for Nursing (1991). These were discussed in Chapter 3. Addi-tionally, some states have developed statements of competencies for graduates of the nursing programs in those states. Similarities and patterns have emerged from all of these statements. The outline of theoretical knowledge and functioning in regard to the nursing process seems to be the most consis-tent. The most divergent opinions seem to be in the area of specific skill or task competency.

Employers' Expectations Regarding Competencies

Employers often ask for further clarification of competence. Have these grad-uates only the necessary theoretical knowledge regarding the skill? Have they actually performed the skill? If so, was it in a practice laboratory only, or was it in a patient care situation? Does competence mean that the new graduate can function independently, or will some supervision still be needed?

Further complicating the picture is the confusion surrounding competen-cies of the graduates of the three types of nursing education programs. Al-though statements by a variety of organizations have distinguished among lev-els of functioning, many employers do not differentiate expectations. Some employers state that new graduates from different types of programs have not clearly demonstrated differences in competencies. This has created confusion in the minds of nurses, employers, and the public over the role of the regis-tered nurse prepared in each type of educational program.

What is expected of the new graduate varies in different health care agencies and in different geographical areas. Expectations are affected by var-ious factors in the community such as whether there are nursing programs in that community and whether new graduates come from one or from many different schools. The acuity of the patient care load and the types of services offered by the agency may also affect expectations.

Based on the NCSBN job analysis study (Chornick et al., 1993), agencies that employ newly graduated registered nurses expect them to demonstrate the following competencies:

1. *Possess the necessary theoretical background for safe patient care and for decision-making.* Many employers believe that new graduates of today are very competent in this area. For instance, the new graduate should understand the signs and symptoms of an insulin reaction, recognize it when it occurs, and know what nursing actions should be taken. The new graduate must know when an emergency or complication is occurring and secure medical help for the client when that is needed.
2. *Use the nursing process in a systematic way.* This includes assessment, analysis, planning, intervention, and evaluation. New graduates should be able to develop plans of care as well as follow plans such as care pathways that have been developed by the agency.
3. *Recognize own abilities and limitations.* To provide safe care, the nurse must identify when a situation requires greater expertise or knowledge

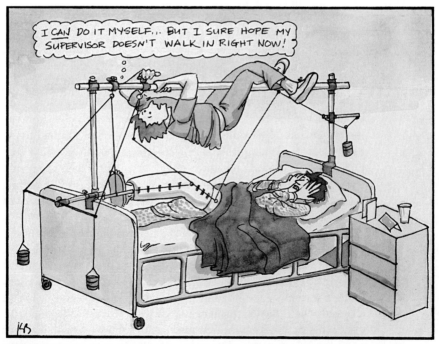

FIGURE 11–1 New graduates are expected to know both their own abilities and when to seek appropriate help.

and when assistance is needed. Employers may be able to assist if nurses ask for help and direction but cannot accept the risk to patients created by nurses who do not know their own limitations.

4. *Use communication skills effectively with clients and coworkers.* In every setting there are clients and families who are anxious, depressed, suffering loss, or experiencing other types of emotional distress. The nurse is expected to respond appropriately to these individuals and to facilitate their coping and adaptation. Effective communication skills are essential to the functioning of the entire health care team. Often the nurse is expected to help coordinate the work of others and this cannot be done without effective communication skills.

5. *Understand the importance of accurate and complete documentation.* Employers generally recognize that the new graduate must be given time to learn the documentation system used in the facility. However, the new graduate is expected to recognize the need for recording data. It is anticipated that the nurse would keep accurate, grammatically correct, and legible records that provide the necessary legal documentation of care.

6. *Understand and have a commitment to a work ethic.* This means that the employee takes the responsibility of the job seriously and will be on time, takes only the allowed coffee and lunch breaks, and will not take "sick days" unless truly ill. It also means that the new graduate recognizes that nurses may be needed 24 hours a day, 365 days a year, and that this may require sacrifices of personal convenience, such as working evening shifts or on holidays.

7. *Possess proficiency in the basic technical nursing skills.* This is an area in which a wide variety of expectations may be present. In most settings proficiency in the basic skills required to support activities of daily living is expected. These skills include such things as transferring, giving baths, and performing general hygienic measures. In some settings nurses will be carrying out these tasks, whereas in different settings they will be directing or teaching others who do them, such as nursing assistants or family members. In either case, proficiency is essential to evaluating the care provided.

The tasks that are reserved for the registered nurse represent the area of widest diversity in the identification of essential skills. The settings in which nurses practice are diverse and therefore technical skills may be needed in one setting and not in another. Some facilities provide extensive orientation programs in which every skill is checked before the new graduate is allowed to proceed independently. Other employers expect the new graduate to perform the skill if able or to ask for help if unable to be independent. Often employers are flexible in their expectations, so that it may be acceptable if an individual seems to have proficiency in a reasonable percentage of skills. Other employers have a list of skills in which proficiency is mandatory, although speed may not be expected. Also, there may be a difference between what the employer would wish and what the employer will accept.

8. *Functioning with acceptable speed.* This is another area in which expectations vary greatly. Most employers state that they expect the new graduate will be slower; however, they may vary in how much slowness is acceptable and how soon they feel that slowness should be overcome. Generally, an orientation period is planned, although with the pressures on health care agencies, this has often been shortened considerably. An acceptable speed of function is reflected by ability to carry out a usual registered nurse assignment within the shift. Thus, if the usual patient assignment for a registered nurse is the care of six to

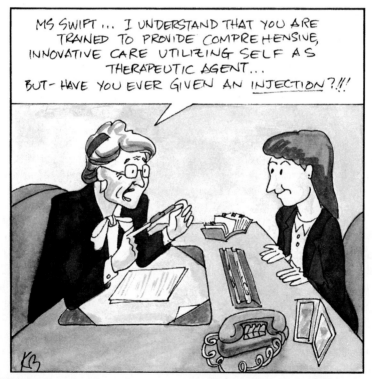

FIGURE 11–2 Employers are often concerned about an applicant's specific technical skills.

eight moderately ill patients, the new graduate is expected to accomplish this by the end of the orientation period.

Personal Career Goals

In caring for patients, you are involved in the process of goal setting. Many nurses recognize the value of this in patient care but never transfer the concept to their personal lives. Nursing as a profession offers many career options. Without carefully setting goals, you might drift for years.

FOCUSING YOUR GOALS

You may want to focus on a broad area of clinical competency, such as pediatric nursing, or on a more restricted area, such as neonatal care. Clinical areas available for concentrated effort become more varied as health care becomes more complex. Emergency care, coronary care, neurologic and neurosurgical nursing, and specialties in the care of persons with ear, nose, and throat disorders are just a few of the clinical possibilities. Nurses specialize in aerospace nursing, enterostomal therapy, and respiratory care as well as operating room nursing and postanesthesia care. Opportunities for additional education and for practice in most clinical specialties are now available for any experienced registered nurse, regardless of the person's initial educational background.

Some specialty areas are in the primary care field, such as the woman's health care specialist, the family nurse practitioner, and the pediatric nurse practitioner. Increasing numbers of these programs require a baccalaureate degree for entry, but some admit registered nurses with experience in that specialty area.

Another approach may be to focus your goals on the setting in which care is delivered, such as acute care, long-term care, or community care. As health care needs expand, these separate realms of care delivery are all demanding more specialized knowledge. Even within the individual area of focus differences are present. For example, within the community are ambulatory care settings, public health nursing agencies, occupational health nursing departments, and day care facilities.

Yet another way of focusing your goals is according to functional categories. Although nurses are initially thought of as direct care providers, they are needed in many other positions. For example, there is need for those who would move into supervisory and administrative capacities, those who teach, and those who conduct nursing research. Nursing also lends itself to writing, to community service, and even to political involvement.

You may decide to set your goals in relation to all three types of foci. That is, you might identify a clinical area, a care setting, and a functional category.

SETTING YOUR GOALS

The first step in setting personal career goals is a thorough self-assessment. Determine how your abilities and competencies correspond to your own expectations as well as to those of the employers. Other factors to explore are your likes and dislikes and the situations or types of work you particularly enjoyed as a student. Also, it is important to recognize the area in which you were most comfortable. Were there areas in which you or your instructor felt that you were an above-average student? Consider your health and personal characteristics in relationship to types of work. Do you have physical restrictions? Do you prefer working independently or with others? How do you respond to close supervision or to relative freedom in the job setting? Do you work well with long-term goals and a few immediate reinforcements, or do you need to see results quickly? Another factor to consider is your own geographic mobility; would you be willing to move or travel as part of a job? Both your personal responsibilities and preferences operate in this arena.

As you plan ahead, you need to examine many of the options offered by nursing. What types of jobs and opportunities are open to you? What education and personal abilities are needed in these areas? Are you interested? Does the education you have meet the educational requirement? Are avenues for additional education available to you? All of these considerations are important as you plan for the future.

Career goals need to be both short and long term. They will help you to plan your future constructively. This does not mean that goals are static. Just as patient goals must be realistic, personal, and flexible, so must your own goals.

Short-term goals will encompass what you want to accomplish this month and this year. What do you want to do and what do you want to be in the immediate future? For example, one recent graduate stated that her short-term goal was to have 2 years of solid experience in a busy metropolitan hospital.

Long-term goals represent where you want to be in your profession 5 to 10 years from now. The long-term goal of the graduate referred to above was to work in a small, remote community in which she would have the opportunity to function autonomously.

Although both long- and short-term goals will be revised as your life evolves, they will guide you in making day-to-day decisions more effectively. In today's world of rapid health care change, you may need to keep your goals somewhat broad and flexible. Be ready to consider alternative goals and a variety of pathways to one goal. These approaches will be of value as you enter a system in transition.

MAINTAINING AND ENHANCING YOUR COMPETENCE

Every nurse has an obligation to society to maintain competence and continue practicing high-quality, safe care. Continuing education may occur through learning on the job, through reading of professional publications, or through attending classes. There are television courses, programmed instruction programs, and examinations related to journal articles. Any of these avenues may be appropriate, depending on the circumstances. Some nurses may want to advance through specialty or higher education. Included in your goal setting should be an approach to maintaining and enhancing your competence.

Making Goals Reality

Philosophical questions regarding goals must be resolved by practical approaches. As a new graduate, your first goal simply may be to get a job in nursing (especially if you live in one of the areas of the country that has more limited opportunities for registered nurses).

Whatever the situation, you are more likely to realize your goals if you are prepared to present yourself in the best possible way to a prospective employer. Many of you have held different jobs in the community as students and as adults. You may be familiar with and competent in the job search process. Others of you have never applied for the kind of job that truly could be considered the beginning of a career. Different expectations are held by both employers and prospective employees in such a situation.

LETTER OF INQUIRY OR APPLICATION

Writing a letter requesting an interview is an excellent way to approach many prospective employers. You can present yourself positively through a well written letter. In addition, a letter may be dealt with at the recipient's convenience, whereas a telephone call may interrupt a busy schedule. There are fewer chances for misunderstanding if your request is in writing and if you receive a written reply.

Before you write your letter, you should make sure you have information about the prospective employer. What kind of facility is this? What types of clients do they serve, and what special services do they offer? It makes a poor impression to write to a prospective employer stating your goal is to work in pediatrics if that facility does not provide any pediatric services.

Another part of your advance planning is identifying how you will focus your letter on your special qualifications and what you want to highlight. You will want to focus on the skills or accomplishments related to the position you want.

Your letter should be no more than one page in length but be planned to present all essential information. Introduce yourself and your purpose for writing in the first paragraph so that the reader immediately has an understanding of the subject. You may want to briefly state your reasons for applying for a position with this particular employer. The more specific the reasons, the better the impression you are likely to make.

Briefly highlight your qualifications for the position. This should not be a simple recitation of what is in your resumé but should either present the information in a slightly different light or add pertinent detail that is not in the resumé. You might include personal qualities that would make you an effective employee in the position.

In the final paragraph, make a summary statement indicating why you want to work for this employer and ask for an appointment for an interview. Be sure to indicate the times you can be available and how and where you can be contacted. Thank the person for considering your application, and close.

Another point to remember is that the letter's appearance as well as its content represents you. You will be judged on spelling, grammar, clarity, and neatness as well as on the letter's content. Your letter of application should be written in standard business form. Make it brief and clear. Ask a friend or family member to check your first draft if you have any questions about its correctness (see accompanying display).

THE RESUMÉ

A resumé is a brief overview of your qualifications for a position. Its purpose is to provide the employer with a way to quickly identify whether you have the basic qualifications for a position and to present you in the most positive light to be considered for the position in which you are interested. In most instances you will want to include your resumé with your initial letter. In addition, you may take your resumé with you and leave it with the employer at the end of your interview.

The appearance of your resumé is important because it presents your initial image to the prospective employer. You will want its appearance to reflect a competent, professional image. It is not necessary to have a professionally produced resumé. Nursing employers, when asked, have indicated that it neither adds to nor detracts from their impression to read a resumé that has been produced by some professional printing method. The important point is that it be a somewhat formal, standard, informative document that is neatly typed without errors.

Your resumé should be on standard-sized, white or off-white, good quality paper so that it is easy to handle, file, and read. A resumé that is individually typed or printed (or reproduced well enough so that is appears to be) usually will be more positively received than a carbon copy or a poor-quality photo-

Sample Letter of Application

Margery Hoskins
1625 13th Ave. N.E.
Seattle, WA 98105

June 8, 1995

[Individual's Name]
[Health Care Agency Name]
[Street Address]
[City, State/Province Zip/Postal]

Dear [Individual's Name]:

I am interested in working as a <u>Registered Nurse</u> in your perioperative department. I am a <u>skilled operating room technician</u> with over <u>10</u> years of experience to offer you. I have now completed my associate degree in nursing. I will take my NCLEX examination on June 10 and expect to have my license by July 1. I enclose my resume as a first step in exploring the possibilities of employment with [name of agency].

My most recent experience was working for an orthopedic surgeon. I was responsible for <u>assuring that the operating room was set up to facilitate his effective function, acting as scrub technician, and providing some surgical assistance.</u> In addition, <u>I worked collaboratively with the operating room staff and perioperative nurses.</u>

As a <u>Registered Nurse</u> with your organization, I would bring a <u>focus on quality and effective problem solving.</u> Furthermore, I work well with others and recognize the value of team work.

I will call you in a few days to arrange an interview at a convenient time for you. If you wish to contact me, I can be reached at the telephone number listed on my resume. Thank you for your consideration.

Sincerely,

Margery Hoskins

copy. If you have access to a computer and word processing, you will find it valuable to create a resumé and save it to a disk. In this way, you will be able to easily revise it and you may even be able to tailor it to an individual job situation. There are inexpensive software programs especially designed to facilitate the production of a well organized and formatted resumé.

To achieve legibility, use wide margins, spacing, indentation, and numbering to separate different sections and topics. You might want to underline or bold print important items or highlight them with an asterisk or bullet to draw swift attention. When an employer is reviewing many such documents, anything that facilitates review and makes you stand out is an advantage.

The content of your resumé is critical. It always begins with your name, address, and telephone number (including area code). If you will be moving, indicate the date the move will be effective and provide an alternate method of contacting you after that date. A permanently settled relative or friend who would be willing to forward your mail would be appropriate. Employers are not permitted to ask about age, marital status, and dependents, and you do not need to include this information.

You should include a personal goal or objective. This may include both a short-term goal such as "employment as a registered nurse on a general medical unit" and a longer-term goal such as "with eventual move to employment in coronary care." Be sure that your goal is realistic and does not imply that you are not really interested in a beginning level position. If you state that your goal is to be a nurse recruiter and you do not have the experience for this kind of position, your application may be discarded. If you state that you want to work in maternity nursing and the only position available is in medical–surgical nursing, you may not be considered for the medical–surgical position that you would have accepted although it was not your first choice.

You will want to include information regarding your licensure and other credentials. Indicate the date your license will be effective and whether you have a temporary permit to work as a nurse. Your nursing license or permit number should be listed. Indicate when you expect to take your licensing examination and have a license.

Work experience is a critical aspect and should provide a complete employment history with no unexplained gaps in time. For example, if you spent 15 years as a homemaker since your last employment, include those dates and state "homemaker" after them. For each job you held include address, dates employed, position, and duties. The prospective employer would be especially interested in a previous nursing assistant position or any other position that demonstrates your knowledge of or experience in some area of health care or the assumption of responsibility.

If you have had only one or two part-time jobs during your educational program, it would be appropriate to include them in detail. However, if during your educational program you held 15 part-time jobs, it is appropriate to list significant ones that offered valuable experience. In one line write, "Various part-time jobs to finance schooling: clerk and waitress. Individual names provided on request." Include the overall dates for this period.

Educational background should form another section and cover your nursing education and any specialized courses or postgraduate work you have done. It is appropriate to note any college-level work. Do not include high school information unless you entered your nursing program directly from high school. Then you might indicate your high school and graduation date on one line of your educational information.

In each group of information list the most recent items first. The most common approach is to group information in the categories just mentioned. See accompanying display for an example of this type of resumé.

Some individuals choose to group employment information into skill or functional categories. This is more common when you have had several positions and you want to emphasize the responsibilities you have had within those positions. We suggest that you use active verbs to describe skills. Words such as supervised, designed, managed, developed, analyzed, coordinated, documented, planned, delegated, created, completed, and operated give life to your resumé and create interest in the reader. See the accompanying display for an example of this type of resumé.

If you had experiences in an educational area that especially relate to the position for which you are applying, you might individualize your resumé by briefly identifying these special experiences. For example, you might have had a senior leadership practicum on an orthopedic unit and this would be particularly relevant to an application for a nursing position in orthopedics. If you had a practicum in the facility or agency to which you are applying, indicate this in some way. Your familiarity with their policies and procedures would be a valuable asset. If you attended any special workshops, include those as a separate section.

Volunteer or community work and awards and honors form two sections when you have these experiences. You might also want to add a section for special skills such as computer familiarity or experience with special types of equipment. Choose the items you list under volunteer and community work carefully. If you are 40 years old, the fact that you were student body president in high school would probably be considered irrelevant. However, if you went from high school directly into a nursing program, this information could be important in demonstrating your leadership ability. Your participation in any community organizations such as the Parent Teacher Association and service in any leadership roles would be significant to an employer.

In some instances you may want to list briefly the skills or abilities gained from a particular volunteer activity. For example, if you worked as a volunteer for a Planned Parenthood clinic, you might specify that your duties included individual client counseling in relation to family planning methods. Simply stating that you were a volunteer might not communicate the level of responsibility you assumed. This is an area that you might want to individualize to target the particular skills you think are important to the position for which you are applying.

List awards and honors that would demonstrate your competence or leadership ability. You may omit this section if you feel that you have nothing pertinent to enter.

References are typed on a separate page and given to the prospective employer if they are requested. Be selective in choosing the people you will list as references. Consider the people who know you and would be able to speak positively of you to a future employer and who would have credibility with the

Resumé of a Recent Graduate—Example A

JAMES L. VASQUEZ
1298 Avenida Diaz
LaQuinta, CA 92253
(619) 524-4321 (H)

Objective: A beginning REGISTERED NURSE position that will provide the opportunity for professional development and delivery of quality nursing care.

Special Skills and Abilities

- Work effectively in a multicultural environment
- Bilingual Spanish/English
- Strong work ethic and experience in working multiple shifts/floating positions

Professional Experience

1992 to Present
Manor Care Center
Palm Desert, CA
Nursing Assistant, Certified: Maintained function and dignity of dependent elderly adults by providing direct care, strong interpersonal relationships, and effective collaboration with nursing and allied health staff.

1982 to 1992
Northrup Corporation
Los Angeles, CA
Machinist: Directed team in meeting time and quality standards for technical equipment production.

Education

1992 to 1995
College of the Desert
Palm Desert, CA
Associate in Science-Nursing, June 1995

Organizations

1992 to 1995
National Student Nurses Association
College of the Desert, Palm Desert, CA
Treasurer

Awards

1992
Golden Acorn Award
Cactus Valley Elementary School PTA, LaQuinta, CA

Resumé of a Recent Graduate—Example B

Margery J. Hoskins
1625 15th Ave. N.E.
Seattle, WA 98105
(206) 526-1234 (H)

Objective: To obtain a position as a REGISTERED NURSE in a perioperative setting where the emphasis is quality care and patient/customer satisfaction.

Functional Summary

- Experienced in perioperative care and management
- Skilled in all orthopedic procedures
- Effective manager of equipment and time for fiscal responsibility
- Team work focused

Professional Experience

Dr. Jason Hoeksler, Orthopedic Surgeon   1989 to Present
Seattle, WA
  Surgical Technician: Orthopedic Surgical Technician and Assistant

Seattle Medical Center   1985 to 1989
Seattle, WA
  Surgical Technician: General Surgical Technician

Education

Shoreline Community College   1993 to 1985
Seattle, WA
  Associate in Applied Arts & Sciences—Nursing, June 1995

Seattle Central Community College   1983–1985
Seattle, WA
  Surgical Technician Certificate, June 1985

Awards Received

Margaret Mallett Memorial Scholarship   1994
Employee of the Year—Seattle Medical Center   1988

employer. Seek the person's permission before giving the individual's name as a reference.

Most commonly you should provide as one reference someone who has known you personally for a relatively long time and who could attest to your ability to relate with others and to such attributes as personal integrity. A second reference should be an instructor or supervisor from your basic educational program. This person would be able to affirm your ability in the nursing field. A third reference should be someone who has employed you and who can describe your work habits and effectiveness as an employee. Include full names with title (if any), addresses, and telephone numbers so that the employer will be able to contact the references easily. When seeking permission to use someone as a personal reference, you might outline what you would like the person to emphasize if contacted; for example, "If you are contacted, I would particularly like you to provide information about my work habits and effectiveness as an employee."

THE INTERVIEW

The interview should be a two-way conversation in which you will be gaining as well as giving information. Think through the situation before going to the interview and outline information that you want to obtain and questions that you want answered. Writing out your questions so that they are clearly stated and so that you do not forget items in the tense atmosphere that often exists in an interview situation is advantageous.

Time spent reflecting on your personal views in advance will be valuable during the interview. Remember that an interview is a chance to sell yourself to an employer, a chance to present yourself as a valuable addition to their nursing staff, and an opportunity to determine how you will fit into that work setting.

When planning for an employment interview, consider your appearance, your attitude and approach, and what the content of the interview will be. Your personal appearance is likely to evoke some type of response from the interviewer. Consider what you would like that response to be and dress appropriately. This would mean that what you wear when applying for one type of job might be inappropriate when applying for another type of job. For example, if you were applying for a position at a hospital, you would wear businesslike clothing, such as dress pants and shirt or a suit or dress. Being neat and well groomed contributes to a businesslike atmosphere. If you were applying for a position in a walk-in health care clinic that offered services to persons who are uncomfortable in a traditional environment, it might be appropriate to wear the casual clothing worn by the workers at the clinic. You need to make a conscious decision about the impression you want to create. Although some may wish that appearances had no effect on the opinions of others, remember that, in reality, appearance often does make a significant difference.

Take a copy of your resumé with you to the interview. In addition, be prepared with the names, addresses, and telephone numbers of all references, and your Social Security number. Take along a black pen to fill out any forms and a note pad to make personal notes of important information. This can increase your self-confidence if you have forms to fill out or if questions about statements on your resumé arise during the interview.

Plan to arrive at an interview early. This gives you time to check your appearance and focus your thoughts. When you arrive at an interview, be sensitive to the problems and concerns of the interviewer. If it is apparent that unplanned events are demanding the interviewer's attention, state that you are aware of the difficulty and ask whether it would be more convenient if you made another appointment. Your sensitivity to the interviewer's cues are evidence of your sensitivity to patients' cues.

Your manner in the interview is also important. Although the employer expects an applicant to be nervous, he or she will be interested in whether your nervousness makes you unable to respond appropriately. Follow common rules of courtesy. Wait to be asked to sit down before you take a chair. Avoid any distracting mannerisms, such as chewing gum or fussing with your hair, face, or clothes. Be serious when appropriate, but do not forget to smile and be pleasant. The interviewer is also thinking of your impact on patients, visitors, and other staff members.

When you prepare your responses, try to anticipate possible questions from the interviewer. Role-playing an interview situation with a friend or relative may help you to feel more confident in your responses. Another technique is to visualize the interview situation in your mind and mentally rehearse responses to questions.

In most instances be sure to answer questions that are asked rather than skirting them. However, if the interviewer asks a question that is illegal, such as age or marital status, you might want to redirect the question to address what appears to be the concern of the interviewer. For example, in response to a question about your age you might say "Perhaps you believe that I appear to be young and inexperienced. I want to assure you that I have demonstrated my maturity and responsibility both in my nursing education and in my position with (name of employer)." In response to a question about marital status or children, you could reply "Perhaps you are concerned about how long I plan to stay in my first position? I want to assure you that whatever my personal situation, professionally, I am looking for a position in an organization where I can be a long-term employee and plan for advancement within the organization."

An interview usually covers a wide variety of subjects. The interviewer may direct the flow of topics or may encourage you to bring up the ones that concern you. Applicants who focus initial attention on the issues of wages and benefits may be viewed as more concerned about themselves than about nursing. Therefore, if you are asked to present questions, ask nursing-related questions first. Demonstrate that you are concerned about how nursing care is given and by whom, where responsibility and authority lie, the philosophy underlying care, the availability of continuing education, and where you would be expected to fit into their overall picture. However, before you leave be sure to cover such topics as hours, schedules, pay scales, and benefits.

POST-INTERVIEW LETTER

After your interview, you should write a brief thank-you letter to the person who interviewed you. In that letter, thank the individual for the time and attention to your questions and concerns. Restate any agreement you feel was reached. For example, "I understand that I am to call your office next week to learn whether I have been scheduled for an interview with the maternity unit manager." Close your letter with a positive comment about the organization. Even if you are not offered a job or do not choose to work at that facility, you are leaving a positive impression. You can never tell when that will be important to you in the future (see accompanying display).

RESIGNATION

When you decide to leave a nursing position, it is important that you provide the employer with an appropriate amount of time to seek a replacement. The more responsible your position, the more time the employer will need. For a staff nursing position you should strive to provide a month's notice unless an urgent matter requires that less notice be given. Notice of resignation should be in a letter that is directed to the head of your department, often to the Director of Nursing. Copies should be sent to other supervisory people, such as the head nurse and the supervisor.

The letter of resignation is important in concluding your relationship with the employer on a cordial and positive basis. The feelings left behind when you resign will influence letters of recommendation and future opportunities for employment with that agency. Give a reason for your resignation as well as the exact date when it will be effective. If you have accrued vacation or holiday time and want to take the time off or be paid for it, clearly state that. Comment about positive factors in the employment setting and acknowledge those who have provided special support or assistance in your growth.

If you are resigning because of problems in the work setting and want to note them, do so in a clear, factual, unemotional way. Avoid attacking anyone personally and do not make broad, sweeping negative comments. Try to make

Sample Interview Follow-Up Letter

3496 Maple Lane
Sioux City, IA 51103

June 15, 1994

Margery Morris RN
1980 Stone Blvd.
Sioux City, IA 51103

Dear Ms. Morris:

Thank you very much for the time you spent with me in an interview for a Registered Nurse position at St. Luke's Medical Center. I understand that at this time you are unsure of whether you will conduct a new graduate nurse orientation in July. I appreciate your willingness to keep my application on file and notify me at the time you determine your needs. You indicated that I would need to be interviewed by a unit manager for a specific position before being offered employment.

My tour of your facility convinced me that I would be proud to be a member of the St. Luke's staff. The obviously positive morale and the emphasis on continuing education that I saw demonstrated that this is a place where one can grow and develop.

As you directed, I will call your office in four weeks to ascertain the status of my file.

Sincerely,

Constance M. Nichols

---

the letter a clear and reasonable statement of your position as a professional (see accompanying display).

Problems of Transition
From Student to Professional

For many of you, graduation from a nursing program and becoming a registered nurse is the realization of a long-cherished goal. You have spent years preparing for this status and now it is here! What you have viewed as an ideal state, freed from financial pressures that you felt as a student, liberated from the tyranny of the examination, may prove to be quite different from what you had expected. Let us consider some of the problems that may occur as you make this transition from student to professional.

Sample Letter of Resignation

Michael M. Phinney
4210 Center Ave.
Riverdale, IL 60627

June 15, 1994

Ms. Monica Jackson, Director of Nursing
Thornton Medical Center
16630 So. State
Riverdale, IL 60627

Dear Ms. Jackson:

It is with some regret that I notify you of my intent to resign effective August 15, 1996. As you are aware, I have been planning to return to school and continue my education. I have been accepted at the University of Illinois and will be beginning classes this fall.

Although returning to school means that I can move forward in my career, I recognize that this agency has provided me with a firm foundation for the future. The support of the experienced staff, the atmosphere that has encouraged me to develop increased skill, and the friendships I developed here have all contributed to my professional growth.

I wish to thank you and all of the staff for the excellence of the experience I gained here.

Sincerely,

Michael M. Phinney

c: Jennifer Watson RN, Unit Manager 3 West

REALITY SHOCK

One problem confronted by the new graduate is the seeming impossibility of delivering quality care within the constraints of the system as it exists. You may feel powerless to effect any changes and may be depressed over your lack of effectiveness in the situation.

Marlene Kramer was the first to call the feelings that result from such a situation *reality shock* (Kramer, 1979). She noted that the new graduate often experiences considerable psychological stress and that this may exacerbate the problem. The person undergoing such stress is less able to perceive the entire situation and to solve problems effectively.

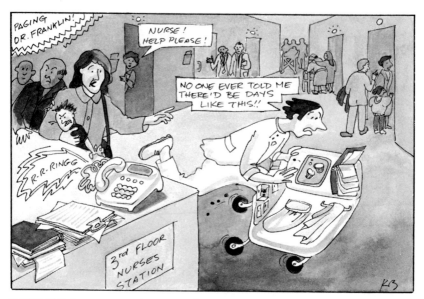

FIGURE 11–3 Some new graduates are disillusioned by the working conditions that they find on their first job.

Causes of Reality Shock

With all of the uncertain expectations and demands, the new graduate often feels caught in the middle. As a student, you may think that you are expected to learn a tremendous amount in an alarmingly short time. The expectations may seem high and in some ways unrealistic. Then, as a new graduate suddenly thrust into the real world, you may feel insecure and think that your educational program did not adequately prepare you for what is expected of you. On one hand you are expected to function like a nurse who has had 10 years of experience, but on the other hand your new ideas may not be considered because you have so little experience. You may become frustrated because you do not have time to provide the same type of care you gave as a student. For example, you may not have adequate time to deal with a patient's psychosocial problems or teaching needs.

As a student, you are taught that the "good nurse" never gives a medication without understanding its actions and side effects and that evaluating the effectiveness of the drug is essential. As a staff nurse, you may find that the priority is getting the medications passed correctly and on time and that there is little or no time to look up 15 new drugs. As for evaluation, that becomes a dream. How can you evaluate the subtle effects of a medication in the 2 minutes spent to pass the medication to a patient you do not know? The individually and meticulously planned care that was so important to you as a student may become a luxury when you are a graduate. Often the focus is on accomplishing the required tasks in the time allotted, and it is efficiency in tasks that may earn praise from a supervisor.

Bradby (1990) suggests that reality shock is part of the passage from novice to experienced nurse. She suggests that it be treated as a normal transitional process with a focus on the growth that can occur.

Effects of Reality Shock

When reality shock occurs some nurses become disillusioned and leave nursing altogether. Others begin to "job hop" or return to school, searching for the perfect place to practice perfect nursing as it was learned. Some push themselves to the limit, trying to provide ideal care and criticizing the system. This may result in their being labeled nonconformists and troublemakers. Still others give up their values and standards for care and reject ideals as impossibly unrealistic expectations that cannot be fulfilled in the real world. These persons simply mesh with the current framework and become part of the system.

Finding Solutions for Reality Shock

There is an alternative to these nonproductive coping methods. It is possible to create a role for yourself that blends the ideal with the possible, one in which you do not give up ideals but see them as goals toward which you will move, however slowly. To do this you need to be realistically prepared for the demands of the real world.

One way of meeting the challenge is to assess yourself as you approach the end of you educational program. Consider what your competencies are. Think about the eight areas of expectation that were discussed earlier in the chapter:

1. Theoretical knowledge for safe practice
2. Use of the nursing process
3. Self-awareness
4. Communication skill
5. Record-keeping
6. Work ethic
7. Skill proficiency
8. Speed of functioning

Second, gain information about what the employers in your community expect from new graduates. This can be done by talking with experienced nurses, requesting interviews with nursing administrators, meeting with the faculty, and contacting recent graduates who are currently employed. Try to get specific information.

After you have gathered this information, try to correlate it with a realistic appraisal of your own ability to function in accordance with the employer's expectations. If you identify any shortcomings, the time to try to remedy them is before graduation. If you identify a lack in certain technical skills, you might register for extra time in the nursing practice laboratory to increase your proficiency. You could even time yourself and work to increase speed as well as skill. You might consult with your clinical instructor to arrange for experiences that would help you gain increased competence. If you recognize that you consistently have difficulty functioning within a time frame, you might obtain employment in a hospital or other health care facility while still in school; this will give you more experience in organizing work within the time limits that the employer sees as reasonable.

As you plan for your first job, you can examine the psychological challenges to be met. Understanding that you are not alone in your feelings of frustration is often helpful. It may be useful to form a support group of other new graduates who meet regularly to discuss problems and concerns and seek solutions jointly. You can also gain valuable reinforcement from other nurses in your work setting. Many have successfully dealt with the problems you face and are able to provide support and help. This "mentor" relationship is an important one and needs to be cultivated.

When confronted with areas of practice that you would like to see changed, weigh the importance of the issue. Use your energies wisely. The "politics of the possible" is important to you. Learn how the system in which you are employed functions and how to use that system for effective change. You, as a person, are important to nursing, so it is important that you neither burn yourself out nor abandon the quest for higher-quality nursing care; you should be able to continue to work toward improving nursing and bringing it closer to its ideals.

Many hospitals are attempting to help new graduates deal with reality shock. Some are doing it by making orientation programs more comprehensive and by providing an experienced nurse to work as a preceptor to the new graduate. Nurse internships or residencies have been created to provide a planned and organized transition time during which the new graduate participates in a formal program, including classes, seminars, and rotations to various units of the hospital. Some hospitals provide an opportunity for student nurses to work during the summer before the last year of their basic program to become familiar with the hospital and the nursing role. In this type of program the student nurse is employed as a nursing assistant but participates in a planned program that introduces the role of the registered nurse. You may wish to inquire whether hospitals in your area have developed any of these or other programs to assist you when you are a new graduate.

BURNOUT

Burnout is a form of chronic stress related to one's job. This problem arises after you have been in practice for a period of time. It can be identified by feelings of hopelessness and powerlessness, accompanied by decreased ability to function both on the job and in personal life. Burnout primarily occurs in nurses who work in particularly stressful areas of nursing, such as critical care, oncology, or burn units. It also occurs in other areas when staffing is inadequate or interpersonal relationships are strained.

Symptoms of Burnout

Symptoms of burnout include both physical changes and psychological distress. Exhaustion and fatigue, frequent colds, headaches, backaches, and insomnia all may occur. There may be changes in disposition, such as being quick to anger or exhibiting all feelings excessively. As burnout progresses, ability to solve problems and make decisions decreases. This frequently results in an unwillingness to face change and a tendency to block new ideas. There may be feelings of guilt, anger, and depression because one cannot meet the expectations for doing a "perfect job."

In response to these feelings, some nurses quit their jobs and move on to other settings. These other settings may not even be in nursing. Others remain in their jobs but develop a personal shell that tends to separate them from real contact with clients and coworkers. The person may become cynical about the possibility of anyone doing a good job and may function at a minimal level.

Causes of Burnout

Many causes of burnout have been discussed in the literature. Prominent among them is the conflict between ideals and reality. Just as this is a problem for the new graduate, it is also a problem for the experienced nurse. In trying to achieve the ideal, the nurse drives harder and harder and becomes critical of environment and of self. Nurses see themselves as being responsible for all things to all people and often take on more and more responsibility, thus increasing their own stress level.

Another cause of burnout is the high level of stress that results from practicing nursing in areas that have high mortality rates. Continually investing oneself in patients who die can take a tremendous toll on personal resources. In addition, the demand is constant for optimal functioning.

Inadequately staffed institutions may also place great stress on nurses. The patients are in need of care, the nurse has the skills to provide the care, and yet the patients do not receive good care. The nurse typically tries to accomplish more, staying overtime, skipping breaks and lunch, and running throughout the shift. Despite this effort, there is little job satisfaction because the things that are left undone or that are not done well seem to be more apparent than all the good that is accomplished.

Preventing Burnout

Burnout can best be prevented by mounting a stress-reduction effort involving the nursing staff, supervisory personnel, the hospital administration, and other health care workers. The most important aspect seems to be bringing burnout into the open and acknowledging the existence of the problems. This alone helps the individual nurse move away from the feelings of separation and alienation that often accompany burnout. Whatever the problems, they seem less frightening if they are defined as "normal" and if the individual nurse does not see himself or herself as the only person not performing as the "perfect nurse."

A second step is to provide for group discussions during which nurses can share feelings and specific concerns in an accepting atmosphere. This sharing may lead to concrete plans to reduce the stress created by the setting. For example, if one source of stress is conflicting orders between two sets of physicians involved in care, a plan might be developed whereby the nurses no longer take responsibility for the conflict but refer the problem to some authority within the medical hierarchy. This type of resolution is possible only when the problem of burnout is being addressed by the whole health care team.

Giving nurses more control over their own practice often decreases stress. This action is limited by the constraints of the setting, but it may involve flexible scheduling, volunteering for specific assignments, and participating in committees that determine policies and procedures.

Rotating nurses out of high-stress areas before they become "burned out" may allow them to rebuild resources and return to the job with enthusiasm. This can be done only if there is no stigma or blame attached to the need to rotate and if other nurses are available for replacement. In patient care areas that are known to be stressful, it is helpful to have a counselor available for nurses. Consulting with this counselor should be viewed by the staff as a positive step and not as an admission of some lack or fault. The counselor needs to be someone who understands the setting and who has the skills to assist people in coping with stress.

As an individual nurse, you also can take actions to prevent burnout. These are the same general actions that are designed to control stress in any aspect of life. Paying attention to your own physical health is an important preventive measure. This includes maintaining a balanced program of rest, nutrition, and exercise. Another important point is not to subject yourself to excessive changes over short periods because changes increase stress. You may decide, for example, not to move at the same time you change to a different shift. A period of "wind down" or "decompression" after work helps you to avoid carrying the stress of the workplace into your private life. This period may be physical exercise, reading, meditation, or any different activity. The activity you choose should not create more demands and increase stress. An important resource is someone who is willing to listen while you ventilate your feelings and talk about your problems. Sometimes this is a family member or personal friend, but it may be more appropriate for this to be a coworker.

Burnout is a serious concern in the nursing profession, but there are strategies for managing it. If you are in a high-stress situation, you need to plan for prevention before you become burned out.

Sex Discrimination in Nursing

The two major areas in which there is concern about sex discrimination in nursing are the issue of comparable worth and discrimination against men in nursing.

COMPARABLE WORTH

Nursing has been, and still is, a profession composed predominantly of women (see Chapter 1). Laws exist in many states that prohibit explicit sex discrimination in salary for a given job. For example, if both men and women are hired by an airline as flight attendants, they must be compensated on the same basis. This principle has been expanded to encompass jobs that are essentially the same work, although the titles may differ. The janitor and the maid may have different titles, but if they have essentially the same tasks, then they must be paid on the same basis.

The next step that many women would like to see accepted is the principle of compensation based on comparable worth. Jobs may be studied and assigned points or rank based on educational requirements, skills required, level of responsibility, and authority. Those with the same points or rank are considered to be of comparable worth although the actual substance of the work may differ. Alaska has a law barring discrimination in pay for work of comparable character.

Many women believe that differing jobs of comparable worth are not compensated equally because of sex discrimination. Most jobs that are found to score high in education, skill, and responsibility and yet have low salaries are jobs that have historically been held by women. Nursing is one example of such a job. Secretaries and teachers are other occupational groups that have traditionally had low wages relative to the level of responsibility required. Groups of women have brought suit against employers charging sex discrimination based on failure to provide equal pay for jobs of comparable worth.

DISCRIMINATION AGAINST MEN

Men in nursing have also expressed concern about sex discrimination. Their concern is not monetary but is related to being allowed to practice in all areas of nursing and being accepted within the profession. Antimale sexism in the United States was discussed by Kus (1985), who pointed out that society stereotypes men just as feminists have criticized that it stereotypes women. He makes a strong case for the importance of nurses examining the stereotypes they hold about men. Stereotypes narrow our thinking and interfere with people being able to develop to their fullest potential. It is appropriate for women in nursing to examine their own behavior and identify whether they have been guilty of perpetuating outmoded stereotypes of the nurse and supporting a type of discrimination toward men that they would fight to eliminate for women.

In some facilities or areas men are not allowed to care for women patients, or if they are allowed to care for women, restrictions are placed on them in terms of obtaining consent for care from each patient. Those who support the limitations on the practice of men in nursing state that it is a matter of providing for the modesty and privacy of the female patient. This position was upheld by a court decision in favor of a hospital that refused to assign a man to a nursing position in labor and delivery (Arkansas, 1981). The argument was made that the patient did not have free choice of a nurse but rather was assigned a nurse for care, and therefore the restrictions were appropriate.

In an article in the *American Nurse*, Ketter (1994) presents the situations of men who have felt discrimination in the workplace based on their gender. One of these men has filed three complaints with Equal Employment Opportunities Commission (EEOC) regarding discrimination in employment in obstetric/gynecologic settings in the 3 years he has been in nursing. His case is expected to end up in federal court.

Those who oppose limitations on the practice of men in nursing state that as a professional, whether man or woman, the nurse should always consider the privacy and modesty of a patient of either gender. This can be done without excluding anyone from providing care in any area. By careful assessment the nurse can determine the true needs of the patient and plan for appropriate avenues to deliver that care. Furthermore, the point has been made that men as physicians have not been excluded from any branch of medicine and this has not created problems. Physicians are not always chosen by the patient either. House staff are assigned, referrals are made to specialty physicians, and many group plans designate a physician to provide care. Female nurses care for male patients in all situations. This has been accepted because women are seen in a nurturing, mothering role that the public associates with nursing.

The American Assembly for Men in Nursing (see Appendix B) provides a forum for the concerns of men in nursing and opposes any limitations on opportunities available to men.

Occupational Safety and Health for Nurses

Nurses have expressed concern regarding safety in the working environment for many years. Employees have a right to expect their employers to provide the safest working environment possible. Some hospitals employ an occupational health nurse to examine the working environment and employment practices to promote health and safety on the job. Nurses themselves, however, have often been lax in recognizing on-the-job hazards and acting for self-protection. This can be likened to the response of those who continue to smoke, regardless of their knowledge of the health hazards of smoking, or those who fail to wear seatbelts, although they know that the statistics show decreased fatalities in automobile accidents when seatbelts are worn. Some people continue to do those things that they know are detrimental to their health and well-being. Unfortunately, nurses are no exception.

INFECTION AS AN OCCUPATIONAL HAZARD

Transmission of infection is a major concern when caring for infected patients. The presence of resistant organisms causes extra concern and makes treatment difficult. All hospitals have an infection control officer, usually a registered nurse, who has the expertise to guide the staff in planning appropriate infection control procedures.

The hidden danger for nurses lies in those patients who have not been diagnosed as having an infection and for whom specific infection control measures have therefore not been prescribed. The incidence of tuberculosis is again on the rise and some is caused by drug-resistant strains of the organism. Although rooms with special ventilation and special masks that are impervious to the tuberculosis organism are available, individuals may be in contact with health care providers long before they are clearly diagnosed. Should nurses in high-risk areas such as the emergency room wear special masks in all patient contact or is this unrealistic? These are important questions to consider.

The acquired immunodeficiency syndrome (AIDS) has created a reevaluation of all approaches to infection control and of health care workers' obligations to provide care for those with communicable diseases. AIDS remains a serious concern for all health care workers. Using universal precautions as described by the Centers for Disease Control and Prevention has become the standard for all health care situations. Nurses must assume responsibility for their own protection through conscientiously carrying out appropriate measures at all times. Employers must be held accountable for providing the supplies and environment to make this possible.

Although the details of infection control are beyond the scope of this text, we would remind you that you hold the key to protecting yourself in many ways. Often health care workers become lax in their attention to the use of gloves or eye protection because these measures are inconvenient. It is your responsibility to maintain the very best of technique for self-protection.

Your employer also has obligations for protecting you from infection. One of the first employer actions toward preventing AIDS and other blood-borne diseases was the provision of "sharps" containers wherever needles were used. Another important employer responsibility is the provision of a supply of gloves and protective eyewear for employee use. Increasing attention is now

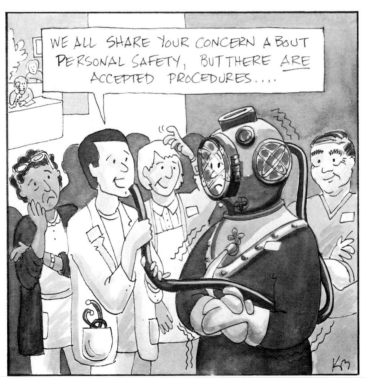

FIGURE 11-4 Personal safety and health in the work environment are important concerns for nurses.

being given to designing needles and other sharp devices in new ways that provide greater protection. For example, a needle with a protective plastic housing is available for use with secondary lines. These needles are unlikely to injure an individual even if they are not handled properly. Needleless intravenous connections are also available. Syringes are available that have a protective cover that the needle retracts into immediately after use. Nurses can request that hospitals provide safer equipment.

Nurses who have frequent contact with blood and blood products and those engaged in intravenous therapy have a special risk for exposure to hepatitis B. Although a vaccine exists to protect against this disease, the vaccine itself is not without side effects; therefore, a discussion with a physician regarding risks versus benefits for you as an individual is appropriate before undertaking immunization. The Occupational Safety and Health Administration (OSHA) has developed standards that require employers to pay for hepatitis B immunization for those employees with significant exposure to blood and body substances that can transmit blood-borne organisms.

HAZARDOUS CHEMICAL AGENTS

Anesthetic gases can increase the risk of fetal malformation and spontaneous abortion in pregnant women who are exposed to them on a regular basis. Standards exist for waste-gas retrieval systems and the allowable level of these gases in the air. Nurses working in operating rooms should seek information on the subject and expect that hospitals will provide a safe environment.

Chemotherapeutic agents used in the treatment of cancer are extremely toxic, and nurses who work in settings where such agents are prepared and administered should seek additional education regarding their administration, not only in relationship to the patient's safety but also in relationship to personal safety. The employer is responsible for providing the equipment needed to maintain safety when handling these agents.

Contact with many medications, especially antibiotics, during preparation and administration may cause the nurse to develop sensitivity. This may not only create transitory problems, such as a hand rash, but may also be a threat if treatment for a serious infection is compromised at some later date. Other medications are absorbed through the skin and may produce an undesirable effect. Nurses who understand this hazard will handle all drugs with discretion and be careful not to expose themselves to these agents.

Cleaning agents and disinfectants used in the hospital may also be hazardous if used improperly. Employers are now required by OSHA to maintain a list of all chemicals used in the work environment, along with information on their possible effects, and the appropriate treatment if individuals are accidentally exposed to them.

BACK INJURIES

Because nursing includes providing direct care to incapacitated individuals, back injuries are a common occupational hazard. Back injuries in general are a serious concern because they interfere with the working life of people in their most productive years.

Some institutions provide instruction in lifting, transfer, posture, body mechanics, other back-saving strategies to help prevent injury. You need to be aware of the potential for back injury and examine your own work habits. Some nurses feel that they must accomplish certain tasks even if the necessary assistance is not available and therefore carry out actions of danger to themselves. Nurses must learn to be assertive in regard to their own safety.

Key Concepts

▷ Throughout the history of nursing there have been changing employment patterns from a focus on the home and the community to a focus on acute care institutions.

▷ In today's health care world the percentage of nurses employed in acute care settings is beginning to diminish as more and more community settings are established for the delivery of care.

▷ Competencies needed by the newly licensed registered nurse can be categorized by criticality and by frequency.

▷ Employers have expectations in eight basic areas: theoretical knowledge for safe practice and decision-making, ability to use the nursing process, self-awareness, communication skills, understanding of the importance of documentation, commitment to a work ethic, proficiency in specified technical skills, and speed of functioning.

▷ Developing a successful career pathway involves setting personal short- and long-term goals including a plan for maintaining and enhancing your own competence.

▷ To obtain a nursing position you will need to develop a professional resumé, be able to write appropriate letters to employers, and interview effectively.

▷ Reality shock occurs when an idealistic new graduate enters the real world of practice and has difficulty with the expectations and demands found there. You can prepare for this transition by attending to your own expectations and developing personal strategies for coping.

▷ Burnout is a stress response experienced by nurses and others who work in occupations that make many emotional demands. Burnout may be alleviated by planned actions, but it may be necessary to change job settings when stress accumulates.

▷ Nurses see sex discrimination in the workplace manifested as wage discrimination against women and job opportunity discrimination against men.

⇨ Occupational safety and health are special concerns for nurses because of the nature of the illnesses that they contact, the toxicity of some chemicals in the nursing environment, and the potential for back injury.

CRITICAL THINKING ACTIVITIES

1. Write out your short- and long-term professional goals with a brief plan on how you can achieve these goals. Think critically about the obstacles you will need to overcome to reach these goals. How will you deal with the obstacles?
2. Create an effective resumé and samples of letters to employers.
3. With a group of nursing students, develop personal strategies for managing reality shock. Discuss your rationale for any strategy you propose.
4. Compare burnout with the stress response you have studied in relationship to client care.
5. Review the advertisements for nursing positions in three current journals and analyze them for gender bias.
6. Research the occupational health program offered by a local employer of nurses. Evaluate that program in relationship to health hazards in the workplace of which you are aware.

References

Arkansas judge rules male nurse out of labor/delivery. Am J Nurs 81(7):1253, 1981

Bradby M. Status passage into nursing: Another view of the process of socialization into nursing. J Adv Nurs 15(10):1220–1225, 1990

Chornick N, Yocom CJ, Jacobson J. 1992–1993 Job Analysis Study of Newly Licensed, Entry-Level Registered Nurses. Chicago: National Council of State Boards of Nursing, 1993

Ketter J. Sex discrimination targets men in some hospitals. Am Nurse 26(4):3, 24, 1994

Kramer M. Reality Shock. St. Louis: CV Mosby, 1979

Kus RJ. Stages of coming out: An ethnographic approach. West J Nurs Res 7(2):177–194, 1985

National League for Nursing. Educational Outcomes of Associate Degree Nursing Programs: Roles and Competencies. Publication No. 23-2348. New York: National League for Nursing, 1991

Further Readings

Alward R, Monk T. The Nurse's Shift Work Handbook. Washington, DC: American Nurses Publishing Co., 1993

A guide to national/international, travel, and home health nursing opportunities. Am J Nurs 94(1):72, 1994

Brady J. Memoirs of a traveling nurse. Am J Nurs 94(1):74, 76, 1994

Buerhaus PI, Dang D, Lehman DL, et al. Analysis of state and local hospital employed RN labor markets. Nurs Econ 11(4):223–228, 258, 1993

Busy nurses need stressbusters. Am Nurse 26(2):5–6, 1994

Butts BJ, Witmer DM. New graduates: What does my manager expect. Nurs Management 23(8): 46–48, 1992

"Career Guide." Nursing, monthly feature

Career Planning Guide. New York: National Student Nurses Association, annual publication

Foley ME. Change signals need for career security versus job security. Am Nurse 26(2):1, 3, 1994

Fulmer H, Cashman S, Bushnell K. Community-oriented primary care: A model for the future. Am Nurse 26(2):19, 1994

Job Focus. American Journal of Nursing, monthly feature

Joinson C. Coping with compassion fatigue. Nursing 22(4):116, 118–119, 120, 1992

Kairns DM. Protect yourself: Set boundaries. RN 55(3):19–22, 1992

Ketter J. Retraining programs benefit staff nurses. Am Nurse 26(4):1, 3, 1994

Lender KL. When you're stretched to the limit. RN 53(7):53–55, 1990

Lindquist KD. Finding the perfect match. Healthcare Trends Transition 1(1):6–8, 1989

Lovejoy RL. When are you entitled to worker's compensation? RN 53(3):81–83, 1990

Mannion J. Change From Within: Nurse Intrapreneurs as Health Care Innovators. Washington, DC: American Nurses Publishing Co., 1990

RN Nursing Opportunities. RN Magazine, annual publication

Schmidt PL, Schoville R, Williams M. From expert to novice. Am J Nurs 93(9):53–56, 1993

Serow WJ, Cowart ME, Chen Y, Speake DL. Health care corporatization and the employment conditions of nurses. Nurs Economics 11(5):279–291, 1993

Sullivan P. Stress and burnout in psychiatric nursing. Nurs Standards 8(2):36–39, 1993

Survival Skills in the Workplace: What Every Nurse Should Know. Washington, DC: American Nurses Publishing Co., 1990

Tammelo AD. Don't be afraid to blow the whistle on incompetence. RN 53(6): 61–66, 1990

Travel nursing: Get up and go! Nursing '93 23(12):60–62, 1993

12

Understanding Nursing Employment Settings

Objectives

After completing this chapter, you should be able to

1. Describe the various settings in which newly registered nurses may begin practice.

2. Describe the three general classifications of health care agencies.

3. Discuss the early development of hospitals and nursing homes and the factors affecting that development.

4. Describe the health care delivery provided in ambulatory care settings and in community agencies.

5. Explain the roles of the governing board, the administrator, the medical staff, and the nursing administrator in a health care agency.

6. Outline the use of clinical ladders as opportunities for nurses.

7. Discuss the purposes of a mission statement, policies and procedures, standards of care, and quality improvement processes in a health care agency.

8. Define terms used in describing organizational structure including channels of communication, chain of command, centralized structure, decentralized structure, and organizational chart.

9. Compare the various patterns of nursing care delivery and how they are integrated into different care environments.

Ellis JR, Hartley CL: NURSING IN TODAY'S WORLD:
CHALLENGES, ISSUES, AND TRENDS, 5th ed.
© 1995 J.B. Lippincott Company

The majority of all nurses are employees of health care institutions and organizations. Relatively few are engaged in private practice. This means that as a new graduate you will need to function within an organization. Some understanding of health care organizations and their historical development as well as a brief introduction to organizational function will help you to assume that role with more comfort and effectiveness.

Types of Agencies Employing Newly Registered Nurses

There are a wide variety of employers in nursing. Not all employ newly graduated nurses; some have positions only for those with experience or advanced education. However, the situation has changed dramatically from the time when everyone assumed that *all* entry-level nurses would work in acute care hospitals. Those planning to move to other fields were expected to spend a minimum for a year or two in acute care first. When this was the assumption, nursing education focused almost exclusively on the acute care hospital as a learning environment. This further ensured that most graduates would feel most comfortable seeking employment in the acute care setting.

As health care has made revolutionary changes, more and more care has moved to settings outside the acute care hospital. The number and variety of long-term care facilities has risen dramatically. These include rehabilitation centers, nursing homes, assisted-living settings, and group homes.

Clinics, offices, and other ambulatory care settings are carefully examining roles of various health care providers and recognizing that the effective use of registered nurses may provide high-quality care at a cost lower than that provided when the physician does not have the support of professional nursing in addressing the needs of clients.

Home care nursing now encompasses a much wider spectrum of patient care needs than previously. Some home care clients require a high degree of skill but represent a relatively stable population, who are able to maintain their status at home as long as adequate support is available. Others have acute problems requiring high-intensity services. For example, hospice care enables dying persons to remain at home.

Businesses are recognizing that nurses may fill many roles. The role of the occupational health nurse in providing information on health promotion and preventive care receives increasing emphasis. Experienced nurses are employed by insurance companies as case managers and care reviewers.

Although many nurses continue to be employed in acute care hospitals, an increasing number of nurses are working in ambulatory care areas such as day surgery. Day treatment, special teaching clinics, and other outpatient services are more commonly found as part of the acute care hospital. Some hospitals have had rehabilitation services for years, but now some are moving into what is called "transitional care," that is, the convalescent or recovery period between acute care hospitalization and discharge home.

Classification of Health Care Agencies

Because the health care industry is so large, so diverse, and so complex, it is difficult to understand. Generally agencies providing care are classified in one of three ways. It should be remembered that any one of these classifications is somewhat arbitrary and any agency may be placed in more than one classification.

CLASSIFICATION ACCORDING TO LENGTH OF STAY

One way of classifying agencies is according to length of stay. This would include short-stay surgical centers, acute care hospitals and long-term care facilities. Short-stay facilities provide services to patients who are suffering from acute conditions that usually require less than 24 hours of care. In some areas the average length of stay for obstetric patients is now less than 24 hours, making short-stay obstetric units a reality. Acute care hospitals, in general, care for patients staying fewer than 30 days. However, the average length of stay for all diagnoses has been declining steadily over the past few years and has become significantly less since the implementation of diagnosis-related groups (DRGs) in 1983. In many hospitals the average stay after general surgery is 3 to 5 days. Thus the differentiation between short-stay and acute care inpatient has blurred.

Long-term care facilities include those that offer services to patients with major rehabilitation needs, chronic disease, or mental illness. The average length of stay extends over several months. State institutions for the mentally ill are usually considered long-term hospitals as are the facilities the federal government operates for veterans in need of rehabilitation. However, long-term rehabilitation may also be located on one unit of an acute care hospital.

CLASSIFICATION BY TYPE OF SERVICE

Health care agencies may also be classified according to type of service provided. The most common type is the general hospital that offers medical, surgical, obstetric, emergency, and other services. Specialty hospitals offer only a particular service such as that provided by psychiatric hospitals, women's hospitals, or children's hospitals. Specialty hospitals tend to be less common than general hospitals.

A term frequently used when referring to hospitals is *community hospital*. They are called community hospitals because they serve the general needs of the specific community for hospital services. Raffel and Raffel (1989) state that community hospitals constitute 83% of the total number of hospitals in the United States and account for 90% of all hospital admissions each year. Tertiary care hospitals are usually associated with a university or are part of a large medical center. These hospitals have specialized types of care such as burn centers, bone marrow transplant centers, and research-based oncology as well as general care. Tertiary care hospitals are expected to provide services for a wide geographic area, not simply their own community.

Long-term care facilities likewise might offer different types of services. The residential facility for young adults with severe disabilities such as cerebral palsy may focus on life skills development and occupational training. The inpatient hospice focuses on respite care, symptom management, and terminal care. The rehabilitation center focuses on individuals with needs related to restoration of function. Some long-term care facilities now focus on individuals with continuing high-intensity needs, such as those who remain permanently dependent on a ventilator.

Subacute care is a growing type of service that may be offered in special units of hospitals or in long-term care facilities. Sometimes termed *transitional care*, this care is seen as a "middle-ground" between the high acuity needs of those in the acute care hospital and the more traditional long-term care patient. Stays in short-term subacute units are up to 30 days in length. Some units focus on intermediate lengths of stay that usually range from 31 to 90 days as people recover enough to move into a home setting or stabilize their needs so that they can be met in a nursing home. Still other subacute units offer care that can extend up to 2 years (Burns, 1993). The units that offer primarily medical services are most commonly located in hospitals, whereas those that offer primarily rehabilitative services are more commonly located in long-term care facilities (Taylor, 1994).

Community health care agencies offer in-home care by a variety of health care professionals including nurses, physical therapists, respiratory therapists, social workers, and home health care aides. Some community agencies focus on direct care services and others focus on health promotion.

CLASSIFICATION ACCORDING TO OWNERSHIP

The final method of classifying health care agencies is according to ownership. Agencies may be classified as government or public when owned and operated by a governmental agency. Proprietary agencies (also known as private for profit) are usually part of a corporation owned by stock holders. Voluntary agencies are those operated by nonprofit groups such as religious bodies, community boards, and other nonprofit groups.

Public, or government, agencies may be owned and operated by federal, state, or local governments. The federal facilities usually serve the needs of a special group of individuals such as veterans, military personnel, Native Americans, or inmates in federal prisons. State mental facilities and hospitals operated by the state as part of the state university medical school are other governmental institutions. Cities, counties, and hospital districts also operate both acute care and long-term care agencies.

Proprietary agencies are investor owned and are operated for the financial gain of the individual or group that owns the facility. Historically, some proprietary hospitals were owned and operated by a small group of physicians, but over the years these have often been sold to community groups. In the past few years there has been a significant trend toward the acquisition of health care enterprises by investor-owned corporations and the formation of multiunit, for-profit systems. Examples would be The Hospital Corporation of America, which is based in Nashville, and Humana, Incorporated of Louisville. Both of these groups own more than 80 hospitals and operate a number of others. Not all investor-owned institutions are general hospitals. In the long-term care field, Beverly Enterprises is an example of a corporation that owns and operates many nursing homes.

Nonprofit or voluntary institutions are owned and operated by community associations, fraternal groups, or religious organizations. More than 50% of the nation's short-term hospitals fall into this classification. The term *nonprofit* may be something of a misnomer in the sense that all facilities must make a sufficient income to continue to exist, to maintain facilities and services, and to plan for capital improvement and development. Those that are classified as nonprofit put any profit to work in the facility. The majority of acute care hospitals have always been nonprofit or governmental although there are many for-profit institutions. The majority of nursing homes are proprietary although some are operated by religious or fraternal groups.

Acute Care Hospitals

The modern hospital may be viewed as the hub or center of the health care delivery system. These facilities are central to the health care of the community. They also provide education to a wide variety of health care workers and, in many cases, are centers for research and its dissemination. Hospitals are using their status and position in health care to enter into cooperative agreements and alliances with other types of providers, insurance companies, and even other hospitals. To better understand the hospitals of today, you will find it useful to look at their history and development.

THE DEVELOPMENT OF HOSPITALS IN THE UNITED STATES

The history of hospitals in the United States can be traced back to the mid-1700s when most cities had built *almshouses*, also called poorhouses, to provide food and shelter for the homeless poor. These structures became homes to the aged, disabled, mentally ill, and the orphaned. Also operating at this time were *pesthouses*, which were built to isolate people with contagious diseases, especially those who contacted the disease while aboard ship. In these facilities were persons suffering from cholera, smallpox, typhus, and yellow fever as well as the more common communicable diseases of the community such as scarlet fever. Pesthouses might open and close as the need dictated.

Neither the almshouses nor the pesthouses represented an institution from which most individuals would want to seek or receive care. They were crowded, unsanitary, and poorly heated and ventilated. Cross-infection was common and mortality was high. Those with the financial means were cared for in their homes.

The first hospital in the United States was the Pennsylvania Hospital in Philadelphia built in 1751 (see Chapter 1). The New York Hospital in New York City was to follow in 1773, Massachusetts General Hospital in Boston in 1816, and New Haven Hospital in New Haven, Connecticut in 1826.

These early hospitals cared for people with acute illnesses and injuries but did not admit the mentally ill. Therefore, during the same period, a number of governmental hospitals were established to house the mentally ill. The first such facility was established as a department of the Pennsylvania Hospital in 1752. The second was founded in Williamsburg, Virginia, in 1773. By 1840, eight hospitals to treat the mentally ill had been established. The forms of treatment of patients in these early mental hospitals is legend, often being cruel and inhumane. Some of you may have studied about Dorothea Dix, a soft-spoken schoolteacher, who campaigned vigorously for and brought about much reform in the area of mental health treatment.

The early hospitals left much to be desired. They were dirty, rank with infection, and poorly ventilated. Linen was used for several patients before it was laundered. Draining, suppurating wounds were common. The stench was overwhelming, and it is said that nurses used snuff to make working conditions more tolerable (Kalisch and Kalisch, 1986). Nursing was not an attractive career, and most of the nursing care was delivered by women who could find no other source of employment—alcoholics, prostitutes, and convicted criminals. They had no formal training for their roles nor were any standards for care applied.

FACTORS AFFECTING THE DEVELOPMENT OF HOSPITALS

Six major developments can be cited that represented major forces in the continued development of hospitals and patient care. Each one played a unique role in the changes.

The Advance in Medical Science

The first of these major developments related to advances in medical science. By the end of the colonial period two medical schools had been established in the United States. Before that time physicians learned their skills through an apprenticeship with a practicing physician. As medicine became more of a science, advances occurred. One of the most significant was the discovery of anesthesia and the rapid advances in surgery that were to follow. The germ theory also did much to advance the practice of medicine because it was soon followed by the development of agents or techniques that would sterilize or serve as antiseptics. The growth of hospitals in the United States was a direct result of these advances that made hospitals safer and more desirable. The discovery of sulfa and antibiotics in the mid-1930s and mid-1940s, respectively, heralded even greater changes.

The Development of Medical Technology

The development of specialized medical technology was a natural successor to the advances in medical science. The first hospital laboratory was opened in 1889, and x-rays were used in diagnosis in 1896. The electrocardiogram (ECG) was discovered in 1903 and the electroencephalogram (EEG) was discovered in 1929 (Haglund and Dowling, 1988).

Changes in Medical Education

Advances in medical education also had a significant impact on the development of health care in this country. The Flexner Report was completed in 1910, and it led to changes in the structure and content of curricula in medical schools. It also expanded the role of hospitals to include education and research and resulted in internships and residencies for medical students. Education of physicians and nurses in hospital-based programs has been supported through federal funding.

Development of the Health Insurance Industry

The growth of the health insurance industry is another factor responsible for the development of hospitals. Although there were some antecedents, most sources indicate that the first hospital insurance plan was initiated at Baylor

University Hospital in 1929 to serve the need of schoolteachers of Dallas, Texas (Raffel and Raffel, 1989). The approach used there was to form the model for Blue Cross plans around the country.

Today figures vary as to what percentage of the population is protected against costs of medical care by some type of insurance. They range from 85% to 90%. Concern continues to be voiced for the 35 million or so individuals who have no protection (Raffel and Raffel, 1989).

Greater Involvement of the Government

The government's role in health care delivery has also had an impact on the development of hospitals. In early times the government was involved primarily at a local level building almshouses and facilities for the insane. By 1935, the government was providing grants-in-aid to assist in the establishment of public health and other programs to furnish health assistance to citizens. In 1946, the Hill-Burton Act resulted in the construction of many hospitals and other health facilities. The initiation of Medicare and Medicaid in 1965 made another significant impact on the health care industry because the legislation contained support for capital construction and development in hospitals through the manner in which reimbursement occurred.

The Emergence of Professional Nursing

The last, but certainly not the least, force significantly influencing the growth of hospitals was the development of professional nursing. Following in the wake of work done by Florence Nightingale in England (see Chapter 1), the first school of nursing opened in the United States in 1873. By 1898, there were 400 schools with 10,000 graduates. Haglund and Dowling (1989, p 165) cite two ways in which the advances in nursing contributed to the growth of hospitals. First, they "increased the efficacy of treatment, cleanliness, nutritious diets, and formal treatment routines" that resulted in patient recovery. Second, they resulted in considerate, skilled patient care that made hospitals acceptable to all people, not just the poor. The role of the nurse and nursing influences the health care delivery system more today than ever before.

The Long-term Care Facility

Long-term care provides assistance with activities of daily living and health care for people of any age who are physically or mentally unable to provide adequate self-care. These conditions may extend over a limited period of time (such as during recovery from a major surgery) or may last a lifetime (such as

cerebral palsy). Care involves coordination between the entire multidisciplinary team to provide counseling, nursing care, rehabilitation, nutritional support, social services, and perhaps special education programs. Long-term care
facilities include nursing homes, chronic disease hospitals, psychiatric hospitals, tuberculosis hospitals, and psychiatric and mental retardation facilities.
The majority of long-term care facilities are nursing homes that care primarily
for the elderly.

THE NURSING HOME TODAY

According to Collopy, Boyle, and Jennings (1991), there are more than
19,000 nursing homes in the United States, of which approximately 75% are
proprietary, 20% are nonprofit, and 5% are government operated. The average annual cost per resident ranges from $28,000 in the Northeast to $20,000
in the South. An estimated 51% of this cost is paid directly by the elderly and
their families, about 44% by Medicaid, 2% by Medicare, and 1% by private
insurance, and other government resources pick up the remainder.

The fastest growing age group in the United States are those 85 years of
age and older. It has been estimated that one in four citizens will spend some
of their lifetime in a nursing home, very often the last years. Women outnum-
ber men in these facilities, with the population composed of 75% women and
25% men. The age of elderly nursing home residents ranges from 65 to older
than 100, with the average age about 84.

HISTORY OF THE NURSING HOME

Like our acute care facilities, the nursing home has a rather harsh beginning.
In the 19th century almshouses and poorhouses were constructed by the government to shelter the destitute elderly. These facilities attracted a strange
mixture of residents, including those who needed asylum and detention, as
well as the poor, the chronically disabled, and the mentally ill. The morality
that prevailed at the time tended to see poverty and disability as indications of
an undisciplined, improvident, and even profligate life. A person who was
housed in a "county poorhouse" often had no family to provide care and assistance and no funds and endured a certain social stigma. In time these
almshouses became the community dumps for all of society's cast-offs. These
early facilities for the country's dependent elderly offered the same grim sur-
roundings of the early hospitals. They were unsanitary, overcrowded, and
poorly ventilated. Residents were expected to work to assist with their keep if
they were able. Care was provided by individuals who sought employment
there as a last resort. Appropriations to manage these facilities were meager
because the majority of the citizens had no identification with these institu-

tions that housed the poor and the transient, who probably had no previous history of contributing to the community.

As the United States grew as a society, various groups became concerned about the conditions that existed in the poorhouse. Gradually, patients tended to be separated according to condition and the mentally and chronically ill were reassigned in different hospitals. Nursing homes began to evolve under different sponsorship as churches and fraternal organizations started homes to care for their elderly members. As a result of the Social Security Act of 1935, private (for-profit or proprietary) nursing homes emerged during the 1930s. Raffel and Raffel (1989, p 205) state, "The original exclusion of benefits for patients in public institutions (since repealed) apparently stemmed from congressional concern about conditions in county poorhouses and a desire to get them closed."

In the postwar period, the Hill-Burton Act of 1948 that supported hospital construction was expanded to include voluntary (nonprofit) nursing homes and some states also developed grant programs. Since 1950, government funding for nursing home care has increased steadily and culminated in the 1965 Medicaid program, which now covers 40% of all nursing home costs (Collopy et al., 1991). Governmental regulation of nursing homes has become increasingly involved and complex.

As changes in funding occurred and as short-term acute care hospitals became increasingly specialized, the role of the nursing home changed. It was affected by the deinstitutionalization movement in the 1950s and 1960s that saw large numbers of elderly discharged from mental hospitals. Nursing homes began to assume the role of providing specialized care for the elderly. By the 1960s, this role was well established, but the nursing home industry was subjected to constant reports of substandard and negligent care and, in some instances, charges of absolute abuse of patients and misuse or embezzlement of their funds. This resulted in even greater scrutiny and regulation by the government.

CARE IN NURSING HOMES

Although the nursing home of today suffers from the negative image of the past, it offers a far different environment than it did even 10 years ago. Maintenance of function, independence, autonomy, and rehabilitation are all goals of nursing homes. There is concern with the living environment as well as the health care environment. Some nursing homes have entire wings of individuals receiving posthospital convalescent care and rehabilitation that will enable them to return to independent living in the community. Units designed for the cognitively impaired provide special facilities that allow for the residents' tendency to wander without the need for restraints and barriers to mobility. The level of autonomy expected of nurses in nursing homes where physicians visit monthly is often surprising to those who have always worked in acute care hospitals where physicians visit patients daily.

Recent years have witnessed the development of retirement communities that can take one of several forms. They may be self-contained towns, retirement villages, retirement subdivisions, retirement residences, or continuing-care communities (Matteson and McConnell, 1988). These communities provide a variety of levels of care to the residents based on the resident's need. In an assisted-living arrangement, the resident can maintain maximum independence, seeking help as it is needed. Most of the facilities also maintain a convalescent center, and services such as occupational therapy, physical therapy, and dental care may also be available. The one limiting factor may be the cost of access.

OTHER LONG-TERM CARE SETTINGS

Rehabilitation centers often focus around a specific health care problem. For example, there are centers for those with spinal cord injuries and other centers focusing on head injuries or cerebral vascular accidents. Although many of these agencies prefer nurses who have taken advanced courses in rehabilitation nursing, many employ nurses with different backgrounds. Many health care settings focus on rehabilitation principles as a part of all care. This may provide background for entering practice in rehabilitation nursing.

Ambulatory Care Settings

The practice of having an ill person leave home and travel to an office or clinic to receive care is a fairly recent phenomenon in human history. When transportation was by foot or by horseback, the ill person was often unable to go anywhere. The care provider, whether physician, midwife, or nurse, traveled to where the patient was located. As physicians began to see more individuals and used equipment in their examinations, the practice of having patients come to an office gradually took hold. In our modern society, the time of the care provider is prized and having individuals come to the care provider eliminates the hours spent traveling. As hospitals developed, more and more emphasis was placed on hospitalization for ill people. Now the trend is moving back away from institutional settings and more and more care is being given in offices, clinics, and day procedure units. All of these settings use registered nurses.

PRIMARY CARE OFFICES

Primary care offices have been the traditional mainstay of basic care for most individuals. Today the federal government considers general practitioners, family practice specialists, pediatricians, internal medicine specialists, and obstetricians as primary care providers. These are the physicians people contact initially for their health problems. One of the major changes in health care has been the decrease in the solo practice office and the growth of group and organizational practice models. Advanced practice nurses and physician's assistants are working in many of these settings. Nurses in these settings may have responsibility for answering questions on the telephone as well as working with patients in the office.

WALK-IN CLINICS

Walk-in clinics treat those with emergent conditions that do not require the high technology resources of the emergency room. These may be referred to as immediate care facilities or emergency centers. They have grown as people have found it increasingly difficult to gain access to traditional health care settings within the time constraints of their lives. Gradually many walk-in clinics have added services such as sports physical examinations for school-age children, pelvic examinations, and Pap tests. As these clinics have matured, some are beginning to act as primary care settings, advertising the willingness of staff doctors to become "family doctors." Walk-in clinics have relatively small nursing staffs; therefore each nurse must have a wide variety of skills and be able to function with a high degree of autonomy.

Community Agencies

Agencies providing care in the community include public health agencies, traditional home care agencies, and home hospice care.

PUBLIC HEALTH AGENCIES

Public health departments are operated as agencies of the government. In general, their focus has been on broad community issues, communicable disease, and infant/child health. Although public health nurses originally did a great deal of individual family visiting, there are now fewer funds for that and they focus more specifically on those who are high risk and those whose health affects the entire community. Nurses hired by public health agencies are required to have baccalaureate degrees in nursing.

TRADITIONAL HOME CARE AGENCIES

Home care agencies provide a broad spectrum of care to individuals in their homes. Some home care agencies focus on providing short-term visits for those who need assistance after a hospital stay or acute illness. Others focus on those who will need ongoing home care for years, such those on dialysis or ventilator support in the home. Some of these agencies provide nursing care for full shifts in the home to provide support and respite for family caregivers.

HOSPICE HOME CARE

Hospice care has gained great momentum as a way to provide maximum quality of life to terminally ill people. Nurses working with hospice patients and their families are part of a multidisciplinary team that may include the physician, clergy, occupational and physical therapists, home health aides, social workers, and volunteers. They work with symptom management and the psychosocial processes that accompany end-of-life events and issues.

COMMUNITY MENTAL HEALTH CENTERS

Community mental health centers were established to allow those with psychiatric problems to remain in their own communities. Evidence supports the belief that psychiatric clients who remain in their communities on an outpatient basis, with family and community ties intact, have more successful treatment outcomes. For those who must be hospitalized, the community mental health center provides a resource so that early discharge from the hospital setting is possible. Another advantage is that people seek help more readily when it is available within the community. These centers usually employ a variety of mental health workers including psychiatrists, clinical psychologists, social workers, marriage and family counselors, psychiatric nurses, and community workers. Services may include individual counseling and therapy, group or family counseling, evaluation, and referral.

In actual practice, community mental health centers have not been adequately funded to meet the many and varied needs of those with mental health problems. The mentally ill often are not eligible for care that can maintain their health but are eligible for care only when they have become acutely ill. Some people are not eligible for help because of the complex rules and regulations governing funding. Still others do not continue with prescribed treatment and thus relapse, but legal constraints do not allow involuntary treatment. Although this recognition of the rights of the mentally ill has been important, there also is concern that society is expecting people to make rational decisions about their own best interests when they are not mentally capable of understanding the consequences of their own actions. The entire area of community mental health has many problems and challenges.

DAY CARE CENTERS FOR THE ELDERLY

Day care centers have been established for elderly people who could not safely be alone throughout the day. There they receive a variety of social and health services while continuing to live in their own or a family member's home. Various maintenance and rehabilitative services usually are available, including exercise classes, medication education and supervision, recreational activities, mental health care, and an opportunity to interact with other people. Some of these centers provide "drop in" or intermittent services for those who need one aspect of the program. Others provide care each day for those who need continuing supervision while family members are at work or school.

Administration of Health Care Agencies

The organizational functioning of health care institutions is not always as clear cut as that of business and industry. Lines of authority and responsibility may vary considerably depending on the size of the facility and the services it renders. The discussion that follows outlines the most common structures.

THE GOVERNING BOARD

Typically health care institutions are governed by a board of directors, a board of trustees, or commissioners. Members of the governing boards may be elected or appointed but usually are influential members of the community who have been successful in their other endeavors. Recently there has been a tendency to have boards composed of individuals with specific management skills, such as business executives, bankers, attorneys, and similar professionals. The governing board sets policy and deals with matters of finance and long-range planning. Recently they have also been accountable for the monitoring of quality control, although this is delegated to the medical staff. They hire an administrator and other key personnel who have responsibility for operating the hospital. Medical matters are usually deferred to the medical staff.

THE ADMINISTRATOR

The administrator has the responsibility for the day-to-day management and supervision of the organization and for implementing the policy established by the board. The administrator has the overall responsibility for managing finances, hiring and supervising personnel, and coordinating organizational activities. In large facilities, assistant administrators may assist with these duties. Although some administrators have had no formal preparation for these responsibilities, today many health care agency administrators have been educated for that role with a master's degree in hospital or health administration. Some smaller hospitals may have a nurse as the administrator, especially in Roman Catholic hospitals run by one of the various nursing orders. The administrator of a nursing home must possess a credential approved by the state. The administrative position may be assigned one of a number of titles, including president, chief executive officer, executive director, or even superintendent.

THE MEDICAL STAFF

Health care providers wishing to bring their patients to a particular hospital must apply for *staff privileges*. The bylaws of the organization describe how this process is managed, but it usually involves making application to the medical board and verifying qualifications in terms of education and professional expertise.

Staff privileges may fall into a number of different categories, including active staff, associate staff, courtesy staff, consulting staff, and honorary staff. Usually each hospital has a *chief of staff*, an elected position held by one of the members of the medical staff for a given period of time. Physicians are responsible for monitoring the quality of care provided within the hospital and operate through a number of medical committees. In large hospitals there may be a "chief" for each of the specialty services such as medicine, surgery, obstetrics, and psychiatry.

Admission to the medical staff has been a barrier to practice for nurse midwives, nurse anesthetists, and other advanced registered nurses. Many of these individuals believe that they need the ability to admit patients although care for the acutely ill person may need to be transferred to an appropriate physician after admission.

A nursing home will typically have a medical director who is responsible for medical policy and procedure. In very large institutions this may be a full-time position, but in many it is a part-time responsibility. Each resident must have a personal physician who provides medical supervision and reviews medical care at least monthly. The medical director may serve as the personal physician for some of the residents in the nursing home.

THE NURSING DIRECTOR OR ADMINISTRATOR

The top nursing position within any health care institution is that of the nursing director or administrator. Because of the responsibilities associated with this position, its importance within the organization, and the number of employees under this person's supervision (nursing is the largest department in any hospital), the trend in the past few years has been to use the title nursing service administrator or assistant administrator for nursing services. The title for this position might also be vice-president for nursing. In nursing homes the most common title is director of nursing. In most of these instances the nursing administrator occupies a position on the organizational chart similar to other assistant administrators.

The administrator for nursing services is ultimately responsible for the nursing care provided within the institution. This person generally controls the budget for nursing services and is responsible for organization and staffing of the nursing units. There has been a strong push in recent years to require that nursing service administrators have a master's degree in nursing. Many master's programs in nursing offer a nursing service administration pathway, and an increasing number are offering a combined nursing and business master's program. In some instances, persons filling this role have master's degrees in business administration in addition to their basic preparation in nursing at a baccalaureate level.

MIDDLE MANAGERS

Middle managers are those individuals with administrative functions at the levels between the highest level nursing administrator and the staff nurses. Traditionally each unit had a *head nurse* or *unit manager* and units were grouped together under a *supervisor*. On the evening or night shift there might be *shift supervisor*.

A common occurrence in today's health care environment is the *restructuring* of the organization. Restructuring refers to changing the organizational pattern of the agency. Many agencies are attempting to decrease the number of middle managers and reduce the number of levels between the staff and the higher administration. In some settings there is no longer a unit manager. Instead, all of the nurses on the unit work together in decision-making about the unit. Everyone then feels involved and accountable. Staff nurses in this environment receive strong recognition of their expertise and decision-making abilities.

Some problems may be associated with this type of restructuring. Nurses may feel that they have added responsibility and authority, but no time to carry out these new duties. Communication may be difficult because there is no central authority figure. Decisions may be made slowly because the process becomes more cumbersome.

CLINICAL LADDERS

Clinical ladders are mechanisms developed to recognize and reward nurses who remain in direct patient care. Historically, the nurse who looked for advancement was required to move away from patient care into administrative positions. As nursing has developed an increasingly responsible and autonomous profile in health care institutions, nurses have sought ways of recognizing the expertise of those in direct care.

Most clinical ladders establish a pathway with titles and higher levels of pay for those who have demonstrated proficiency in patient care. Sometimes the clinical ladder requires a certain amount of continuing education in a specialty field or certification in a specialty. Peer evaluations, supervisor evaluations, and self-evaluations may be part of the process of obtaining advancement on a clinical ladder. Through this process the nurse is encouraged and supported in developing greater expertise.

Establishing and Implementing Organizational Goals

All organizations must have methods and provisions for establishing their goals and objectives and for implementing them. These often begin with the establishment of broad policies for operation and continue through the development of a mission statement, philosophy of care, and goals and objectives.

THE MISSION STATEMENT

Health care institutions, like other major organizations, usually have developed *mission statements*. Mission statements are broad declarations of the purpose of the organization. A typical mission statement for a community hospital might read as follows: "Cleaver Community Hospital exists to provide high level health care and services to the citizens of Cleaver County." Mission statements will vary depending on the nature, purpose, and setting of the institution. The mission statement of a university hospital heavily involved in education and research will reflect those commitments. A small community hospital that refers many of its critical patients to a nearby metropolitan hospital will probably not have statements in its mission about research and, in fact, may not be involved in research activities.

The mission statement is implemented through the philosophy of care and goals of the organization. The *philosophy of care* outlines what the organization believes about the care to be delivered to consumers. In other words, the philosophy is a statement of belief. Philosophies of care might include such statements as "Cleaver Community Hospital believes that each individual, regardless of race, religion, economic status, or chosen life-style is entitled to personalized, quality care provided with respect for the dignity of the individual."

The philosophy of care, in turn, is implemented through *goals and objectives*. Broad goals and objectives may outline and describe the activities of the organization as a whole. Usually some goals and objectives address more specifically the endeavors of a particular care unit. If the hospital has a hospice unit, the goals and objectives of that department will likely be quite different from the goals and objectives outlined for the institution's birth center.

POLICIES AND PROCEDURES

A *policy* is a designated plan or course of action for a specific situation. The responsibility and authority for developing policies for any agency rests with the governing board. The governing board delegates to the administrator the responsibility for determining that these policies are implemented and followed. Policies are written and copies are maintained in a policy manual. Usually there is a policy manual in each major department or unit within the agency. Depending on the area in which you are employed, you will find varying needs for referring to the policy manual in your role as a recently licensed registered nurse. As you might anticipate, the need for special policies related to occurrences in an emergency department, delivery room, or a critical care unit will be greater than those of a general medical or surgical unit of a hospital. Special unit policies are sometimes termed *protocols*. For example, the protocol for the patient receiving epidural analgesia would include a designation of the monitoring that must be done and who is responsible for that monitoring.

Procedure manuals are also found in each unit or department. Procedure manuals spell out how a particular nursing activity is to be completed and is often related in a number of steps. For example, you may find a procedure for changing the dressing on a central intravenous line, for administering oncologic agents, and for doing a host of basic care procedures such as catheterizations.

Nurses have been given increasing responsibility for affecting and developing institutional policies and procedures. They are serving as representatives to various committees responsible for developing and monitoring policies and procedures. Policies for an individual unit that are within the guidelines of general policy may be developed and adopted by the personnel on that unit. This might include a policy of how scheduling requests are handled. Policies or protocols that relate to specific patient care needs may be reviewed by an appropriate committee of the medical and nursing staff before final acceptance. Newly developed policies that are broad in scope must move up the chain of command and be approved by the governing board, but nurses' input at the grassroots level is becoming more common.

STANDARDS OF CARE

Standards of care are found on many different levels. At their broadest, standards of care are developed by the American Nurses Association or one of a number of specialty nursing organizations (American Nurses Association, 1991). These apply across the nation and are broad and general in nature. Nurse practice acts contain language that describes the standard of practice that applies to all nurses within the state.

Each agency may also develop standards of care for patients with selected health care problems. These standards of care may take the form of generalized nursing care plans designed to cover the most commonly occurring health problems encountered in the setting.

QUALITY IMPROVEMENT

Quality improvement (QI), total quality management (TQM), and continuous quality improvement (CQI) all refer to programs being introduced into many health care organizations as a mechanism to assess and improve care. This is seen by many as the next step after quality assurance programs have been established. *Quality assurance* often has involved ensuring that basic standards for care have been met. *Quality improvement* helps an organization move beyond these basic standards to an ever-expanding view of quality care. Plans for QI are mandated by the accrediting organization, the Joint Commission for the Accreditation of Healthcare Organizations (JCAHO).

The first step in QI is defining what the individual organization means by quality of care. This involves consulting consumers as well as providers of health care. Consumers may describe difficult-to-measure qualities such as attitudes toward consumers by employees in the institution. Practical concerns may be expressed by consumers such as timeliness in meeting appointments and accessibility of care providers when consumers have questions. Professionals often have other attributes in mind when they speak of quality care. These attributes may include addressing concerns of the whole family as well as those of the individual patient.

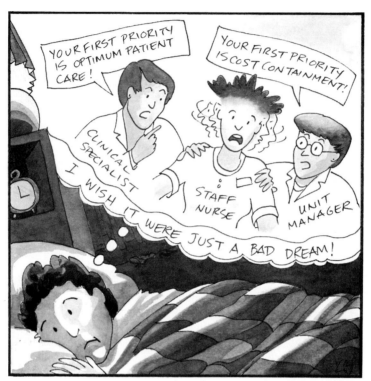

FIGURE 12–1 The first step in quality improvement is to define what the organization means by quality of care.

Whatever the concerns, QI identifies goals and objectives that represent higher standards of care. After these higher goals and objectives are identified, the next step is developing plans to move toward them. Through QI, health care providers are striving to create a care delivery system that is responsive and caring and that demonstrates the highest standards possible in light of today's health care system.

Understanding Organizational Structure

Hospitals, nursing homes, and large clinics are bureaucratic organizations. By that we mean that they operate and are administered through a number of departments and subdivisions with appointed individuals having responsibility for carrying out various defined functions. The structure determines responsibility and authority. Often the routines established and the communication paths to be followed are rather inflexible but are established to provide order and structure to the organization. Bureaucracy in hospitals is also a product of their history with its strong military and religious influence. The bureaucracy of hospitals has often been transferred to other health care agencies.

Students entering into any environment should have some understanding of its structure. The following section outlines some of the more commanding aspects of the hospital organization. Students are encouraged to gain greater depth in this area in books devoted entirely to the topic.

THE ORGANIZATIONAL CHART

Characteristically, agencies are organized into departments that are generally established based on the function or purpose they serve within the organization. Each will have a described set of tasks to be accomplished by the persons employed in that area. Thus, in a typical hospital, you see admitting departments, maintenance and housekeeping departments, medical records departments, outpatient departments, nursing departments, and so on. Nursing homes may have some of the same departments, but they do not have the diagnostic and treatment services that are such a major part of a hospital. Ambulatory clinics may have a different type of structure in which each department relates to a particular medical specialty with a cross section of various health care providers in each department. Which departments are present, the size of these departments, and the specific domain under which they are situated within the organization will depend on the purpose and size of the institution.

The relationship of one department to another is defined in terms of *organizational structure* and is usually depicted in an *organizational chart*. The number of levels on any chart is determined by the need within the organization to assign authority and responsibility. The greatest authority exists at the top of a pyramid-shaped chart and decreases as you move toward the base. Persons having jobs within the organization that are located at the top of the organizational chart are considered administrators, executives, or "the management," and those closer to the base are considered employees or staff. Often located between these two levels is an area known as "middle management," composed of a group of individuals who coordinate and control activities of specified groups of workers to accomplish the directives established by the executives.

The organizational chart may take one of several forms, reflecting the type of administration operating within that organization. If the organization has chosen to have a *narrow span of control*, that is, has placed the responsibility for overseeing the activities of the organization in the hands of a few indi-

(*text continues on page 434*)

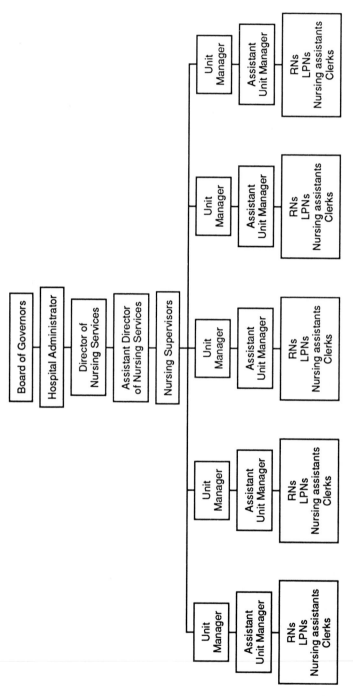

FIGURE 12–2 Centralized (tall) organizational structure of nursing service.

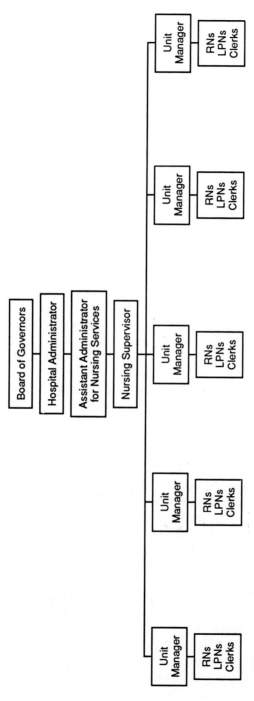

FIGURE 12-3 Decentralized (flat) organizational structure of nursing service.

viduals, it is said to have a *centralized* or *tall* organizational structure. If, however, the organization has chosen to have a *broad span of control*, then it places responsibility in the hands of a larger number of individuals and is said to have a *decentralized* or *flat* organizational structure.

Of course, many organizations develop variations of these basic structural patterns. In some instances a local institution may have what appears to be a simple structure, but it is complicated by its relationship to a large corporation that manages many health care institutions. You will want to investigate the structure of any organization in which you seek employment.

CHANNELS OF COMMUNICATION

The structure of the organization also spells out the *channel of communications*. Channels of communication run up and down the organizational chart, moving from one level of responsibility and authority to the next. Thus, the nursing administrator communicates instructions to the assistant nursing administrator, who will communicate the message to the nursing manager, who communicates with the nursing staff. In return, the staff communicate messages to their nursing manager who communicates with the assistant administrator and so forth. It is generally considered improper and inappropriate to skip or bypass any of the levels in this communication process. It is not appropriate for the staff nurse to communicate a concern to the assistant administrator without first sharing it with the nursing manager.

CHAIN OF COMMAND

Paralleling the channel of communication is the *chain of command*, which describes the path of authority and accountability from the individuals at the top of the organization to those at the base of the organization. It is also referred to as the *organizational hierarchy*. Typically the nursing administrator gives instructions to and evaluates the performance of the assistant administrator, who in turn gives direction to and evaluates the performance of the nursing manager, and so forth throughout the organization. Working from the base of the organization to the top, we frequently use the language "reports to." Thus, the staff nurse reports to the nursing manager and the nursing manager reports to the assistance administrator, who reports to the nursing administrator. Again, the length of the "chain of command" and the number of different "reports to" will depend on the size of the organization, being fewer in small organizations and greater in large facilities.

One problem in some complex organizations is that individuals may find that they are responsible to more than one supervisor. As long as these two supervisors share goals and priorities, this may pose few problems. If, however, these supervisors have differing priorities, the employee may feel stressed by the conflicting expectations.

JOB DESCRIPTIONS

The responsibilities of all jobs or positions within the organization are spelled out in *job descriptions*. Job descriptions are written statements, usually found in policy manuals, that describe the responsibilities to be assumed by individuals hired into any of the jobs or positions within the organization. Thus, the job description of the staff nurse explains what that individual will do, the job description of the nurse manager outlines that person's responsibilities, and the job description of the admitting clerk will describe the role that person plays within the organization. These job descriptions should form the foundation for the evaluation of the individual working in that role.

One of the major issues affecting all employees in health care today is the issue of *work transformation*, which has been defined as restructuring work roles and the organization itself to more effectively carry out the mission of an organization. Embedded in this concept are restructuring the patient care delivery positions themselves, reducing the number of managers, and using self-managed work teams. As this process occurs, there is an increasing emphasis on worker flexibility, cross-training, and the breaking down of barriers to individual performance (Boston and Vestal, 1994). As this has occurred, many traditional job descriptions have become outmoded and the emphasis has been on developing an open system. Many nurses are concerned that some of these changes will result in less effective patient care, whereas others see the changes as opportunities to develop wider skills and abilities.

Patterns of Nursing Care Delivery

The nursing department of any health care institution carries major responsibility for the quality of nursing care delivered. Throughout the years, the structure of the delivery of that care has taken a number of different formats. Among the factors influencing the delivery pattern selected are the type of patients served, the type of care provided, the cost of the care, and the number and education of potential employees.

In the following section we describe the typical implementation of various patterns of care delivery. It is important for you to know and remember as you read through these descriptions that there are variations and adaptations made within different facilities of any pattern of care. We have outlined what each pattern typically looks like, but you might find it practiced just a little differently where you are employed.

THE CASE METHOD

The case method was the first system used for the delivery of nursing care in the United States. A nurse worked with only one patient and was expected to meet all of that patient's nursing needs. Often the nurse lived in the patient's home or might "special" that patient in the hospital. If working in the patient's home, the nurse often had other household duties associated with carrying out nursing care, such as cooking for the patient. This one-to-one relationship had many advantages as far as care was concerned, but the nurses worked long hours and were poorly paid. Advancing technology and changes in cost made this type of care delivery impractical in the hospital.

THE FUNCTIONAL METHOD

The functional method of care delivery emerged during the Great Depression of the 1930s. This method allowed for the care of increased numbers of patients in hospitals and for the advancing technology. The division of nursing responsibilities varied from hospital to hospital depending on the number of nurses, nursing students, and nonlicensed assistive personnel available. Typically, with the functional method specific tasks were assigned by the head nurse to the various persons employed on the unit according to the level of skill required for performance. A "temperature nurse" took temperatures; a "treatment nurse" cared for wounds, dressing changes, and other treatments to be administered; and a "medicine nurse" would give all of the medications, chart them, and provide a list of replacement needs to the head nurse. A nurse might have been assigned more than one of these responsibilities if there were fewer patients or fewer nurses. The head nurse gave "report" to the next shift of nurses who would care for the patients.

The system was economical and efficient, but it had the disadvantage of fragmenting care. No one person was responsible for planning the patient's care. Staff members charted the aspect of care for which they were responsible. Communication among the different persons who cared for the patient was lacking, and often the patients had no idea who was in charge of their care. Another problem that has arisen in functional care has been the equating of procedures or tasks with nursing care. When this happens no recognition is given to the need for time to analyze data, to critically examine possible alternatives, or the need to talk with the patient in greater depth to gather data. Unfortunately, today we see many hospitals returning to functional approaches in an effort to contain costs.

TEAM NURSING

The concept of team nursing was introduced in the early 1950s. This approach to patient care is based on having a group of people of different levels of skill assigned to a group of patients. Typically the rooms in a hospital unit are divided between or among nursing teams each led by a registered nurse, who is basically responsible for overseeing the care delivery to the assigned group of patients by the "team."

The team is composed of other registered nurses, nursing students, practical nurses, and nursing assistants, to whom the "team leader" delegates or assigns responsibilities as appropriate. The team works together, with members performing those tasks for which they are best prepared. Often the team leader gives all medications and delegates responsibilities to other members of the team. The team leader gives report to the team that follows on the next shift. A central aspect of its function is the team conference in which the

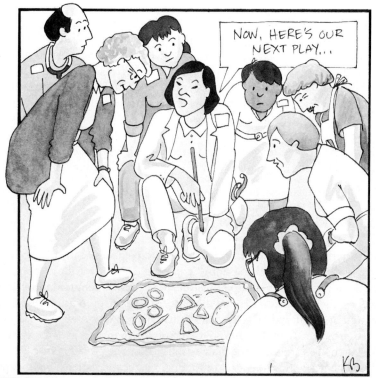

FIGURE 12–4 Team conferences, planning, and communication are critical elements of team nursing.

team members plan patient care together with the team leader responsible for seeing that this occurs.

The potential for high-quality care is present in team nursing, but the time required for team conferences and the necessity for constant communication can interfere with achieving the ideal. There remains the concern that patients may not be able to identify the persons responsible for their care. Nurses may also feel some frustration at the lack of autonomy. Without team planning and communication, team nursing may become in reality just a variation of functional nursing.

Team nursing is again becoming prevalent in health care. With pressure for cost containment, many facilities are decreasing the number of registered nurses and adding more unlicensed assistive personnel. Nurses must evaluate the skills of those with whom they work, delegate appropriate aspects of care, and supervise the delivery of nursing care as well as provide their own level of skilled care.

TOTAL PATIENT CARE

During the late 1970s and early 1980s, many hospitals returned to a total patient care type of assignment, in which a registered nurse or licensed practical (vocational) nurse is assigned for all care needs. The assignment is based on the needs of the patient. This nurse cares for a group of four to six patients, depending on how acutely ill each patient is. This returns a greater sense of control to the nurses, giving them a greater sense of autonomy and fostering a greater sense of involvement in patients' outcomes. This type of care focuses on the total person rather than on a collection of tasks or procedures. By maintaining a broad range of skills, the nurse can enjoy the satisfaction that comes from seeing and being involved in the whole spectrum of care.

PRIMARY NURSING

In a pattern of primary care, which came into popular use in the 1980s, one nurse is assigned by the head nurse or nursing coordinator the responsibility for the care of each patient from the time the patient is admitted through that patient's discharge planning and discharge. The primary nurse is responsible for initiating and updating the nursing care plan. An associate nurse works with this same patient on other shifts and on the primary nurse's days off. The associate nurse carries out the plan established by the primary nurse. The obvious benefit for the patient is continuity of care, and patients often express satisfaction in knowing who is responsible for their care. Nurses often find greater job satisfaction because they have more autonomy and control of the care given. More nurses are required for this method of care delivery, and it is more expensive than other methods.

One of the problems associated with primary nursing is the role of the primary nurse. In most facilities every nurse serves as the primary nurse for a few patients and as the associate nurse for the patients of primary nurses on other shifts. Sometimes the nurse finds it difficult to follow plans made by another if there is disagreement. The patient's condition may also change, requiring the plan to be changed without consulting the primary nurse. Another concern is the level of expertise and commitment required of all nurses. Because there is no team leader to help coordinate efforts, patient care will suffer if a nurse is not fully competent to perform everything needed. Some hospitals have required that all primary nurses have baccalaureate degrees in nursing. Nursing service administrators in hospitals that have used the primary nurse pattern of care delivery have also expressed concern that nurses have forgotten how to delegate responsibilities. In a work environment in which the nurse provided all care, there was no opportunity to decide who might best carry out various patient care activities if more than one individual was involved in giving that care.

CASE MANAGEMENT

Case management is a process of monitoring an individual patient's health care for the purpose of maximizing positive outcomes and containing costs. A key to case management is the identification of a critical pathway for care and treatment that includes specific timelines and standard protocols.

The case manager is an individual assigned responsibility for this process. The case manager may follow the patient from the diagnostic phase through hospitalization, rehabilitation, and back to home care. The case manager ensures that plans are made in advance for the next needed step. Through this longitudinal relationship, the case manager assists with decision-making and helps to ensure that the patient receives care that will achieve the most positive outcomes in the most efficient manner. This process helps to eliminate costly delays in progress. For example, one case manager for cardiac surgery patients identified a common problem that was creating lengthened hospital stays. By consulting with the surgeons, a preventive approach to this problem was identified and the average length of stay for these cardiac patients was decreased. This resulted in a significant cost saving to the hospital and a significant increase in well-being for the patients.

Registered nurses are the group of health care professionals who most often act as case managers. Case management goes beyond primary nursing to responsibility for managing the patient's interaction with the entire health

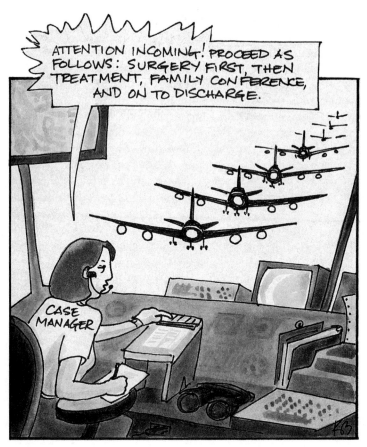

FIGURE 12–5 The case manager may follow the patient from the diagnostic phase through hospitalization, rehabilitation, and back to home care.

care system and may not include the provision of any direct care. In some settings social workers also act as case managers. Case managers may be employed by third-party payers (such as insurance companies) or by health care agencies such as hospitals or long-term care facilities.

In some instances case management means including a third party into the patient–physician decision-making process. The case manager from an insurance company may be consulted at the start of the diagnostic process for approval for high-cost diagnostic studies. This case manager must be familiar with the indications for the use of these technologies and when less costly alternatives would provide adequate information. It is within the responsibility of the case manager to suggest a second opinion or further diagnostic studies.

Preadmission certification may also be performed by the insurance company's case manager. The physician contacts the case manager to obtain prior approval for hospitalization and surgery. In these instances the case manager has the authority to suggest nonhospital treatment if that would achieve the same outcome for the patient. When hospitalization is approved, the case manager begins planning for discharge needs.

During hospitalization, the case manager follows the patient's progress, helps to coordinate various services needed, and supports discharge planning that shortens hospitalization. After discharge, the case manager continues to follow the patient's progress to ensure that desired outcomes are being attained.

Case managers employed by hospitals typically follow a patient from the time admission is planned through the time of discharge. This case manager might plan the admitting process to ensure that all preadmission work-ups are completed and that the patient is being admitted at the appropriate time to facilitate follow-through on problems. For example, the hospital case manager might ensure that a patient having a certain series of diagnostic tests be admitted on Monday because the tests can be performed within 5 days only if no weekend intervenes. Some hospitals are extending their case managers to plan for post hospital care as well (Lumsden, 1994).

Case managers are also helping employers to establish wellness programs that seek to contain health care costs by decreasing the need for services. Blood pressure management, stress management, stopping smoking, and exercise classes may significantly decrease costs of health care for a large corporation. By setting up programs for identification and treatment of those who have substance abuse, there are ultimate savings in major medical costs.

Case managers in private practice may focus on a particular group of clients; for example, the geriatric case manager focuses on managing care for the older client. The private case manager is paid by the client or family, usually based on the hours of service provided. The case manager may help the family to identify all of the options for care and treatment, ask questions to obtain greater understanding of the overall problem, and work with the family in the decision-making process. Private geriatric case managers have been particularly helpful to midlife children trying to plan care for elderly parents who live in a distant city.

Problems for case managers include opposition from physicians who see the role as an infringement on their historical rights of autonomy in decision-making. Providers may also believe that the case manager is more concerned with the "bottom line" of cost than with what is best for the individual. In the same vein, accusations are sometimes made that quality is sacrificed to cost containment through case management. Some companies have challenged the theory that case management always results in cost savings. When nurses are carefully overseeing patient care, they may identify additional health care needs as well as facilitating care for known needs. These newly identified needs may then require additional services.

Nurses dramatically change their roles when they assume responsibility for case management. They have increased autonomy and power. They relate more effectively to the business community, and as they do this they are becoming more familiar with health care financing and the many constraints on the system. Case management is a growing arena in which nurses are making significant contributions to health care.

Integrating Care Delivery in Nursing

Patterns of care delivery may be integrated in a wide variety of methods in different settings. The needs and organizational pattern as well as the public expectations will influence the approach chosen by the individual health care agency.

INTEGRATING CARE DELIVERY IN ACUTE CARE

Acute care hospitals are developing many different patterns of care delivery that often combine aspects of the traditional patterns. As work is restructured, nurses in one unit may focus on one type of care delivery while those in another area focus on another. Even on the same unit, the pattern of care delivery may differ from days to nights and from weekdays to weekends. The individual nurse must understand and be able to function whatever the needs of the moment.

Hospital emergency rooms often use functional approaches to care. Emphasis is on efficient assessment and immediate treatment. The goal is stabilization or resolution of the emergency situation and not on meeting nonemergent needs. Because of the demands for rapid assessment and critical judgment, nurses need experience and additional education. Team nursing may be used on general medical–surgical units. Total patient care is frequently used in critical care units while primary nursing is common on obstetric units. Because of the intensity of care needed by each patient, the individual nurse may be assigned to only one to two patients and provide all of their care. However, even here, some facilities are introducing assistive personnel.

Acute hospitals of today often demand a great deal of their nurses. Nurses must often develop the skills to work in more than one specialty area. They must be proficient in basic care skills but may often need to delegate this aspect of care. More sophisticated monitoring and documenting systems are creating new roles and responsibilities within the agency. The development of collaborative management systems often requires the participation of nurses in higher level decision-making and in monitoring and evaluating systems in ways that were not previously considered part of the role of the staff nurse.

INTEGRATING CARE DELIVERY IN LONG-TERM CARE

Functional nursing is used in many nursing homes because of its economy and efficiency. The registered nurse may be in charge. The licensed practical nurse may be assigned to give all medications, and the nursing assistants may do all direct personal care. In the long-term care setting, where both staff and residents are there over a long period of time, some of the disadvantages of functional care may be overcome. A specific registered nurse may be assigned to assess each resident and plan appropriate care. That same nurse may be responsible for updating nursing care plans monthly and for assigning and supervising the nursing assistants. The staff may be stable enough to know the residents well and communicate with each other effectively. The resident and family may know all of the staff well enough to be aware of who is in charge. Unfortunately, not all long-term care settings have the resources for this kind of planning and communication.

The Omnibus Budget Reconciliation Act of 1987 (OBRA '87) put in place a nationwide standard for minimum educational preparation of nursing assistants for nursing homes that receive reimbursement through Medicare or Medicaid. As a nurse in long-term care, you would need to be familiar with this education and what level of skill can be expected of the assistive personnel. Licensed practical (vocational) nurses are often given a much higher level of responsibility in long-term care settings. They often are responsible for all medications and treatments and may be in charge of units in some settings. Although OBRA '87 also required greater registered nurse supervision, the standards are still minimal.

The registered nurse in the long-term care unit has responsibility for managing the care of a large group of patients integrating effective care into the pattern that has been established by the agency. This would include managing the living environment, focusing on rehabilitation and maintenance of function, collaborating with the interdisciplinary team, and assuming responsibility for overall assessment and planning. Long-term care also has record-keeping requirements that are nationally standardized.

INTEGRATING CARE DELIVERY IN AMBULATORY CARE

In clinics and offices, nurses have varied roles. They may need to develop competencies in areas that "belong" to other health care professionals in the institutional setting. In office settings nurses frequently draw blood, complete simple laboratory tests, perform ECGs, and demonstrate other technical skills commonly done by other personnel in inpatient settings. In recommendations made regarding the health care workforce for the year 2000, the development of multiple competencies such as those seen in the office nurse are seen as essential (O'Neil, 1993).

Another important role of nurses in ambulatory care settings is related to triage. *Triage* involves determining the priority for care among differing clients. The ambulatory care nurse may do this through telephone interviews as well as assessment of the person who comes to the office. Critical thinking and judgment are essential in this role.

In many office settings, nurses assume responsibility for patient teaching in regard to treatment plans, medications, and other health-related matters. As physicians are pressured to support cost-effective ambulatory care, more are considering the responsibilities that they can delegate to nurses.

Some ambulatory care settings provide clients with treatments or therapies such as intravenous medications. Nurses in these settings develop long-term relationships with clients.

Because there are fewer registered nurses to provide mentoring in ambulatory settings, most employers in these agencies prefer to hire experienced registered nurses. However, this too is changing. As more ambulatory care occurs in large group practices or clinic settings, more opportunities are available in settings where there will be supervision for the beginner.

INTEGRATING CARE DELIVERY IN HOME CARE AGENCIES

A variation of the case method is used in most home care agencies. In these situations, the nurse is assigned the "case" and cares for the individual through the entire time care is provided by the agency. Although this is not 24-hour-a-day care, it does encompass the totality of the client's care needs. When more than one individual needs care, the same nurse may provide care for the entire family. Home health care by registered nurses is influenced by the requirements of insurance companies and Medicare in regard to reimbursement. The registered nurse in home health provides skilled assessment, teaching for independence, and treatments that require the skill of a registered nurse. In the modern home health agency, the nurse who is assigned the case may also be responsible for coordinating the efforts of other health care providers such as home health aides.

Key Concepts

⇨ Many different types of agencies now employ registered nurses; these include long-term care settings, acute care hospitals, ambulatory care centers, home care agencies, health care businesses, and others.

▷ Health care agencies are classified according the length of stay, the type of service provided, and the ownership of the agency.

▷ The organizational chart provides a diagram of lines of authority, channels of communication, and the chain of command within an organization. Job descriptions are a valuable resource for determining responsibility and accountability; however, the trend is toward restructuring and transforming jobs to be more multiskilled.

▷ An organization's mission statement is used to provide overall purpose and direction. Within the organization, policies and procedures and standards of care help to guide individuals. Quality improvement is a process designed to identify ways to improve care and service and institute systems that support high quality.

▷ The administrative structure of a health care institution usually includes a governing board, an administrator or chief executive officer, an administrator for nursing, and the medical staff. Clinical ladders have been developed in some settings to reward nurses who remain at the bedside.

▷ Nursing care is delivered in a variety of ways. The case method, functional method, team, total patient care, primary nursing, and case management are all used in differing ways to accomplish the desired outcomes of care.

▷ Acute care hospitals have a long history. The development of hospitals was affected by advances in medical science, the development of medical technology, changes in medical education, the development of the health insurance industry, government involvement, and the emergence of professional nursing.

▷ Long-term care facilities provide many types of care. Nursing homes provide care for those without the ability to manage activities of daily living and who need ongoing care. Rehabilitation centers provide for return to maximum independence for the individual.

▷ Ambulatory care settings provide care on an outpatient basis. This may range from simple office calls for common illnesses and health promotion activities such as immunizations to the performance of ambulatory surgery.

▷ Home care agencies offer services within the home that assist individuals to avoid institutional care settings.

CRITICAL THINKING ACTIVITIES

1. Investigate a health care agency in your community. Find out about its average length of stay, types of services offered, and ownership type. Analyze its overall contribution to the health care in your community.
2. Based on your view of the needs within your community, write a mission statement for an acute care hospital.
3. Compare the various patterns of nursing care delivery with the pattern being used in a facility where you currently have clinical experience. Analyze the needs in that setting and evaluate whether another pattern of care delivery would be as effective.
4. In a nursing home, examine the MDS forms and the RAPs currently being used. Evaluate the MDS as to whether it provides a comprehensive assessment process. Evaluate the RAPs for their consistency with current standards of nursing care.

References

American Nurses Association. Standards for Clinical Nursing Practice. Washington, DC: American Nurses Publishing Co., 1991

Boston C, Vestal KW. Work transformation. Hospitals and Health Networks 68(7):50–54, April 5, 1994

Burns J. Subacute care feeds need to diversify. Modern Healthcare 23(50):34–36, December 13, 1993

Collopy B, Boyle P, Jennings B. New directions in nursing home ethics (A Hastings Center Report Special Supplement, March–April) Hastings Cent Rep 21(2):1–16, 1991

Donahue MP. Nursing: The Finest Art. St. Louis, CV Mosby, 1985

Haglund CL, Dowling WL. The hospital. In Williams SJ, Torrens PR: Introduction to Health Services, 3rd ed. New York: John Wiley & Sons, 1984:160–211

Kalisch PA, Kalisch BJ. The Advance of American Nursing. Boston: Little, Brown, 1986

Lumsden K. Beyond four walls. Hospitals and Health Networks 68(5):44–45, March 5, 1994

Matteson MA, McConnell ES. Gerontological Nursing: Concepts and Practice. Philadelphia: Harcourt-Brace-Jovanovich, 1988

O'Neil EH. Health Professions Education for the Future: Schools in Service to the Nation. San Francisco: Pew Health Professions Commission, 1993

Raffel MW, Raffel NK. The U. S. Health System: Origins and Functions, 3rd ed. New York: John Wiley & Sons, 1989

Taylor, KS. Clamor over subacute care creates adversaries/new partners. Hospitals and Health Care Networks 68(6):102, March 20, 1994

Further Readings

Aiken LH. Charting the future of hospital nursing. Image 22(2):72–78, 1990

Chaska NL. The Nursing Profession: Turning Points. St. Louis, CV Mosby, 1990

Flood SD, Diers D. Nurse staffing, patient outcomes and cost. Nurs Management 19:34–43, 1988

Krieger G, Sullivan J. The case for case management. J Occup Health Safety 1:92, 1988

Moccia P. 1989: Shaping a human agenda for the nineties: Trends that demand our attention as managed care prevails. Nurs Health Care 10(1):14–17, 1989

Moxley D, Buzas L. Perceptions of case management services for elderly people. Health Soc Work 8:196–203, 1989

Parker M, Secord LJ. Case managers: Guiding the elderly through the health care maze. *In* Lindeman CA, McAthie M: Readings: Nursing Trends and Issues. Springhouse, PA: Springhouse Corporation, 1990:271–274

Parker M, Secord LJ. Private geriatric care management: Providers, services and fees. Nurs Econ 6(4):165–168, 1988

Smith J. Changing traditional nursing home roles to nursing care management. J Gerontol Nurs 17(5):32–39, 1991

13 Organizations for and About Nursing

Objectives

After completing this chapter, you should be able to

1. Discuss the reasons for the existence of the large numbers of nursing organizations.

2. Identify the purposes of the major structural units of the American Nurses Association (ANA) and how they carry out the activities and programs of the ANA.

3. Explain the purposes of the International Council of Nursing, the American Nurses Foundation, and the American Academy of Nursing.

4. Identify the major structural units of the National League for Nursing (NLN) and how these serve to support its purposes, programs, and activities.

5. Differentiate the criteria for membership in the NLN and the ANA.

6. Outline the activities of the National Student Nurses' Association.

7. Describe the organizations representing licensed practical nurses.

8. Discuss the major purpose of each specialized organization presented in the chapter.

Ellis JR, Hartley CL: NURSING IN TODAY'S WORLD:
CHALLENGES, ISSUES, AND TRENDS, 5th ed.
© 1995 J.B. Lippincott Company

A student once said that it seems that every time nurses identify a problem, their first action is to form a new organization. Although this may be something of an exaggeration, it contains some bit of truth. When you are first introduced to the great number of nursing and nursing-related organizations, it may all seem confusing and their purposes and functions may seem duplicative.

The existence of the large number of diverse organizations for nurses is, in many ways, a reflection of nursing itself. The profession offers a wide variety of employment opportunities to its members with distinct and varied contributions and interests in health care. As nurses become committed to a particular specialty group, there is a tendency to want to advance the purposes and interests of the people working in that area. For example, operating room nurses would have more common interests and concerns with other operating room nurses than they would with nurses involved in hospice care. And nurses involved in hospice care would prefer to share concerns with one another than perhaps with critical care nurses. Allowing for the fact that there are more than 2.2 million nurses in the United States, it seems reasonable that there are many different areas of nursing interest and therefore a number of different nursing organizations.

The formation of the large number of nursing organizations has resulted in concern regarding the overlapping of function and interrelationships among some of the organizations. Unfortunately, often there has been a spirit of competition rather than one of cooperation among groups in the past. Because nurses traditionally have not had high incomes, the decision of whether to join none, one, or several organizations has often been an economic as well as a philosophical issue.

Nursing organizations have recently put forth a concerted effort to promote cooperation. Nurses, as a whole, seem to be better informed about the various organizations, and they generally receive better salaries than in the past. However, this has not resulted in significantly greater participation by professional nurses in their organizations. Some people specifically do not join because of philosophical differences, but many nurses seem to be apathetic and do not recognize the importance to the profession of nurses acting together. Others, because they are combining job with family and home responsibilities, feel they do not have time or energy to become involved. Nurses need to recognize the potential for power that they possess as a group. As the nation moves toward health care reform, this was never a more critical issue.

American Nurses Association

The ANA, the professional association for registered nurses, had its origins in a meeting of nursing leaders at the World's Fair in Chicago in 1890. Through their suggestions and efforts, in 1896 the alumnae organizations of 10 schools

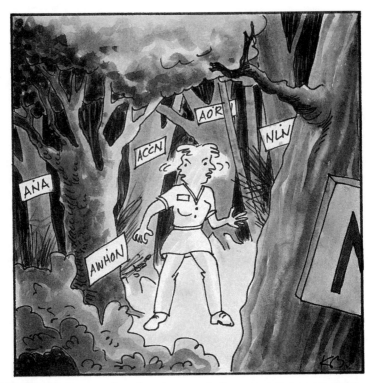

FIGURE 13-1 The large number of nursing organizations may seem overwhelming.

of nursing sent delegates to form a committee to organize a professional association. The resulting organization was called the National Associated Alumnae of the United States and Canada. The name was changed in 1899 to the Nurses' Associated Alumnae of the United States and Canada. In 1901 Canada was dropped from the title because the state laws of New York (where the organization was incorporated) did not allow for representatives from two countries. The name American Nurses Association was adopted in the United States in 1911 and Canadian nurses formed their own organization.

MEMBERSHIP

The ANA has been identified as the organization for registered nurses. As such, it has always had as its primary interest the concern of the nurses it represents. Throughout history, the organization has been active in issues relating to licensure (see Chapter 4), collective bargaining (see Chapter 9), nursing education (see Chapter 2), and a host of other concerns facing nurses and nursing. The ANA membership is composed of the 50 state nurses' associations and the 3 territorial constituent units. State nurses' associations (SNAs) are comprised of district nurses associations (DNAs). The individual nurse belongs through the SNA. Prior to 1982, when the federation model was adopted, individual nurses were members of ANA. The change was made believing that SNAs would be able to recruit more members and have greater control. However, because there was no reduction in dues this has not occurred. Each state is free to establish its own membership plans; however, membership is limited to registered nurses. The only exception to this is the admission to membership of some new graduates who have not yet passed state board examinations. It is regrettable that fewer than half of the registered nurses in the United States participate in the organization. Those who do participate are often the leaders in the profession. One reason for the low level of membership is its high cost. Dues to the national association and the state and district associations are paid together, and in most areas of the country they are more than $250 annually. Another reason given for not joining is lack of time to participate in activities. Many nurses have dual responsibilities of job and home and feel they have no time for a professional organization. Other nurses do not see how the benefits available through the association are personally valuable. Some explain that they are just not interested in the issues and concerns in which the organization is involved. Lastly, some nurses do not join because they do not agree with the position of the ANA on major issues. This has been especially true with regard to the role of the SNAs in collective bargaining and with regard to some of ANAs positions on nursing education.

Those who are active in the ANA believe that its work is severely hampered by the low level of membership. The funds of the organization are limited by the number of members. Because some specific programs, such as those involved with collective bargaining, are costly to the state association, there has been a strong move to require nurses to belong to the association if it serves as a bargaining agent. In some states the state association has set a specific percentage of staff that must be members before they will become the bargaining agent.

A current controversy involves differing views regarding the purpose of the professional organization. Many nurses believe that the major concern of the organization should be what it can do for the individual nurse. Others believe that a truly professional approach focuses on what the individual can contribute to the profession through the organization. Some think that the organization should not be an advocate in the realm of economic security, whereas others see this as essential. Another point of controversy is the organization's stand on political issues.

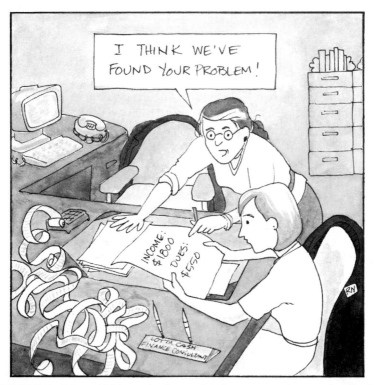

FIGURE 13–2 Deciding which organizations to join is an economic as well as a philosophical decision.

ORGANIZATIONAL STRUCTURE

The basic structure of ANA is a *federated* model. That means that the ANA is an organization whose membership is composed of other organizations; in this case, the SNAs. Figure 13–3 provides an overview of the ANA structure. Activities of the organization are focused into the two broad areas represented by the Congress on Nursing Practice and the Congress on Nursing Economics, established in 1990. The organization also has two institutes. The Institute of Constituent Members on Nursing Practice reports directly to the Congress of Nursing Practice. The Institute of Constituent Member Collective Bargaining Programs consists of one elected representative from each Constituent Member and functions more autonomously with regard to issues related to collective bargaining.

Six councils focus on clinical or functional needs of the organization. Councils are organized around nursing specialties, such as gerontology, mater-

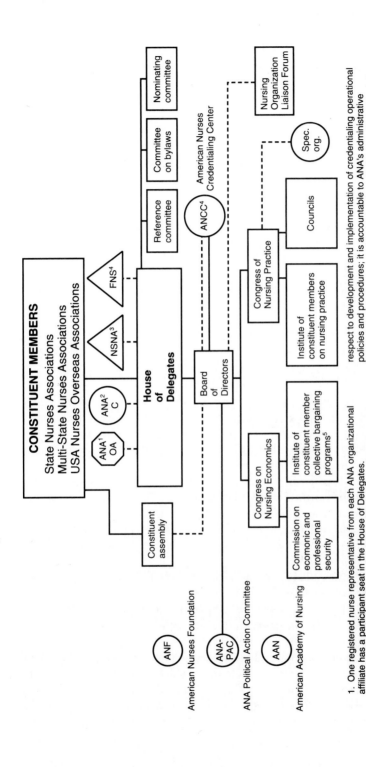

CONSTITUENT MEMBERS
State Nurses Associations
Multi-State Nurses Associations
USA Nurses Overseas Associations

ANF — American Nurses Foundation

ANA-PAC — ANA Political Action Committee

AAN — American Academy of Nursing

Constituent assembly

ANA[1] OA

ANA[2] C

NSNA[3]

FNS[4]

House of Delegates

Reference committee

Committee on bylaws

Nominating committee

Board of Directors

ANCC[4]

American Nurses Credentialing Center

Nursing Organization Liaison Forum

Spec. org.

Congress on Nursing Economics

Institute of constituent member collective bargaining programs[5]

Commission on economic and professional security

Congress of Nursing Practice

Institute of constituent members on nursing practice

Councils

1. One registered nurse representative from each ANA organizational affiliate has a participant seat in the House of Delegates.
2. One representative from each ANA council has a participant seat in the House of Delegates.
3. One representative each from the Federal Nursing Services and the National Student Nurses Association has a courtesy seat in the house of delegates.
4. The American Nurses Credentialing Center is autonomous with respect to development and implementation of credentialing operational policies and procedures; it is accountable to ANA's administrative structure in other aspects. ANA retains the authority to set standards for nursing education, nursing practice, and nursing service.
5. Institute is autonomous with respect to development of operational standards, positions, policies, practices, and all other matters related to constituent member collective bargaining programs; it provides informational reports to Congress on Nursing Economics.

FIGURE 13–3 ANA structure showing accountability and reporting relationships.

nal-child, or medical–surgical nursing practice, and also around special interest groups such as cultural diversity, research, and advanced practice (Board approves, 1993).

Standing committees deal with business and organizational functions of the ANA. These committees are determined by the bylaws and are permanent. The bylaws, finance, and membership promotion committees are examples of standing committees. Special committees and task forces are set up to deal with a particular problem at a particular time. For example, a special task force of the ANA was appointed to develop a statement on scope of practice. This task force reported back to the House of Delegates at the 1987 ANA convention.

The Constituent Assembly includes the presidents and executive directors of the SNAs. This group meets to discuss concerns of common interest, to study issues, and to present a unified voice from the SNAs on topics of national interest. For example, in 1986 it recommended that future membership in the ANA include both professional and technical nurses. This recommendation was presented to the Board of Directors of the ANA (Forum, 1987).

POLICY-MAKING

The SNAs elect individuals from their membership to serve in the ANA House of Delegates. This group meets every year; in even years in the biennial convention and on odd years as a group. The power to set policy and direction for the organization rests with the House of Delegates. Between conventions the Board of Directors of the organization ensures that decisions of the organization are made based on the policies set by the House of Delegates.

The members of the House of Delegates also vote for candidates for all elective offices in the organization. A Board of Directors (15 members) is elected to oversee the functioning of the association. The officers of ANA (president, vice-president, secretary, and treasurer) are also elected and serve on the board.

The ANA has a large, professionally staffed office in Washington, DC. Although the volunteers in the organization are essential, the many and varied tasks could not be accomplished without the full-time staff. Clerical and secretarial staff support the positions filled by professional nurses with special expertise. This is especially true of those positions that require the individual to represent the organization and the interests of nurses to other organizations and individuals. The executive director is the chief administrator of the organization and is hired by the board. Throughout the history of the organization the executive director has always been a nurse with administrative expertise. The executive director works cooperatively and supportively with the president and the board.

The ANA supports work on such policies as the ANA Social Policy Statement (American Nurses Association, 1980). These activities are ongoing efforts to support the advancement of nursing as a profession. The ANA also supports research on topics related to the profession itself, such as the historical patterns of licensure (Snyder and LaBar, 1984).

ACTIVITIES AND SERVICES

The ANA has been referred to many times throughout this book. As a professional association it has been involved in all the issues that nursing has confronted. There has not been universal support within the nursing community for all the activities that the ANA has championed or for the stands that it has taken. With any group as large as nursing, it is perhaps inevitable that there should be a wide range of viewpoints.

Certification

One of the biggest services ANA offers to its members is certification through the American Nurses Credentialing Center. Recognition for expertise in a particular area is provided that is generally based on demonstration of knowledge through testing and clinical practice, although the criteria for certification vary among specialties. Current clinical practice is essential to all. Certification is granted for a period of 5 years after which the certification can be renewed by submitting new evidence of currency and ability. Effective in 1998, as approved by the House of Delegates in 1991, individuals seeking certification as generalists in all specialties will be required to have a baccalaureate in nursing; those seeking certification as specialists or advanced practice nurses will need a master's degree in nursing. These requirements are already in place for many of the specific certification programs.

Legislative Activity

One of the major activities of the ANA relates to legislative activity. The organization often represents the profession in testimony before Congress on numerous issues affecting nursing. Being geographically closer to have greater participation in legislative efforts was the major reason for the relocation of the ANA offices in Washington, DC in 1992. The organization provides testimony for or against legislation that will affect the profession, either directly or indirectly, such as funds for nursing education, collective bargaining issues, concerns for higher education, and human rights issues. It also testifies on health-related issues that will affect the general public, such as the quality of care in nursing homes and health care reform. A newsletter, *Capital Update*, is published monthly and provides information to the reader regarding issues currently being addressed in the capital.

Since 1974, ANA has sponsored a political action committee. Formerly known as N-CAP, the group is now called ANA-PAC. Because tax-exempt organizations such as the ANA must function under certain legal restraints regarding partisan politics, this group is independent of the ANA but related to it. ANA-PAC endorses candidates for office and otherwise becomes involved in political activities. It also takes a major role in educating nurses about politics. It operates primarily through donations and is headquartered at ANA's Washington office.

Economic and General Welfare

A major area of activity of the organization in regard to the economic welfare of nurses is support of collective bargaining. This is also one of the most controversial services of the ANA. The SNAs are the official bargaining representatives in most instances (see Chapter 9). The ANA works with the states and territories to help them institute this role and to develop strategies and techniques for collective bargaining. The ANA serves as the primary source for bargaining for nurses in the employ of federal facilities such as the Veterans Administration institutions. Initially, the major concerns of the economic and general welfare section focused on adequate remuneration for nurses. Today, with nurses' salaries significantly better than in earlier years, the emphasis is shifting to practice concerns.

Insurance and Other Benefits

In addition to its activities, the ANA provides direct services to members. These include access to a group professional liability insurance plan and group insurance for health, disability, and accident coverage. From time to time the ANA also provides access to group travel arrangements and purchasing discounts.

PUBLICATIONS AND EDUCATIONAL MATERIALS

Through its educational services, the ANA produces and distributes a wide variety of educational materials, such as films for nursing, as well as a biennial report entitled "Facts About Nursing." This report provides basic statistical information used by many organizations and individuals. Reports of committees and commissions and special studies supported by the ANA are also published.

The *American Nurse* is the official publication of the ANA; official announcements of ANA business are published in this paper. The paper also contains current news of relevance to nursing and health care, editorials, letters, and classified advertisements. The *American Journal of Nursing* is the official journal of the organization. It is published monthly and contains some current news, but its major focus is professional articles. It is published by the American Journal of Nursing Company in New York City and retains autonomy over its own content. The American Journal of Nursing Company is wholly owned by the ANA.

The organization also publishes many pamphlets and informational resources that are of value to nurses. A complete list of publications is available from the organization.

Organizations Related to the ANA

As the official professional association, the ANA is related to three other organizations in a special way. These organizations operate autonomously from ANA but the ties are close.

INTERNATIONAL COUNCIL OF NURSES

The International Council of Nurses (ICN) is the international organization for professional nursing, with membership composed of national nursing organizations. The ANA, as a constituent member of the ICN, sends delegates to its convention and participates in its activities. The ICN is interested in health care in general and nursing care in particular throughout the world. It works with the United Nations when appropriate and with other international health-related groups, such as the International Red Cross.

The ICN concerns itself with such issues as the social and economic welfare of nurses, the role of the nurse in health care, and the roles of the various national nursing organizations throughout the world and their relationships to their governing bodies. The primary governing body of the organization is the Council of National Representatives, which meets biennially.

The ICN has representatives of 104 national nurses' organizations. The organization is governed by the Council of National Representatives, which consists of all the presidents of the member organizations. Activities of the organization are carried out by its Board of Directors, the officers, volunteer nurse members of constituent organizations, and employed staff, including an executive director. The ICN maintains headquarters in Geneva, Switzerland.

Every 4 years a quadrennial congress is held. This meeting is open to all nurses and to delegates from the national organizations. Concerns addressed at recent congresses focused on such issues as career ladders, educational standards, research, human rights, and nursing's roles in the planning of national health policy.

AMERICAN NURSES' FOUNDATION

In 1955, the ANA established the American Nurses' Foundation (ANF) as a tax-exempt, nonprofit corporation for the purpose of supporting research related to nursing. It is autonomous in financing and governance. The Board of Trustees is composed of members of the Board of Directors of the ANA, other nurse members, and nonnurse members from other health-related fields and from the public.

The ANF maintains a three-pronged approach to supporting research. The first objective is conducting policy analyses to provide nursing leaders and public policy-makers with the information they will need for decision-making. The second objective is related to developing a group of "nurse scholars" who engage in study in such areas as journalism and public policy. Support is directed toward independent study, research, and doctoral and postdoctoral work for these nurse scholars. The third objective is facilitating the research and educational activities of ANA. This includes providing consultation and funding for groups within the ANA that wish to initiate projects.

To accomplish its varied objectives, the ANF solicits gifts and contributions from individuals and organizations. These gifts are tax deductible.

AMERICAN ACADEMY OF NURSING

The American Academy of Nursing (AAN) was established by the ANA in 1973 as an honorary association within the ANA. The original members were chosen by the Board of Directors of the ANA. The AAN is now an independent organization, and new members are selected by those currently in the AAN. Those elected to the AAN are called fellows and may use the title Fellow of the American Academy of Nursing (FAAN). The purpose of this organization is to recognize nurses who have made significant contributions to the profession of nursing.

The National League for Nursing

Another major nursing organization is NLN, which was established in 1952 and is often referred to as "The League."

The forerunner of the NLN was the National League of Nursing Education that was organized under the title of the American Society of Superintendents of Training Schools for Nurses of the United States and Canada. Established in 1893, it was the first nursing organization in the United States.

The name was changed to the National League of Nursing Education in 1912. This organization then fused with six other organizations or committees to form one in 1952. Using the name of the National League of Nursing Education, the other groups that joined together included the National Organization for Public Health Nursing (established in 1912), the Association of Collegiate Schools of Nursing (established in 1933), the Joint Committee on Practical Nurses and Auxiliary Workers in Nursing Services (established in 1945), the Joint Committee on Careers in Nursing (established in 1948), the National Committee for the Improvement of Nursing Services (established in 1949), and the National Nursing Accrediting Service (established in 1949).

For many years the NLN produced the licensing examination for the state boards of nursing. In 1982, the NLN lost its bid for development of the new NCLEX state licensing examinations for registered and practical nursing. Management of licensure testing had provided a major part of the operating budget for the organization. Other avenues had to be developed to maintain fiscal stability. Business operations needed to be separated from internal membership discussions and conflicts.

Therefore, in 1989, after several years of planning, the NLN changed its structure. As part of the change the National League for Nursing, Incorporated became one of two subsidiaries of the larger National League for Health Care, Incorporated (NLHC). The other subsidiary of the NLHC is the Community Health Accreditation Program (CHAP), which was designed, developed, and supported by the NLN, but is expected to eventually become a profit-making organization. The president of the NLN serves as chairperson of the Board of Trustees of the NLHC; the majority of the members of the NLHC board are elected officers of the NLN.

Essentially this moved the NLN into a corporate structure, allowing it to be involved in both for-profit and not-for-profit ventures. Monies from the for-profit areas, such as CHAP, can be returned to the NLN to provide assistance to support its activities. At this time the NLN is reexamining this structure in light of recent legal opinions as to whether it is a necessary to maintain the National League for Health Care to achieve the NLNs goals and objectives relative to profit-making activities.

ORGANIZATIONAL STRUCTURE AND MEMBERSHIP

The new NLN, Incorporated retained its previous activities and responsibilities. The stated mission of the NLN is to advance "the promotion of health and the provision of quality health care within a changing environment by promoting and monitoring effective nursing education and practice through collaborative efforts of nursing leaders, representatives of relevant agencies, and the general public" (Convention '89, 1989, p 387). It continues to offer membership to individuals and agencies and is unique among nursing organizations in its consumer participation. The NLN extends membership to those on the health care team, interested laypersons, institutions concerned with nursing service and nursing education, as well as to registered nurses.

The NLN is governed by a Board of Governors, three of whom are elected officers; president, president-elect, and treasurer. The other members are elected as governors at large, and the final seat is that of secretary, which is filled by the chief executive officer of the NLN. The elected chairmen of each of the councils of the NLN are also members of the Board of Governors. At present there are 11 councils: 4 educational councils and 7 with a practice or multidisciplinary focus:

> The Council of Associate Degree Programs
> The Council of Baccalaureate and Higher Degree Programs
> The Council of Diploma Programs
> The Council of Practical Nursing Programs
> The Council of Community Health Services
> The Council for the Society for Research in Nursing Education
> The Council for Nursing Practice
> The Council for Nursing Informatics
> The Council for Nursing Centers
> The Council for Nurse Executives
> The Council of Constituent Leagues

As you can easily determine by reviewing these titles, they provide representation from the various groups comprising the organization. Agencies may join any of the various councils, and individual members may maintain membership in more than one council should they so desire.

The Council of Constituent Leagues represents the state level organizations of the NLN. A few heavily populated states have more than one constituent league, whereas in less populated areas two states may be combined into one constituent league.

The NLN works in a complementary, rather than competitive, manner with the ANA. Whereas the ANA speaks as the official voice of nurses, the NLN seeks to unite the interests of nursing with those of the community. These two major nursing organizations along with the American Association of Colleges of Nursing (AACN) and the American Organization of Nurse Executives (AONE) form the membership of another group known as the Tri-Council. The Tri-Council is active in uniting and speaking for all nursing on issues and causes that will benefit the public and the profession.

SERVICES PROVIDED BY THE LEAGUE

The NLN provides a number of vital services: accreditation, consultation services, continuing education, evaluation and testing, research, and publishing. In addition, the NLN assumes an active role in ensuring that nursing has input into health policy-making. It provides information to the U.S. House of Representatives and Senate, the Administration, and other policy-makers and keeps the membership alert to key legislative issues. Of current interest is a national health care plan.

Accreditation

Most students are aware of the accreditation services, especially if they are attending an NLN-accredited school. Accreditation, which is voluntary, is one of the oldest services provided. Initially this was done by the National Nursing Accrediting Service, which was merged with other groups to form the NLN. It is currently carried out by the Division of Education and Accreditation Service of the NLN. The goals of accreditation include providing the public with well prepared nurses, guiding students in the selection of a program, ensuring the public of the quality of the school and its faculty, and stimulating the continued improvement in schools. Recently there has been a significant push toward evaluating the "outcomes" of the various educational programs rather than focusing more heavily on the process of education and its structure. The criteria for accreditation developed by each educational council reflected outcome-oriented criteria after June 1991.

Designated by the U.S. Department of Education as the accrediting body for all nursing programs, the NLN currently accredits more than 1500 educational programs. The NLN also provides accreditation to home care and community health programs, which ensures consumers that an agency meets national standards for care.

The schools and agencies seeking accreditation request this service and pay for it. Working with published criteria and guidelines, each school or agency prepares a rather involved self-study. After the self-study is completed, the school or agency is visited by representatives of the NLN. These visitors are either educators from other NLN-accredited schools or community health experts from accredited agencies, whichever is appropriate to the group seeking accreditation. These representatives have been specially selected and prepared to serve as voluntary visitors for the NLN. Their purpose in visiting the school or agency is to assess and evaluate the program and make recommendations about accreditation status. If the program is seeking continuation of ongoing accreditation and the recommendation of the visitors is to renew the accreditation status, the Board of Review does a limited review of the materi-

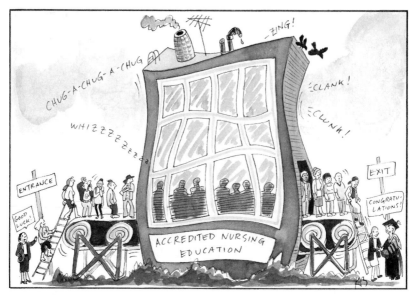

FIGURE 13-4 Accreditation is designed to help ensure that the desired outcomes of education are achieved.

als before voting on accreditation status. If the program is seeking initial accreditation or if the recommendation of the visitors is to deny or defer accreditation or impose other conditions, the program is then reviewed in full by the Board of Review.

The Board of Review is composed of eight nurse educators, one nursing service representative, and one public member, all of whom have been elected by schools that carry accreditation status. The Board of Review meets twice each year for the purpose of reviewing programs. More and more schools and agencies are recognizing the value of NLN accreditation and are participating in the program.

A list of NLN-accredited programs is published each year in *Nursing and Health Care* and is also printed in low-cost pamphlets listing accredited schools.

Consultation

The NLN also offers consultation to schools that are seeking to improve their programs or that are initiating new programs and to health agencies that are seeking to improve services. This consultation usually takes the form of personal visits to the school by paid staff and appointed members, but consultations at NLN headquarters or by telephone are also offered.

Continuing Education

The NLN sponsors continuing education workshops and conferences throughout the country, often repeating a workshop in different locations to spare nurses and others the expense of travel. Subjects are determined in consultation with the councils and are geared to current needs and interests. Curriculum, research, accreditation, testing and evaluation, student recruitment and retention, political awareness and health care legislation, and a nurse executive series are regular subjects for continuing education. The NLN has developed and conducted workshops designed to assist the new graduate with the state licensing examination.

The constituent leagues, which are grouped by regional assemblies, also offer workshops designed to meet the interests of particular areas of the country.

Evaluation and Testing

Students may also be aware of the testing and evaluation services of the NLN because it is the only testing service exclusive for nursing and health-related disciplines. The testing service provides preentrance testing to programs preparing practical and registered nurses as well as to graduate nursing programs. It also prepares achievement tests that can be administered to students who are enrolled in practical and professional programs while in school and proficiency examinations for nursing service personnel. The NLN working with the American Nursing Review also prepares materials and conducts workshops to assist new graduates to prepare for the licensure examination.

Research

When any group needs figures on nursing education, it cites data gathered by NLN's Division of Research. The division is a primary provider of statistics on nursing education, each year surveying all schools of registered and practical nursing for enrollments, admissions, and graduations. It also conducts a yearly survey of newly registered nurses for characteristics of employment. Every 2 years the nurse–faculty census is taken; every 3 years data are gathered on men and minorities in schools of nursing. These data are published in the annual *Nursing Data Book*. The division also publishes the yearly "blue books," which contain essential information on state-approved schools of registered nursing and of practical nursing.

Other Services

The career information service answers the thousands of inquiries that come in every year about nursing education by mail and telephone. The NLN publishes annual lists of accredited schools of associate degree, baccalaureate, master's, diploma, and practical nursing programs, plus a list of doctoral programs and information on scholarships and loans. (Each of these booklets carries a nominal price.)

The Division of Communication monitors the vital signs in Washington, DC and communicates its findings on legislation affecting nursing and nursing education through a monthly column in *Nursing & Health Care* and a quarterly newsletter, *Public Policy Bulletin.* Sometimes NLN spokespersons offer testimony on legislation or rulings significant to the organization. This division also distributes a wide variety of information regarding the organization and publishes a number of texts and references regarding curriculum, ethics, public policy, nursing administration, long-term care, and other topics of interest to nursing.

Throughout this book, and especially in Chapter 2, we have referred to the NLN publications. As a nursing student you are already aware of the monthly magazine *Nursing & Health Care*, the official journal of the NLN. This journal focuses on administrative and educational concepts, better methods of care delivery, expanding roles and practice, and material of nursing theory and research. It does not carry articles on direct patient care or specific clinical material.

As a nursing student you may also have had the opportunity to watch one of many videotapes prepared by the NLN. "Nursing in America: A History of Social Reform" is widely used in nursing programs to celebrate and share with students the extraordinary achievements of nurses as social activists. Videotapes have also been developed that focus on basic skills, such as patient transfer and personal care, and on topics of interest to nursing educators and administrators.

The NLN consistently has pushed for better services for the consumer through improved education of nurses and improved delivery of services. They have continued a push begun in 1982 to improve the public image of the nurse. Students who wish to learn more about the NLN and its functions are encouraged to obtain the pamphlet "This Is the National League for Nursing" (Publication No. 41-1532), available from the NLN in New York (see Appendix B for address).

National Student Nurses' Association

The National Student Nurses' Association (NSNA) is the professional organization for students in schools of nursing and was started in 1952. Although it works with the ANA and the NLN, it is a fully independent organization, run and financed by nursing students. It sponsors its own annual convention.

Although the NSNA is an autonomous organization, it has close ties with the ANA. Members of the NSNA serve on selected committees within the ANA, speak to the House of Delegates at the ANA convention to provide a student viewpoint, and work together with the ANA in regard to current issues.

Each state has a state nursing student association that operates in the same relationship to the state professional organization as the NSNA does to the national organization. State conventions and workshops are held in many states. State issues are addressed by the state association in the same way that national issues are addressed by the NSNA. Local nursing student organizations may or may not exist in individual schools of nursing. These local organizations may be closely tied to the state and national groups, or they may be independent. It is possible for an individual student to join the state and national student nurses' organizations even if no local counterpart exists.

A major project of the NSNA is "Breakthrough into Nursing," which is designed to recruit and maintain the enrollment of minorities in schools of nursing. The project has enlisted nursing students to speak to minority teenagers to interest them in nursing early in their scholastic careers and to act as preceptors and tutors to increase the retention of minority students when they enroll in schools of nursing.

The NSNA is frequently asked to testify before congressional committees when issues relevant to nursing education are being considered. In this role the organization becomes the public voice for all nursing students.

In 1975, the NSNA developed a Student Bill of Rights. This document carefully balances the rights of students with the responsibilities of students. It supports the view of students as competent adults who are engaged in an educational program. The rights outlined relate to the educational program itself, to the rules and policies of the institution, and to freedom in personal life and decision-making.

In the past it was not uncommon for schools of nursing to require membership in the student nurse organization at local, state, and national levels. With increasing emphasis on student rights and freedom of choice, this practice is no longer followed and has led to recruitment problems for many of the nursing student organizations. Students are busy, with full lives and limited funds. Some do not understand that the efforts of the organization benefit them in larger ways not immediately visible. The activities of the student organization cannot occur without a wide membership base for funding and for credibility. Certainly the profession of nursing as a whole and the situation of the individual nursing student would be adversely affected if the NSNA did not remain a viable and active force.

National Council of State Boards of Nursing

Although it is not a nursing organization in the sense of those previously discussed, our discussion would not be complete without mention of the National Council of State Boards of Nursing, Inc. (NCSBN). This organization

N.S.N.A. STUDENT BILL OF RIGHTS

The following Student Bill of Rights and Responsibilities was adopted by the NSNA House of Delegates in April 1975.

1. Students should be encouraged to develop the capacity for critical judgment and engage in a sustained and independent search for truth.

2. The freedom to teach and the freedom to learn are inseparable facets of academic freedom: students should exercise their freedom with responsibility.

3. Each institution has a duty to develop policies and procedures which provide and safeguard the students' freedom to learn.

4. Under no circumstances should a student be barred from admission to a particular institution on the basis of race, creed, sex, or marital status.

5. Students should be free to take reasoned exception to the data or views offered in any course of study and to reserve judgment about matters of opinion, but they are responsible for learning the content of any course of study for which they are enrolled.

6. Students should have protection through orderly procedures against prejudices or capricious academic evaluation, but they are responsible for maintaining standards of academic performance established for each course in which they are enrolled.

7. Information about student views, beliefs, and political associations which instructors acquire in the course of their work should be considered confidential and not released without the knowledge or consent of the student.

8. The student should have the right to have a responsible voice in the determination of his/her curriculum.

9. Institutions should have a carefully considered policy as to the information which should be a part of a student's permanent educational record and as to the conditions of its disclosure.

10. Students and student organizations should be free to examine and discuss all questions of interest to them, and to express opinions publicly and privately.

11. Students should be allowed to invite and to hear any person of their own choosing, thereby taking the responsibility of furthering their education.

12. The student body should have clearly defined means to participate in the formulation and application of institutional policy affecting academic and student affairs.

13. The institution has an obligation to clarify those standards of behavior which it considers essential to its educational mission and community life.

14. Disciplinary proceedings should be instituted only for violations of standards of conduct formulated with significant student participation and published in advance through such means as a student handbook or a generally available body of institutional regulations. It is the responsibility of the student to know these regulations. Grievance procedures should be available for every student. *(continues)*

FIGURE 13-5 NSNA Student Bill of Rights.

15. As citizens and members of an academic community, students are subject to the obligations which accrue them by virtue of this membership and should enjoy the same freedom of citizenship.

16. Students have the right to belong or refuse to belong to any organization of their choice.

17. Students have the right to personal privacy in their living space to the extent that the welfare of others is respected.

18. Adequate safety precautions should be provided by schools of nursing, for example, to and from student dorms, adequate street lighting, locks, etc.

19. Dress code, if present in school, should be established by student government in conjunction with the school director and faculty, so the highest professional standards possible are maintained, but also taking into consideration points of comfort and practicality for the student.

20. Grading systems should be carefully reviewed periodically with students and faculty for clarification and better student–faculty understanding.

(Reprinted by permission of the National Student Nurses' Association, Inc © 1978)

FIGURE 13–5. *(Continued)*

was organized in 1978 to replace the Council of State Boards that had been part of the ANA. The purpose of this organization is to provide a forum for the state boards to act together regarding matters of common concern, especially the development of the licensing examination. There is one delegate from each state board to this council. One reason given for establishing this independent organization rather than remaining within the ANA was to avoid any potential conflict of interest between the legal licensing authority and the professional organization. Although delegates to the 1978 ANA convention expressed dismay over this change, the ANA did vote to develop a liaison with the new council. The actions of this council are particularly important because its membership represents the legal authority for control of nursing education and nursing practice. Although each state board must operate within its own laws, it does have authority to establish many specific rules and regulations. Working together, the state boards hope to promote uniform standards for the nursing profession. One of the agendas items they have addressed is the development of a Model Nurse Practice Act. Much energy recently has gone into the development, validation, and establishment of computerized testing for the licensing examination for both registered and practical nursing.

Organizations Representing Licensed Practical Nurses

Two nursing organizations have as their major thrust advancing the interests of practical (vocational) nursing. These two organizations are the National Federation of Licensed Practical Nurses (NFLPN) and the National Association for Practical Nurse Education and Service (NAPNES).

NATIONAL FEDERATION OF LICENSED PRACTICAL NURSES

The NFLPN is one of the professional organizations for practical nurses. Founded in 1949, its membership is limited to licensed practical and vocational nurses. The NFLPN has worked with the ANA in regard to some of its activities and actively supports the need for the practical nurse in health care. State and local groups of the NFLPN are active in regard to educational issues for the licensed practical nurse and have supported the associate degree as an appropriate educational preparation for the responsibilities of the licensed practical nurse in the current health care system.

NATIONAL ASSOCIATION FOR PRACTICAL NURSE EDUCATION AND SERVICE

This group was organized as the Association of Practical Nurse Schools in 1941. Its purpose was to address the needs of practical nursing education. The name was changed in 1942 to the National Association for Practical Nurse Education and in 1959 added "and Service" to that title. The official publication of the organization is *The Journal of Practical Nursing*, which it has published since 1951 (Kurzen, 1989). It also publishes a newsletter, *NAPNES Forum*, that keeps members alert to activities of the organization. Membership is open to licensed practical/vocational nurses, practical/vocational nursing students, faculty, directors, and others interested in promoting the purposes of the organization. It was the first organization to provide accreditation to practical nursing programs.

Specialized Nursing Organizations

In addition to the nursing organizations already described, there are many other nursing organizations that have a special focus. These groups may have local organizations only in larger population centers; however, nurses may often join the national organization, regardless of whether there is a local chapter.

NATIONAL FEDERATION FOR
SPECIALTY NURSING ORGANIZATIONS

In an effort to have a stronger voice in nursing, in 1981, the National Federation for Specialty Nursing Organizations (NFSNO) was started. This group had its beginnings in a meeting sponsored by ANA in 1972 that brought together representatives from 10 specialty groups to share common concerns and interest.

By 1973, an organization titled the National Federation for Specialty Nursing Organizations and American Nurses' Association was started with 13 members. In 1981, the name was changed to reflect the current title.

The purpose of NFSNO is to foster excellence in specialty nursing practice by providing a forum for communication and collaboration and to assume a leadership position in activities that contribute to specialty nursing practice (Kelly, 1991). You will frequently find local representatives from this organization sitting on statewide groups that are concerned about nursing practice, nursing shortages, or statewide plans for nursing.

NORTH AMERICAN NURSING DIAGNOSIS ASSOCIATION

The North American Nursing Diagnosis Association (NANDA) is open to individuals as well as to group members. The purpose of this group is to work toward a uniform terminology and definitions to be used in regard to nursing diagnosis and to share ideas and information regarding this topic. Individuals identify and research problems nurses manage, prepare documentation, and submit these to NANDA to be included in the consideration process. The individual problems are then reviewed by committees. Those that meet the basic criteria for nursing diagnoses are submitted to the membership, defining characteristics are identified, and conditions that the diagnosis is related to are identified. A national convention held every 2 years is the final forum for debate and discussion of proposed new nursing diagnoses. The general outline of the taxonomy (classification system) was established by a group of nursing theorists and then accepted by the organization.

CLINICALLY RELATED ORGANIZATIONS

Some of the earliest specialty organizations were related to specific clinical practice areas of nursing. A major focus of these organizations is continuing education related to the nursing specialty. Most of these groups also have some mechanisms, such as certification, for recognizing achievement in the field. One of the earliest specialty organizations, founded in 1941, was the American Association of Nurse Anesthetists, a group of approximately 24,000 members of whom 40% are men.

Specialty organizations also include groups that began as auxiliaries to specialty physicians' organizations such as the AWHONN: The Association of Women's Health, Obstetrical, and Neonatal Nurses. This organization was started for nurses affiliated with physicians who were "fellows" of the American College of Obstetricians and Gynecologists. As more members joined and nurses became more active, groups such as this became autonomous (see Appendix B for a listing of the major specialty groups.)

One concern has been the overlapping of purpose and action between the Councils on Practice of the ANA and the corresponding specialty organizations. One attempt to promote more cooperative effort was the creation of the Nursing Organization Liaison Forum (NOLF), which operates as a forum within the ANA.

GROUPS RELATED TO ETHNIC ORIGIN

As the movement for self-determination and preservation of identity arose within ethnic groups in the United States, nurses within ethnic groups began to unite for a greater voice in health care. Some groups are nationally organized. Other ethnic groups may be organized on a more local level. As these groups become more organized and stronger, their interests include the recruitment and support of nursing students from the ethnic group they represent. They also encourage their members to become more politically involved in nursing and nursing leadership.

NATIONAL ALLIANCE OF NURSE PRACTITIONERS

One of the newest nursing organizations is the National Alliance of Nurse Practitioners (NANP), organized in 1986. Its purpose is to promote the health care of the nation by promoting the visibility, viability, and unity of nurse practitioners. Its major activities focus on advancing the role of the nurse practitioner in the health care delivery system including issues related to reimbursement.

HONORARY ORGANIZATIONS

Sigma Theta Tau is an international organization established in collegiate schools of nursing to recognize those with superior ability, leadership potential, and contribution to nursing. Candidates may be asked to join during the senior year of a baccalaureate program or any time thereafter. Sigma Theta Tau has established a nursing library at its headquarters in Indianapolis that has reference abilities to support advanced scholarship and provides the first "on-line" nursing journal that can be accessed by computer. Local chapters may maintain funds to support individual research projects, hold research conferences, and recognize those who have made significant contributions to nursing.

Alpha Tau Delta is a professional nursing fraternity. Students who are enrolled in baccalaureate nursing programs and demonstrate scholarship and personality characteristics in line with the organization's professional goals are eligible for membership.

RELIGIOUSLY ORIENTED ORGANIZATIONS

The National Council of Catholic Nurses and the Nurses' Christian Fellowship (primarily a nondenominational Protestant group) were organized to assist nurses to share concerns and integrate their work and their religious beliefs. These two organizations place special emphasis on meeting the patient's spiritual needs and on dealing with ethical issues.

EDUCATIONALLY ORIENTED ORGANIZATIONS

There has been a great deal of change and development since the 1960s as nursing education has moved from the hospital into the educational setting. During this time there has been an increasing emphasis on educational methods, curriculum development, and research.

Regional Organizations

Within several major geographical regions of the United States, organizations extending membership to schools of nursing, members of the state boards of nursing, and interested individuals were developed to promote interstate and interinstitutional cooperation in seeking pathways to improved nursing education and scholarship. These organizations are the Western Institute of Nursing (WIN), the Council on Collegiate Education for Nursing of the Southern Regional Education Board (CCEN/SREB), the New England Organization for Nursing (NEON), the Midwest Alliance in Nursing (MAIN), and the Mid-Atlantic Regional Nursing Association (MARNA).

National Organization for the Advancement of Associate Degree Nursing

Another relatively new national organization is the National Organization for the Advancement of Associate Degree Nursing (NOAADN). Organized in 1986, this group was the outgrowth of the development of several state organizations that were originated to focus attention on the value of associate degree education in nursing. The first state to initiate an organization was Texas, where the first chapter was started in 1984.

The NOAADN has four purposes: to speak for associate degree nursing education and practice, to reinforce the value of associate degree nursing education and practice, to maintain endorsement of registered nurse licensure from state to state for the associate degree nurse, and to retain the registered nurse licensure examination for graduates of associate degree nursing programs. To fulfill these goals, seven objectives have been incorporated into the bylaws of the organization that relate to activities soliciting support for associate degree nursing, including legislative activity. Membership is open to individuals, states, agencies, and organizations, with varying dues assessed each group.

American Association of Colleges of Nursing

The American Association of Colleges of Nursing (AACN) was formed to assist collegiate schools of nursing to work cooperatively to improve higher education for professional nursing. Membership is restricted to deans and directors of programs that offer a baccalaureate degree in nursing with an upper-division nursing major and that are part of a regionally accredited college or university. Likewise, hospital schools of nursing have formed the National Association of Hospital Schools of Nursing, the aim of which is to support quality education in hospital-based programs.

POLITICAL ACTION ORGANIZATIONS

Specific rules and regulations govern the conduct of individuals and groups in the political realm. A nonprofit professional organization may provide expert testimony in regard to an issue but is prohibited from actively lobbying on the behalf of either legislation or a candidate. As nurses have become more politically active, one of the routes they have chosen has been for the formation of specific political groups. The financing of these groups must not be related to any nonprofit organization, and membership must be voluntary. Political action groups are free to undertake lobbying efforts as well as to work on behalf of candidates. Many individual states have political action organizations for nurses. The ANA-PAC is the ANA's political action group (see Chapter 10 and previous discussion in this chapter).

MISCELLANEOUS ORGANIZATIONS

The Gay Nurses' Alliance was an outgrowth of the movement of homosexual individuals to be accepted without having to disguise their sexual orientation. This group has primarily focused on the issue of gay rights. They also provide a forum for individuals to address the difficulties they may face in the nursing profession.

The American Assembly for Men in Nursing was formed for men who believe that, as a minority in the profession, they need to speak on issues with a united voice. The organization has addressed the issue of discrimination toward men in nursing and seeks to present a view of nursing as a profession in which both men and women can contribute and excel.

Nurses House Inc. provides assistance for nurses in need. It originated from a bequest in 1922 from Emily Bourne, who donated $300,000 to establish a country place where nurses might find needed rest. As the need for a specific residence decreased, those who had become supporters of this endeavor sold the estate and invested the proceeds. Income from the investment and other funds donated by nurses and friends of nurses are used to provide guidance and counseling for nurses with emotional and chemical dependency problems, encouragement to homebound nurses, and temporary financial assistance to nurses who are ill, convalescing, or unemployed. Nurses House seeks members to continue these activities and donations to support them.

Other Health-Related Organizations

There are a great many of other health-related organizations in the United States. Some are open to nurses as members or even have a special forum for nursing interests, and others have more restricted membership. Often the activities of these organizations affect the health care climate in which the nurse works. As you identify these organizations in your own field of employment or specialization, you will need to explore their purposes and goals. Knowledge of these organizations may help you to respond more effectively to their actions.

Key Concepts

- ▷ A wide variety of organizations exist in nursing, a situation that is often confusing to the new graduate as well as the public. These organizations represent nurses as a whole as well as special interest groups in nursing.
- ▷ One of the major nursing organizations is the American Nurses Association whose membership is open to registered nurses only. It is recognized as the voice of professional nursing. It is also active in issues related to the economic welfare of nurses.
- ▷ Another major nursing organization is the National League for Nursing which, historically, has championed for better nursing education. Membership is open to individuals and agencies interested in nursing. The NLN has the responsibility for accreditation of nursing programs throughout the United States.

⇨ The National Student Nurses Association speaks to the interests and needs of nursing students. This is a fully autonomous organization open to nursing students only.

⇨ Two nursing organizations exist expressly to serve the needs of licensed practical (vocational) nurses. These groups are the National Federation of Licensed Practical Nurses and the National Association for Practical Nurse Education and Service.

⇨ Organizations also exist that represent specialty groups in nursing. Members are usually drawn together by their common interests and concerns. The organizations provide continuing education and, in some instances, certification.

⇨ Some organizations, such as Sigma Theta Tau, are honorary in their focus. These groups strive to bring recognition to nurses and nursing.

⇨ A wide variety of other organizations meet the special needs of their membership. This may relate to social interest, ethnic backgroud, or other common denominators.

CRITICAL THINKING ACTIVITIES

1. As a new graduate you have $400 per year to spend on membership in a nursing organization. Which organization would you join? Provide clear rationale based on both economic and professional issues for your choice.
2. In trying to decide which organization to join, how would you go about learning the focus of several groups that capture your interest? What process could you use to ensure that you are joining the group that best serves your needs?
3. If you were to develop a process to reduce the number of nursing organizations, what criteria would you suggest be used for the continuation of existing groups? Provide the rationale for each criterion you suggest using.
4. Do you believe there are too many nursing organizations? Give the rationale for your answer.

References

American Nurses Association. Nursing: A Social Policy Statement. Kansas City, MO: American Nurses Association, 1980
Board approves six councils in new substructure. Am Nurse 25(10):6, 1993
Convention '89. Nurse Health Care 10(7):364–387, 1989
Forum considers nursing scope statement. Am Nurse 19:1, 1987

Kelly, LY. Dimensions of Profession Nursing. Elmsford, NY: Pergamon Press, 1991:598–600
Kurzen CR. Contemporary Practical/Vocational Nursing. Philadelphia: JB Lippincott, 1989
Snyder ME, LaBar C. Issues in Professional Practice: I. Nursing: Legal Authority for Practice.
    Kansas City, MO: American Nurses Association, 1984

Further Readings

ADN educators organize new group to fight for RN license. Am J Nurs 86(7):862, 1986
ANA honors nursing leaders. Am J Nurs 82(8):1142, 1982
Allen A. Tri-Council for Nursing issues statement on assistive personnel for the registered nurse.
    J Post Anesth Nurs 5(4):295–296, 1990
Christy T. The first fifty years. Am J Nurs 71(9):1778–1784, 1971
Convention 1982. ANA votes federation. Am J Nurs 82(8):1246, 1982
Curtin LL. Creating a culture of competence. Nurs Management 21(9):l, 7–8, 1990
Facts About Nursing. Publication No. D-92. Kansas City, MO: American Nurses Association,
    a recurring publication
Foundation awards $62,000 in research grants. Am Nurse 18:18, 1986
Gilliland K, et al. Specialty nursing council: A peer support group for nurses in independent roles.
    Clin Nurs Spec 4(1):38–42, 1990
Gunning CS, et al. Identifying nursing's future leaders. Nurs Outlook 38(2):78–80, 1990
Joel LA. An interview with ANA president Lucille A. Joel: Nursing's eye toward current and
    future health care issues. ANNA J 19(2): 173–177, 1992
Morse M. ANA-PAC Board amends bylaws, elects new officers. Am Nurse 26(2):7–8, 1994
NSNA turns thirty. Am J Nurs 82(7):1024, 1982
Puetz BE. A federation of equals: National Federation of Specialty Organizations. Rehabil Nurs
    14(6):316, 1989
Purposes outlined for new councils. Am Nurse 26(2):10–11, 1994
Quinn S. ICN: Past and present. Int Nurs Rev 36(6):174–175, 1989
Schmidt MS. Why a separate organization for state boards? Am J Nurs 80(4):725–726, 1980
Shaver JLF. What the new council structure means for you. Am Nurse 26(2):10–11, 1994
Sigma Theta Tau International's "Actions for the 1990s." Reflections 16(1):1–2, 1990

State Boards of Nursing

For specific information regarding licensure requirements, regulations, and fees, write or telephone the specific board.

Alabama
State Board of Nursing
RSA Plaza
Suite 250
770 Washington Avenue
Montgomery, AL 36130-3900
(205) 242-4060

Alaska
Board of Nursing
Department of Commerce
P.O. Box 110806
Division of Occupational Licensing
Juneau, AK 99811
(907) 465-2544

Arizona
State Board of Nursing
1651 East Morten Avenue
Suite 150
Phoenix, AZ 85020
(602) 255-5092

Arkansas
State Board of Nursing
University Tower Building
Suite 800
1123 South University Avenue
Little Rock, AR 72204
(501) 686-2700

California
Board of Registered Nursing
400 "R" Street
Suite 4030
P.O. Box 944210
Sacramento, CA 94244-2100
(916) 322-3350

Board of Vocational Nurse and
    Psychiatric Technician Examiners
1414 K Street
Suite 103
Sacramento, CA 95814
(916) 445-0793

Colorado
State Board of Nursing
1560 Broadway
Suite 670
Denver, CO 80202
(206) 894-2430

Connecticut
Department of Health Services, Nurse
    Licensure
150 Washington Street
Hartford, CT 06106
(203) 566-1032/1036

Ellis JR, Hartley CL: NURSING IN TODAY'S WORLD:
CHALLENGES, ISSUES, AND TRENDS, 5th ed.
© 1995 J.B. Lippincott Company

Delaware
Board of Nursing
Margaret O'Neill Building
Box 1401
Dover, DE 19903
(302) 739-4522

District of Columbia
Nurses Examining Board
614 H Street, N.W.
Room 904
Washington, DC 20001
(202) 727-7465

Florida
Board of Nursing
111 Coast Line Drive East
Suite 516
Jacksonville, FL 32202
(904) 359-6331

Georgia
Board of Nursing
166 Pryor Street, S.W.
Suite 400
Atlanta, GA 30303
RN (404) 656-3943
PN (404) 656-3921

Hawaii
Board of Nursing
Box 3469
Honolulu, HI 96801
(808) 548-3000

Idaho
State Board of Nursing
280 North 8th Street
Suite 210
Boise, ID 83720
(208) 334-3110

Illinois
Department of Professional Regulation
320 West Washington Street
3rd Floor
Springfield, IL 62786
(217) 785-0800

Indiana
State Board of Nursing
Health Professions Bureau
402 West Washington Street
Room 041
Box 82067
Indianapolis, IN 46204
(317) 232-2960

Iowa
Board of Nursing
State Capitol Complex
1223 East Court Avenue
Des Moines, IA 50319
(519) 281-3255

Kansas
State Board of Nursing
Landon State Office Building
900 S.W. Jackson Street
Suite 551-S
Topeka, KS 66612-1230
(913) 296-4929

Kentucky
Board of Nursing
312 Whittington Parkway
Suite 300
Louisville, KY 40222-5172
(502) 329-7000

Louisiana
Board of Nursing
912 Pere Marquette Building
150 Baronne Street
Room 912
New Orleans, LA 70112
(504) 568-5464

Board of Practical Nurse Examiners
Tidewater Place
1440 Canal Street
Suite 1722
New Orleans, LA 70112
(504) 568-6480

Maine
State Board of Nursing
35 Anthony Avenue
State House Station #158
Augusta, ME 04333
(207) 624-5275

Maryland
Board of Nursing
4201 Patterson Avenue
Baltimore, MD 21215
(301) 764-4747

Massachusetts
Board of Registration in Nursing
100 Cambridge Street
Room 1519
Boston, MA 02202
(617) 727-9961

Michigan
Board of Nursing
Department of Licensing and Regulation
Ottawa Towers North
611 West Ottawa
P.O. Box 30018
Lansing, MI 48909
(517) 373-1600

Minnesota
Board of Nursing
2700 University Avenue West
#108
St. Paul, MN 55114
(612) 642-0567

Mississippi
Board of Nursing
239 North Lamar Street
Suite 401
Jackson, MS 39201-1397
(601) 359-6170

Missouri
State Board of Nursing
P.O. Box 656
3605 Missouri Boulevard
Jefferson City, MO 65102
(314) 751-0681

Montana
Board of Nursing
Division of Professional and
  Occupational Licensing
Arcade Building, Lower Level
111 North Jackson
P.O. Box 200513
Helena, MT 59620-0513
(406) 444-4279

Nebraska
Board of Nursing
Department of Health, Bureau of
  Examining Boards
P.O. Box 95007
Lincoln, NE 68509
(402) 471-2115

Nevada
Board of Nursing
1281 Terminal Way
Suite 116
Reno, NV 89502
(702) 786-2778

New Hampshire
New Hampshire Board of Nursing
Division of Public Health Services
Health and Welfare Building
6 Hazen Drive
Concord, NH 03301-6527
(603) 271-2323

New Jersey
Board of Nursing
P.O. Box 45010
Newark, NJ 07101
(201) 504-6430

New Mexico
Board of Nursing
4253 Montgomery N.E.
Suite 130
Albuquerque, NM 87109
(505) 841-8340

New York
State Education Department
Division of Professional Licensing
  Services
Cultural Education Center
Room 9B30
Albany, NY 12230
(518) 474-3843

North Carolina
Board of Nursing
P.O. Box 2129
Raleigh, NC 27602
(919) 782-3211

North Dakota
Board of Nursing
919 South 7th Street
Suite 504
Bismarck, ND 58504
(701) 224-2974

Ohio
Board of Nursing
77 South High Street
7th Floor
Columbus, OH 43266-0316
(614) 466-3947

Oklahoma
Board of Nurse Registration and Nursing
  Education
2915 Classen Boulevard
Suite 524
Oklahoma City, OK 73106
(405) 525-2076

Oregon
Board of Nursing, Ste 465
800 N.E. Oregon Street #25
Portland, OR 97232
(503) 731-4745

Pennsylvania
Board of Nursing
Department of State
Box 2649
Harrisburg, PA 17105-2649
(717) 783-7142

Rhode Island
Board of Nurse Registration and Nursing
   Education
Cannon Health Building
Room 104
3 Capitol Hill
Providence, RI 02908
(401) 277-2827

South Carolina
Board of Nursing
220 Executive Center Drive
Suite 220
Columbia, SC 29210
(803) 731-1648

South Dakota
Board of Nursing
3307 South Lincoln Avenue
Sioux Falls, SD 57105-5224
(605) 335-4973

Tennessee
Board of Nursing
283 Plus Park Boulevard
Nashville, TN 37247-1010
(615) 367-6232

Texas
Board of Nurse Examiners—Registered
   Nurse
9101 Burnet Road, Suite 104
Box 140466
Austin, TX 78714
(512) 835-4880

Board of Vocational Nurse Examiners
9101 Burnet Road
Suite 105
Austin, TX 78758
(512) 835-2071

Utah
Division of Professional Licensing
Board of Nursing
160 East 300 South
P.O. Box 45805
Salt Lake City, UT 84145-0802
(801) 530-6628

Vermont
Board of Nursing
Redstone Building
26 Terrace Street
Montpelier, VT 05602
(802) 828-2363

Virginia
Board of Nursing
6606 West Broad Street
4th Floor
Richmond, VA 23230-1717
(804) 662-9909

Washington
Washington State Nursing Quality
   Assurance Commission
P.O. Box 1099
Olympia, WA 98507-1099
(206) 753-2206

West Virginia
Board of Examiners for Registered
   Nurses
101 Dee Drive
Charleston, WV 25311-1620
(304) 558-3596

Board of Examiners for Practical Nurses
Embleton Building
922 Quarrier Street
Suite 506
Charleston, WV 25301
(304) 348-3572

Wisconsin
Board of Nursing
Box 8935
Madison, WI 53708
(608) 266-3735

Wyoming
Board of Nursing
Barrett Building
2nd Floor
2301 Central Avenue
Cheyenne, WY 82002
(307) 777-7601

U.S. TERRITORIES

American Samoa
American Samoa Health Service
    Regulatory Board
LBJ Tropical Medical Center
Pago Pago, American Samoa
(684) 633-1222 ext. 206

Guam
Board of Nurse Examiners
P.O. Box 2816
Agana, Guam 96910

Northern Mariana Islands
Board of Nurse Examiners
Public Health Center
P.O. Box 1458
Saipan, Northern Mariana Islands 96950
(011-670) 234-8950

Puerto Rico
Office of Regulations and Certification
    of Health Professionals
Attn: Board of Nurse Examiners
Call Box 10200
San Juan, PR 00908
(809) 725-8161

Virgin Islands
Board of Nursing
Medical Arts Complex
Suite 13
P.O. Box 4247
Charlotte Amalie, St. Thomas, VI 00803

Nursing-Related Organizations

	Year Established	Membership Eligibility	Publications (monthly unless otherwise noted)
Overall Professional Organizations			
American Nurses Association (ANA) 600 Maryland Ave. SW Suite 100 West Washington, DC 20024-2571	1896	RNs only	American Journal of Nursing, The American Nurse (for others, write for list)
International Council of Nurses (ICN) 3, place Jean Marteau 1201 Geneva 20, Switzerland	1900	National professional nurse organizations	International Nursing Review
National Federation of Licensed Practical Nurses, Inc. 3948 Browning Pl., Suite 205 PO Box 18088 Raleigh, NC 27619		All LPNs or LVNs	
National Federation of Specialty Nursing Organizations (NFSNO) 875 Kings Highway West Deptford, NJ 08096		Specialty nursing organizations	

(continued)

Nursing-Related Organizations *(Continued)*

	Year Established	Membership Eligibility	Publications (monthly unless otherwise noted)
National Student Nurse Association (NSNA) 55 West 57th Street New York, NY 10019	1953	Officially enrolled students of RN and RN baccalaureate programs	*Imprint* (5 times/yr)
National League for Nursing (NLN) 350 Hudson Street New York, NY 10014	1952	Individuals and agencies interested in the profession of nursing and delivery of nursing care	*Nursing and Health Care* (for others, write for list)
Organizations Related to Scholarship and Leadership in Nursing			
American Academy of Nurses (AAN) c/o American Nurses Association 600 Maryland Ave., SW Suite 100 West Washington, DC 20024-2571	1973	Members elected by current members, based on contribution to nursing Use title "Fellow" (FAAN)	*Nursing Outlook* (bimonthly)
Alpha Tau Delta 5207 Mesada St. Alta Loma, CA 91737	1921	Students in baccalaureate programs in nursing	*Captions of Alpha Tau Delta* (biennial)

Organization	Year	Eligibility	Publication
Sigma Theta Tau International 550 West North Street Indianapolis, IN 46202-3163	1922	High achievers: senior students in baccalaureate, master's and doctoral programs; outstanding RNs with baccalaureate or higher degree	*Image, Reflections* (newsletters, both quarterly)
Groups Related to Ethnic/Racial Origin			
American Indian Nurses Association (AINA) PO Box 1588 Norman, OK 73071	1972	Student nurses and RNs of American Indian ancestry	*Newsletter of the AINA* (bimonthly)
Association of Black Nursing Faculty (ABNF) in Higher Education, Inc. 1708 N. Roxboro Rd. Durham, NC 27701		Nursing faculty members of African-American background and those interested in their issues	
National Black Nurses Association, Inc. 1012 Tenth Street, NW Washington, DC 20001	1971	African-American RNs	*Journal of National Black Nurses' Association* (twice yearly)
National Association of Hispanic Nurses 1501 Sixteenth St., NW Washington, DC 20036	1976	Hispanic nurses, associate/all nurses	Newsletter (quarterly)
Phillipine Nurses Association of America, Inc. 459 Joan Street South Plainfield, NJ 07080		Filipino nurses and those interested in their issues	

(continued)

Nursing-Related Organizations *(Continued)*

	Year Established	Membership Eligibility	Publications (monthly unless otherwise noted)
Educationally Oriented Associations			
American Association of Colleges of Nursing (AACN) One Dupont Circle, NW Suite 530 Washington, DC 20036-1110	1969	Collegiate program with upper-division major in nursing	*Journal of Professional Nursing* (bimonthly) *AACN Newsletter* (10 times/yr) (for others, write for list)
Commission on Graduates of Foreign Nursing Schools (CGFNS) 3600 Market St., Suite 400 Philadelphia, PA 19104-2651			
Council on Collegiate Education for Nursing for the Southern Regional Education Board (SREB) 1340 Spring Street, NW Atlanta, GA 30309	1963	Colleges and universities in the southern states that have nursing programs	Write for list
Mid-Atlantic Regional Nursing Association (MARNA) 350 Hudson Street New York, NY 10014	1981	Agencies preparing persons in health care and that deliver health care	*Marnagram* (quarterly)

Organization	Founded	Membership	Publication
Midwest Alliance in Nursing, Inc. (MAIN) 2511 East 46th Street, Suite E-3 Indianapolis, IN 46205	1979	Agencies engaged in providing direct nursing care or teaching persons to provide direct care	MAINlines (bimonthly newsletter)
National Association for Practical Nurse Education and Service, Inc. (NAPNES) 1400 Spring Street, Suite 310 Silver Springs, MD 20910	1941	All persons interested in LPN/LVN education	Journal of Practical Nursing (quarterly) NAPNES Forum
National Council of State Boards of Nursing (NCSBN) 676 N. St. Clair Suite 550 Chicago, IL 60611-2921	1978	State/territorial licensing boards	Issues
National Organization for Associate Degree Nursing (NOADN) 1730 N. Lynn St. Suite 502 Arlington, VA 22209-2004	1985	Open	Advancing Clinical Care
North American Nursing Diagnosis Association (NANDA) 1211 Locust St. Philadelphia, PA 19107	1976	RNs	Nursing Diagnoses

(continued)

Nursing-Related Organizations *(Continued)*

	Year Established	Membership Eligibility	Publications (monthly unless otherwise noted)
New England Organization for Nursing (NEON) Hewitt Hall, University of New Hampshire Durham, NH 03824	1964	Colleges and universities in the New England states that have nursing programs	Write for list
Western Institute of Nursing (WIN) PO Drawer P Boulder, CO 80302	1957	Colleges and universities in the western states that have nursing programs	Write for list
Occupational or Specialty-Related Organizations			
American Academy of Ambulatory Care Nursing North Woodbury Road, Box 56 Pitman, NJ 08071	1974	RNs in administration of ambulatory nursing	
American Academy of Nurse Practitioners Capitol Station LBJ Bldg. PO Box 12846 Austin, TX 78711			
American Association of Critical Care Nurses (AACN) 101 Columbia Aliso Viejo, CA 92656-1491	1969	RNs, LPNs, student nurses	*Heart and Lung Journal* (bimonthly) *Focus on Critical Care* (bimonthly)

Organization	Founded	Membership	Publications
American Association for the History of Nursing, Inc. PO Box 90803 Washington, DC 20003	1980	Anyone interested in the history of nursing	*The Bulletin* (4 times/yr)
American Association of Legal Nurse Consultants 500 N. Michigan Suite 1400 Chicago, IL 60611			
American Association of Neuroscience Nurses (AANN) 224 N. Des Plaines Suite 601 Chicago, IL 60661	1968	RNs	*Journal of Neuroscience Nursing* (bimonthly)
American Association of Nurse Anesthetists (AANA) 222 South Prospect Ave. Park Ridge, IL 60068-4001	1931	RNs who are certified registered nurse anesthetists (CRNAs)	*American Association of Nurse Anesthetists Journal* (bimonthly) *AANA Bulletin* (bimonthly)
The American Association of Nurse Attorneys (TAANA) 720 Light Street Baltimore, MD 21230-3826	1982	Nurses who are attorneys or are in law school and attorneys in nursing schools	*Inside TAANA* (newsletter, quarterly)
American Association of Occupational Health Nurses (AAOHN), Inc. 50 Lenox Pointe Atlanta, GA 30324	1942	RNs practicing in an occupational health setting	*AAOHN Journal* *AAOH News*

(continued)

B | Nursing-Related Organizations (*Continued*)

	Year Established	Membership Eligibility	Publications (*monthly unless otherwise noted*)
American Association of Office Nurses 109 Kinderkamack Rd. Montvale, NJ 07645			
American Association of Spinal-Cord Injury Nurses 75-20 Astoria Blvd Jackson Heights, NY 11370-1178	1983	RNs and LPNs who practice in diverse SPCI settings	*SCI Nursing* (quarterly journal) Also educational and practice guidelines
American Burn Association Burn Treatment Center Crozier-Chester Medical Center 15th and Upland Avenue Chester, PA 19013	burn patients	Professionals working with	
American College of Nurse Midwives (ACNM) 818 Connecticut Avenue NW Suite 900 Washington, DC 20006	1955	RNs who are certified Nurse Midwives or students in accredited programs	*Journal of Nurse Midwifery Quickening* (newsletter)
American Holistic Nurses Association 401 Lake Boone Trail, Suite 201 Raleigh, NC 27607	1981	Active: RN, LPN/LVN Contributing: all others	*Journal of Holistic Nursing* (annual) *Beginnings* (newsletter)

Organization	Founded	Membership	Publication
American Nephrology Nurses Association (AANA) North Woodbury Road, Box 56 East Holly Avenue Pitman, NJ 08071	1969	RNs, LVNs employed in the field	*Journal of AANA* (6 times/yr) *AANA Update* (newsletter)
American Organization of Nurse Executives (AONE) 840 North Lake Shore Drive Chicago, IL 60611		RNs in administrative positions	
American Psychiatric Nurses' Association 6900 Grove Rd. Thorofare, NJ 08086			
American Public Health Association (APHA) Public Health Nursing Section 1015 15th Street, NW Washington, DC 20005	1972	All persons interested in Public Health Various categories of membership available	*American Journal of Public Health* *The Nation's Health*
American Radiological Nurses Association 10110 Forum Park Drive Houston, TX 77036	1981	Active: RNs employed in radiologic nursing Associate: other RNs and LPNs in radiologic nursing	*ARNA Images* (4 times/yr)
American Society for Long-Term Care Nurses 660 Lonely Cottage Drive Upper Black Eddy, PA 18972-9313	1990	Anyone interested in supporting long-term care	*ASLTCN Journal* (bimonthly)
American Society of Ophthalmic Registered Nurses (ASORN), Inc. PO Box 193030 San Francisco, CA 94119	1976	RNs working in ophthalmology	*Insight* (newsletter)

(continued)

Nursing-Related Organizations *(Continued)*

	Year Established	Membership Eligibility	Publications (monthly unless otherwise noted)
American Society of Pain Management Nurses 11512 Allecingie Parkway Richmond, VA 23235		Student and corporate memberships available	*ASPMN Pathways* (quarterly newsletter)
American Society for Parenteral and Enteral Nutrition—Nurses' Committee 8630 Fenton Street, Suite 412 Silver Springs, MD 20910-3803	1975	Multidisciplinary: professionals working with parenteral and enteral nutrition	
American Society of Plastic and Reconstructive Surgical Nurses, Inc. North Woodbury Road, Box 56 Pitman, NJ 08071	1975	Active: RNs, LPNs working in the field Associate: RNs, LPNs interested in the field	*Journal of Plastic and Reconstructive Surgical Nursing*
American Society of Post-Anesthesia Nurses 11512 Allecingie Parkway Richmond, VA 23235	1980	RNs, LPNs, Anesthesiologists, CRNAs	*Breathline* *Journal of Post Anesthesia Nursing* (quarterly)
American Urological Association Allied 11512 Allecingie Parkway, Suite C Richmond, VA 23235	1972	Active: RNs, LPNs, PAs, technicians Associate: industry, physicians	*AUAA Journal* (quarterly) *Urogram* (newsletter)

Organization	Year	Membership	Publications
Association of Nurses in AIDS Care 704 Stoney Hill Road, Suite 106 Yardley, PA 19067 (215) 321-2371	1988	Nurse, industry, and affiliates interested in promoting health, welfare, and rights of HIV-infected persons	*Journal of the Association of Nurses in AIDS Care* (JANAC) *ANACdotes* (quarterly newsletter)
Association for Professionals in Infection Control and Epidemiology 1016 16th Street NW Washington, DC 20036	1972	Active: professionals in infection control Associate: other	*AJIC* (bimonthly) (for others, write for list)
Association for the Care of Children's Health 3615 Wisconsin Avenue, NW Washington, DC 20016	1965	All individuals interested in children's health	*Children's Health Care* (for others, write for list)
Association of Operating Room Nurses (AORN) 2170 S. Parker Road, Suite 300 Denver, CO 80231-5711	1949	Active: RNs employed in OR or in a related educational program or in research	*AORN Journal*
Association of Pediatric Oncology Nurses Suite 3A 11512 Allecingie Parkway Richmond, VA 23235	1976	RNs	*APON Newsletter* (quarterly) (for others, write for list)
Association of Rehabilitation Nurses 5700 Old Orchard Road, 1st Floor Skokie, IL 60077	1974	Regular: RNs Associate: all interested persons	*Rehabilitation Nursing* (bimonthly journal) Pamphlets

(continued)

Nursing-Related Organizations (*Continued*)

	Year Established	Membership Eligibility	Publications (*monthly unless otherwise noted*)
Association of Women's Health, Obstetric, and Neonatal Nurses (AWHONN) (formerly NAACOG) 700 14th Street NW Suite 600 Washington, DC 20005	1969	RNs and allied health individuals in OGN nursing	*Journal of Obstetric Gynecologic, and Neonatal Nurse (JOGN)* (bimonthly) *AWHONN Newsletter*
Coalition of Nurse Practitioners, Inc. PO Box 123 East Greenbush, NY 12061	1980	Nurse practitioners and students in nurse practitioner programs	*Coalition Communique* (quarterly)
Department of School Nurses of the National Education Association (NEA) 1201 Sixteenth Street, NW Washington, DC 20036	1968	School nurse members of the NEA	*The School Nurse*
Dermatology Nurses' Association East Holly Avenue, Box 56 Pitman, NJ 08071-0056	1981	Active: RNs, LPNs/LVNs involved in dermatology	*DNA Focus* (bimonthly newsletter)
Developmental Disabilities Nurses' Association 1720 Willow Circle, Suite 515 Eugene, OR 97402			

Organization	Founded	Membership	Publication
Drug and Alcohol Nursing Association 660 Lonely Cottage Dr. Upper Black Eddy, PA 18972	1979	Active: nurses caring for clients with drug- and alcohol-related disorders Associate: all others	DANA *Newsletter* (quarterly)
Emergency Nurses Association (ENA) 216 Higgins Rd. Park Ridge, IL 60068	1970	RNs	*The Journal of Emergency Nursing* *Emergency Nursing Core Curriculum*
Flight Nurse Section Aerospace Medical Association Washington National Airport Washington, DC 20001	1964	Designated flight nurses and RNs who are members of Aerospace Medical Association	*Aviation, Space, and Environmental Medicine*
International Association for Enterostomal Therapy (IAET), Inc. 2081 Business Center Drive Suite 290 Irvine, CA 92715	1968	Active: graduates of accredited IAET program	*Journal of Enterostomal Therapy*
Intravenous Nurses' Society, Inc. 2 Brighton Street Belmont, MA 02178	1973	Nurses interested in intravenous therapy	*Journal of Intravenous Therapy*
National Alliance of Nurse Practitioners 325 Pennsylvania Ave, SE Washington, DC 20003-1100		DONS in long-term care agencies	

(continued)

Nursing-Related Organizations (*Continued*)

	Year Established	Membership Eligibility	Publications (monthly unless otherwise noted)
National Association of Directors of Nursing Administration in Long Term Care (NADONA/LTC) 10999 Reed Hartman Hwy., Suite 229 Cincinnati, OH 45242			
National Association for Health Care Recruitment PO Box 5769 Akron, OH 44372	1975	Active: health care recruiters	*Recruitment Directions* (10 times/yr)
National Association of Neonatal Nurses 1304 Southpoint Blvd. Suite 280 Petaluma, CA 94954-6859	1984	Regular: RNs Associate: all others	*Neonatal Network: The Journal of Neonatal Nursing* (bimonthly)
National Association of Orthopaedic Nurses East Holly Avenue, Box 56 Pitman, NJ 08071	1980	RNs, LPNs, LVNs	*Orthopaedic Nursing* (for others, write for list)
National Association of Pediatric Nurse Associates/Practitioners (NAPNAP) 1101 Kings Highway North, Suite 206 Cherry Hill, NJ 08034	1973	RNs with advanced education who are primary care practitioners in pediatrics	*The Pediatric Nurse Practitioner* (newsletter) *The Journal of Pediatric Health Care*

Organization	Year	Membership	Publications
National Association of School Nurses Lamplighter Lane, PO Box 1300 Scarborough, ME 04074	1969	Active: RNs employed by educational institutions Other categories for students, retirees, organizations	*School Nurse Journal* *NAS Newsletter* (quarterly)
National Gerontological Nurses Association 7250 Parkway Dr., Suite 510 Hanover, MD 21076		Other categories for students, retirees, organizations	
National Flight Nurses Association 6900 Grove Road Thorofare, NJ 08086-9447	1981		*Aeromedical Journal* (bimonthly) *Across the Board* (quarterly)
National Nurses Society on Addiction 5700 Old Orchard Road, First Floor Skokie, IL 60077-1057	1983	Regular: RNs Associate: all others	*Annual Review of Nursing and the Addictions* Quarterly newsletter
Nurse Consultants Association, Inc. 414 Plaza Drive, Suite 209 Westmont, IL 60559	1979	RNs with 60% of income from consultant-type sources	Quarterly newsletter Annual membership directory
Nurses Organization of Veteran's Affairs 6728 Old McLean Village Drive McLean, VA 22101			
Oncology Nursing Society 501 Holiday Drive Pittsburgh, PA 15220		Nurses interested in oncology	

(continued)

Nursing-Related Organizations (*Continued*)

	Year Established	Membership Eligibility	Publications (*monthly unless otherwise noted*)
Society for Vascular Nursing (SVN) 309 Winter Street Norwood, MA 02062	1982	Active: currently licensed nurses	*SVN Journal* (quarterly)
Society of Gastroenterology Nurses and Associates, Inc. 1070 Sibley Tower Rochester, NY 14604	1974	Individuals employed as gastrointestinal nurses or assistants	*Gastroenterology Nursing* (bimonthly)
Society of Otorhinolaryngology and Head-Neck Nurses, Inc. 116 Canal St., Suite A New Smyrna Beach, FL 32168	1976	RNs actively working in ORL/head-neck nursing	*ORL-Head and Neck Nursing* (4 times/yr) *Update* (quarterly newsletter)
Transcultural Nursing Society College of Nursing Madonna University 36600 Schoolcraft Rd. Livonia, MI 48150	1979	Nurses and nonnurses	Biannual newsletter

Organization	Year	Membership	Publication
World Federation of Neuroscience Nurses P.O. Box 3703 Parramotta, NSW 2150 Australia		Professional nurses working in neuroscience	
Miscellaneous			
American Assembly for Men in Nursing PO Box 31753 Independence, OH 44131	1971	All men in nursing	*Interaction*
National Nurses for Life 1998 Menold Allison Park, PA 15104			
Nurses Christian Fellowship 6400 Schroeder Road PO Box 7895 Madison, WI 53707	1948	Christian students and RNs	*Journal of Christian Nursing* (quarterly)
Nurses Educational Funds 555 West 57th Street New York, NY 10019	1911	Donors welcome	Semiannual newsletter
Nurses Environmental Health Watch c/o 181 Marshall St. Duxbury, MA 03443			
Nurses' House, Inc. 350 Hudson Street New York, NY 10014	1925	Payment of annual contribution	

Index

and women's health care, 361
workplace advocacy programs of,
336–337
American Nurses' Credentialing
Center, 59, 99, 146, 147, 455
American Nurses' Foundation (ANF),
458
American Organization of Nurse Exec-
utives (AONE), 460, 489
American Psychiatric Association, 274
American Red Cross, 51
Americans with Disabilities Act
(1990), 361
American Society of Superintendents
of Training Schools for Nurses of
the U.S. and Canada, 458
Americas, the, health care in, 21–22
Amniocentesis, 242, 244–245, 276
ANA-PAC, 456, 472
Anencephaly, 244, 269–270
Anesthetists, nurse, 377
certification of, 142, 146
expanded role of, 128
Antidepressant drugs, 274
Application. See also Goals, career
for admission to diploma program,
54
for employment, 386–387, 388, 408
Apprenticeship
diploma education as, 53
early nursing as, 12
Aquinas, St. Thomas, 207
Arbitration. See also Collective
bargaining
binding, 324
in labor disputes, 323–324
Art, nursing as, 7
Articulation, in nursing education, 14,
75, 100
Artificial insemination, 250, 252, 276
Art therapists, 293
Asklepios, 10
Assault. See also Legal issues
defined, 181
example of, 181–182
Assessment, in ethical decision-
making, 216
Assignments, adapting to, 185–186

Assisted-living settings, 412
Assistive devices, 292, 296
Associate degree, 52. See also Educa-
tion, nursing
Associate degree programs, 49, 62
ANA position paper on, 90
characteristics of, 62–63
at community colleges, 62–65
competencies of, 63, 97
comparison of, 68–69
concerns facing, 63–65
creation of, 37
and grandfather clause, 95
"Associate nurse," 94
Association of Colleges of Nursing, 350
Association of Collegiate Schools of
Nursing, 36, 459
Association of Operating Room Nurses
(AORN), 92, 491
Association of Practical Nurse Schools,
468
Association for Practitioners in Infection Control, 145
Association of Rehabilitation Nurses,
92, 491
Association of Women's Health,
Obstetric and Neonatal Nursing
(AWHONN), 92, 142–143, 470,
492
Assyria, health care in, 19
Attitudes. See also Beliefs; Values
authoritarian, 213
paternalistic, 213 (see also Paternal-
ism)
and right to refuse treatment, 265
social and cultural, 208
Audit, process of, 227–228
Australia, nursing education in, 141
Authority
chain of command, 434–435, 445
in organizational charts, 431–434,
445, 453
and substandard care, 218
Autonomy
ethical decisions concerning, 204,
232
of nurses in nursing homes, 421
Avalon Foundation, 38

Information, privileged, 173, 191
Informed consent, 173
  advance directives, 175
  legal requirement for, 174
  and mentally incompetent, 177–178
  minors and, 177
  for nursing measures, 176
  in Patient's Bill of Rights, 201, 202
  responsibility for, 174
  withdrawing consent, 177
Injunction, in labor disputes, 325–326
"Injunctive relief," 127
Inquiry, letter of, 386–387, 388, 408
Institute of Medicine study, 41
Institute of Nursing Sisters, 29
Institute of Society, Ethics, and the
  Life Sciences. See Hastings Center
Institutional policies, 154–155
Institutions. See also Agencies, health
  care; Goals, organizational;
  Organizational structure
  as health care providers, 293, 297,
    313–314
  inadequately staffed, 401–402
  nonprofit, 415
  policies and procedures, 428–429,
    445
Insurance, provided by ANA, 456. See
  also Health insurance; Liability
  insurance
Insurance industry, 299–300, 314
  and hospital development, 417–418
  nurses employed by, 378, 412
Intensity measures, 312
Intensive care units, 5, 229
Interactive programs, 101
International Congress of Nurses
  (ICN), 141
International Council of Nurses
  (ICN), 457, 481
  code of ethics of, 13–14
  Code for Nurses of, 198, 216
International nursing licensure, 141
Internships, for nursing graduates,
  78–79
Interstate endorsement, 96
Interview. See also Goals, career
  letter following, 395, 396

participating in, 394–395
preparation for, 393
requesting, 386
Irish Sisters of Charity, 29
Islamic law, 196

J

Jehovah's Witnesses, 176, 178, 264
Job descriptions, 435, 445
"Job hopping," 399
Johnson, Dorothy E., 8
Johnson, Eddie Bernice, 353
Joint Commission on Accreditation of
  Healthcare Organizations
  (JCAHO), 227, 304
Joint Committee on Careers in Nurs-
  ing, 459
Joint Committee on Practical Nurses
  and Auxiliary Workers in Nursing
  Services, 459
Journal of Practical Nursing, The, 468
Judicial decisions, and ethical issues,
  211, 232. See also Courts
Justice
  as ethical concept, 204, 232
  social equity and, 208, 232

K

Kaiser Permanente Health Care organ-
  ization, 300–301
Kalisch, Beatrice and Phillip, 32–33,
  34
Kant, Immanuel, 206, 268
Kellogg, W. K. Foundation, 38, 41, 141
Kennedy Institute Center for
  Bioethics, 237
Kenny, Sister, 34
Kidney dialysis, 210
King, Imogene M., 8
Knights Hospitallers of St. John, 25
Knowledge
  scientific method and, 12
  specialized nursing, 11–12
Kohlberg, L., 105, 106

N

Technicians
defined, 290
medical laboratory, 291, 295
respiratory, 292
Technologist
defined, 290
medical, 291, 295
Technology
and ethical issues, 209, 210, 232
and health care, 337
and hospital development, 417, 445
impact on nursing of, 5–6
in nursing education, 101–102
and rationing health care, 275
Technology Assessment, U.S. Office of,
and right-to-die issues, 263
Telecommunication systems, 74
Teleological theory, 206
Television
in classroom, 102
nurses on, 32–33
Test Pool Examination, State Board,
87, 130–131
"Test tube baby," 249
Theology, 10. See also Religion
Theory
defined, 105
ethical, 206–209
Theory, nursing
in baccalaureate education, 60
development of, 106–107
increased emphasis on, 105–108, 109
Third-party payments, 13
access to, 365
case managers employed in, 440
changes in, 304
of insurance companies, 305
Third Reich, 246
Thompson School, 51
Titling
in nurse practice acts, 125
problem of, 93–94
Torts
defined, 158
intentional, 158
and liability, 163–166
Total patient care, 438, 445
Total Quality Improvement (TQI), 337

Total Quality Management (TQM),
429
"Toward Quality in Nursing," 37–38
Traditions, nursing, 42, 44
nursing cap, 42
nursing pin, 42
uniform, 43–44
Transfer credit, 71
Transition, problems of, 396
burnout, 401–403, 408
reality shock, 397–400, 408
"Transitional care," 413, 414
Transplantation issues. See Organ
transplantation
Travelbee, Joyce, 107
Triage, 444
Tri-Council, 350, 460
Truth, Sojourner, 32
Truth-telling, and health care
providers, 272–274, 277
Tuberculosis, 405
Tubman, Harriet, 32
Tuition costs, 66, 104. See also Educa-
tion, nursing
"Twenty Thousand Nurses Tell Their
Story," 37
"Two-on-two" approach, to nursing
education, 64, 70–71

U

Uniform, nursing, 43–44
Uniform Anatomical Gift Act (1971),
267
"Union busting," 355, 338
Unionism
argument against, 331
growing acceptance of, 332
Unions, 321. See also Collective
bargaining
Unitary Men, Martha Roger's theory
of, 108
United Network for Organ Sharing,
272
Universal coverage, 366. See also
Health care reform
Universal precautions, 406